Simulated Medical Office Software for Allied Health

Wilburta Q. Lindh | Marilyn S. Pooler
Carol D. Tamparo | Barbara M. Dahl

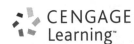
CENGAGE
Learning™

Australia • Brazil • Japan • Korea • Mexico • Singapore • Spain • United Kingdom • United States

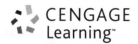
CENGAGE
Learning™

Simulated Medical Office Software for Allied Health

Wilburta Q. Lindh | Marilyn S. Pooler
Carol D. Tamparo | Barbara M. Dahl

Executive Editors:
 Maureen Staudt
 Michael Stranz

Senior Project Development Manager:
 Linda DeStefano

Marketing Specialist:
 Sara Mercurio
 Lindsay Shapiro

Senior Production / Manufacturing Manager:
 Donna M. Brown

PreMedia Supervisor:
 Joel Brennecke

Rights & Permissions Specialist:
 Kalina Hintz
 Todd Osborne

Cover Image:
 Getty Images*

* Unless otherwise noted, all cover images used by Custom Solutions, a part of Cengage Learning, have been supplied courtesy of Getty Images with the exception of the Earthview cover image, which has been supplied by the National Aeronautics and Space Administration (NASA).

For product information and technology assistance, contact us at
Cengage Learning Customer & Sales Support, 1-800-354-9706

For permission to use material from this text or product,
submit all requests online at **cengage.com/permissions**
Further permissions questions can be emailed to
permissionrequest@cengage.com

ISBN-13: 978-1-111-21587-3

ISBN-10: 1-111-21587-1

Cengage Learning
5191 Natorp Boulevard
Mason, Ohio 45040
USA

Cengage Learning is a leading provider of customized learning solutions with office locations around the globe, including Singapore, the United Kingdom, Australia, Mexico, Brazil, and Japan. Locate your local office at:
international.cengage.com/region

Cengage Learning products are represented in Canada by Nelson Education, Ltd.

For your lifelong learning solutions, visit **www.cengage.com/custom**

Visit our corporate website at **www.cengage.com**

Printed in the United States of America

Anthem Education Group and Cengage Learning used multiple textbook resources to create this custom textbook for you. Some resources and supplements referenced within are not included in your course materials and are not required for this class.

CUSTOM TABLE OF CONTENTS

SynapseEHR 1.1:
An Electronic Charting
Simulation Exercise Booklet

By Michelle E. Heller, CMA (AAMA), RMA

INTRODUCTION TO SYNAPSE

SYNAPSE is an electronic charting program that simulates documenting information within an electronic medical record. SYNAPSE exercises incorporate many activities that mimic tasks the medical assistant will perform while working in an electronic medical record (EMR). SYNAPSE uses a variety of techniques to build chart notes, including:

- Entering free text in the chart note

- Clicking drop-down lists to populate information in the chart note

- Using standard templates

SYNAPSE allows students to get a feel of how the EMR works without getting into a great deal of extraneous technical content.

INSTRUCTIONS FOR INITIAL SETUP

1. The Sign-In screen is the first screen that will appear when SYNAPSE opens. You will notice a box labeled "Username" with the word "Student1" and a Password box that already has a password installed. These are the initial settings to get you into the program, so just click OK. You should now be in the main menu.

CHANGING YOUR USERNAME AND PASSWORD

1. You will notice an icon labeled "Change Password." This icon will open a screen to allow you to set up the software using your own name and password. Click the Change Password icon.

2. Enter your first name in the First Name box.

3. Enter your last name in the Last Name box.

4. Enter a username in the Username box. This may be a combination of your first and last name, or a name your instructor will assign you.

5. Next, enter a password. Write down this information so that it is handy in case you forget your username or password. The information is case-sensitive, so pay close attention to whether uppercase or lowercase letters are used.

6. Click the Save icon.

7. Click the Close icon.

8. Click the Quit icon.

9. Reopen the SYNAPSE software.

10. Clear the Username box and enter your username.

11. Clear the Password box and enter your last name.

12. You should now be in the Main Menu.

DESCRIPTION OF THE ICONS USED IN SYNAPSE

SYNAPSE uses a variety of icons that assist the user in navigating through each screen. Next is a description of the various icons found in this program.

Main Menu Screen

The Main Menu screen is the opening screen and contains icons that will allow the user to navigate throughout the software (Figure 1). Each icon represents a different section within SYNAPSE. Icons found on the Main Menu are described next.

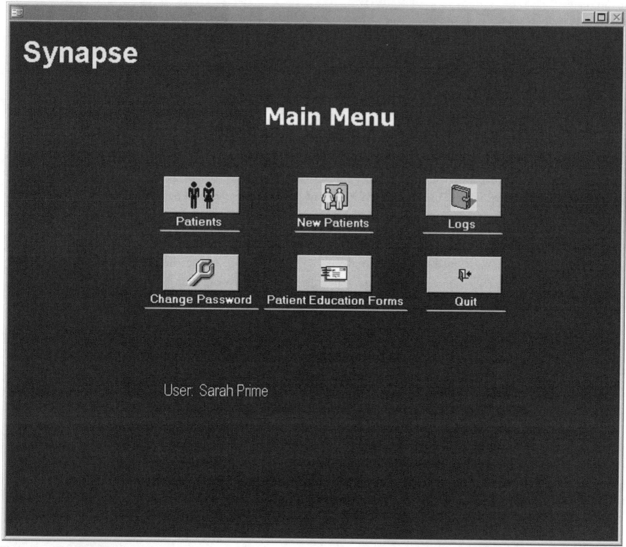

Figure 1   The Main Menu screen

PATIENTS ICON

When clicked, the Patients icon takes the user into a screen that lists all of the established patients in alphabetical order. There are only a few established patients within the software prior to beginning the SYNAPSE exercises; however, the patient population will grow with each exercise. Once a new chart is created, it will be stored in the patient database found on this screen.

NEW PATIENTS ICON

This icon is used when the user wants to create an electronic chart for a new patient. When the user clicks this icon, a series of tabbed screens appear, requesting the following patient information:

- Name and address
- Birth date

- Social Security number

- Telephone number

- Spouse information

- Responsible party information

- Payer information

- Allergy information

- List of the current medications, including over-the-counter medications

Once the chart has been created, the user will click the Demographics icon in the Patient Information Menu to make changes to this information. This screen should be accessed whenever there is a change in the patient's demographic information.

LOGS

The Logs icon takes the user to a screen that houses specific logs typically kept in paper form within the medical office. The following table includes a description of each type of log.

Name of Log	Description	Tracking Purpose
In-House Lab	This log tracks all tests performed in-house or within the medical office.	These logs track results of certain tests performed within the office and aid in tracking lot numbers of various testing reagents, kits, and strips. If the manufacturer sends out a recall notice for a specific lot number of reagents or test kits, the office will know which patients need to be retested.
Quality Control	This log tracks all of the controls used to check the accuracy of various test kits, strips, and instruments used for testing purposes.	The purpose of running lab controls is to confirm that test kits, strips, and lab equipment are working properly. Quality control logs confirm that the office institutes quality control measures, and may be reviewed when the medical office goes through a site evaluation.
Universal Narcotics	This log tracks narcotics that are dispensed or administered in the office.	The purpose of this log is to discourage employees tempted to steal narcotics. This log can also be used in reports to find trends within a specific patient population who use the drugs, or practitioners who prescribe the drugs.
Universal Immunization	This log tracks all immunizations administered in the office.	This log is useful in the event there is a recall on a specific lot number of a vaccine and is also useful for running reports for statistical data.

CHANGE PASSWORD ICON

This icon is used to set up a username and password, or to change an existing password.

PATIENT EDUCATION FORMS ICON

This icon takes the user to a screen that shows a series of educational forms used in the practice. Examples of educational materials include asthma, diabetes, smoking cessation, hypertension, IBS, and many other health-related materials.

QUIT ICON

This icon is used to quit SYNAPSE.

Patient Information Menu Screen

The Patient Information Menu screen is the initial screen within the patient's personal medical record (Figure 2). To get to this screen, the user clicks the Patients icon in the Main Menu. Next, the user clicks the name of the patient whose record is being accessed and clicks the Open Patient Record icon. The patient information screen then appears. A series of icons display in this screen, which allows the user to navigate within the patient's personal medical record. Icons found within this screen are listed next.

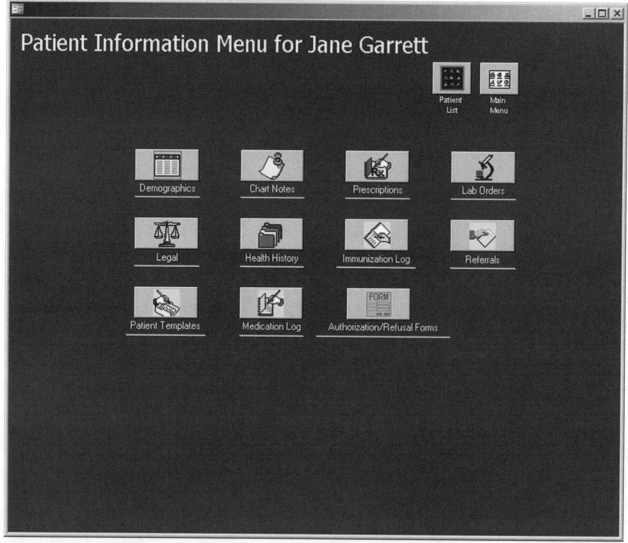

Figure 2   The Patient Information Menu screen

PATIENT LIST ICON

This icon is used to navigate from the current patient's record into the electronic record of another patient.

MAIN MENU ICON

This icon is used to return to the Main Menu, the starting point of SYNAPSE. This icon should be clicked whenever the user needs to document information in the Logs section, retrieve patient education forms, or to quit the program,

DEMOGRAPHICS ICON

This icon is used when the user wants to update the patient's demographic information. It can also be used to update allergy information, medication information, and the chronic problem list; however, these items can also be updated within progress notes. Because this information is private, more offices are now relying on clinical staff members to perform this task while the patient is behind closed doors.

CHART NOTES ICON

All previous chart notes for each patient are housed within this screen. The chart notes screen is also used to create a new office visit chart note or telephone note.

PRESCRIPTIONS ICON

This icon takes the user to the prescription screen. This screen allows the user to view the patient's prescription history and to create and discontinue prescriptions. Medication history should also be updated in the Allergies & Meds table found in the Patient Information screen in order for changes to be reflected in the patient's progress note.

LAB ORDERS ICON

The lab orders screen is used to create a lab requisition when the clinician orders a test. The user can also review the patient's lab history by clicking the Lab History icon found on this screen, and can update lab results by clicking the Update Lab Results icon.

LEGAL ICON

This screen has a list of topics frequently discussed between the clinician and patient that may have legal implications. Any time one of these topics is addressed, it should be documented within the patient's chart. Some of the listed items in this screen include privacy statement information, DNR orders, Power of Attorney information, and more. When patients complete and sign these forms, the forms should be scanned into the record for future use.

HEALTH HISTORY ICON

This icon takes the user into a series of tabs that display questions related to the patient's health. It is here that the user will record information about the patient's family history, hospitalization history, medical history, and social history. The lab and medication history can also be viewed from this section of the record. Any changes made in the lab and prescription screens will automatically populate into these screens.

IMMUNIZATION LOG ICON

This icon takes the user into the patient's personal immunization log. Any time a patient has an immunization performed, it should be documented in this log as well as the universal immunization log, which can be accessed by clicking the Logs icon on the Main Menu.

REFERRALS ICON

This icon takes the user to a referral letter template that can be used when the patient is referred to an outside physician. Names and addresses of physicians whom the practice routinely refers to are stored within this template to further simplify the referral process.

PATIENT TEMPLATES ICON

This icon takes the user to several letter templates that may be used in the medical office. Letter templates include Lab Results Are All Normal, Proof of Appointment, Lab Results (Unable to Reach by Phone), and a Return to Work Excuse. The user just clicks on the appropriate letter and completes the template information. Once the form is completed, it is either printed and given to the patient or sent to the patient, via email when appropriate.

MEDICATION LOG ICON

The Medication Log icon navigates the user to the patient's personal medication log. Any time an injection is administered or an oral medication is dispensed, it is documented within the patient's electronic medication log.

AUTHORIZATION/REFUSAL FORMS ICON

This icon takes the user to immunization consent forms, special procedure consent forms, and a refusal form that is completed when a patient refuses various treatments or tests. When working in the field, these forms will be scanned back into the patient's personal medical record.

SYNAPSE VERSION 1.1 EXERCISES

SYNAPSE is designed to simulate tasks the medical assistant typically performs within the electronic chart. The assignments for SYNAPSE are broken down into modules. Each module represents a portion of a new day in the medical office. Each module will include a variety of activities, including:

- Creating charts for new patients

- Documenting chief complaints and vital signs on existing charts

- Creating lab requisitions and prescriptions

- Documenting within a variety of electronic logs

Data for each new patient is listed within patient data tables. A variety of tasks will be assigned within each module. Modules I through III will end with a list of critical thinking questions that will challenge the user from both a software and clinical viewpoint. Each student should have a blank folder while performing SYNAPSE exercises. Any time the student is asked to print information, it should be printed, labeled, and placed in their SYNAPSE folder. Each module will have a different set of forms to print, so students should separate forms by module number. Module IV is a competency that is graded by the instructor to evaluate the student's comprehension of SYNAPSE. An EMR performance evaluation checklist is found at the end of this appendix, following Module IV.

MODULE I

Today's date: May 14, 2007
Appointments for May 14, 2007:

Patient's Name	Appointment Time	Reason for Appointment	Clinician	MA
Cindy Swaim	9:00 AM	Anxiety	Dr. Heath	Fauna Stout, CMA

Work Assignments

Module I has a total of ten tasks, and it lays the foundation for all other modules because it lists step-by-step instructions for the various tasks. Included throughout the exercises are Help boxes to assist the user what to do if he or she runs into problems while working in particular screens. The following tips may assist the user in finding information quickly when performing future SYNAPSE exercises:

1. Highlight all first-time instructions with a pink marker.

2. Highlight all Help boxes with a yellow marker.

3. Place a large paper clip on the pages that contain first-time instructions or Help boxes.

Task 1-1: Documenting in the Quality Control Log

Every morning, a different person is responsible for opening the lab and turning on the equipment. The person opening the lab also runs controls on various instruments and test kits. Today, it is Fauna Stout's turn to open the lab and run controls, and you will take on the role of this medical assistant.

1. Log in to SYNAPSE.

2. Begin documentation by clicking the Logs icon on the Main Menu screen.

3. Next, click the drop-down arrow under Quality Control Log. There will be a list of test kits or equipment on which you routinely perform controls. Yesterday, Fauna noticed that several of the patients had lower-than-normal glucose levels. Today she performed a control on the glucose unit to make certain it is functioning correctly. Start the documentation by clicking the word "Glucose."

4. Click Open Selected Log located at the top center of the screen.

5. Next, click the update button located at the bottom of the screen (Figure 3). Enter the information listed in Table 1 within the requested fields.

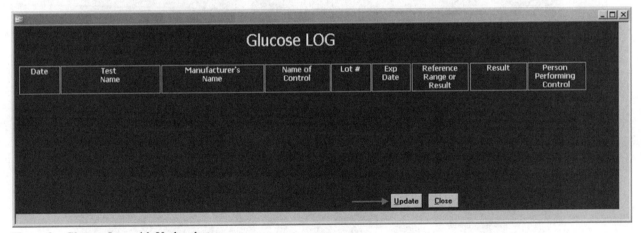

Figure 3   Glucose Log with Update button

TABLE 1   TASK 1-1 INFORMATION

Date	05/14/2007
Test Name	Glucometer Essential
Manufacturer's Name	Jefferson Diagnostics
Name of Control	High Control
Lot #	4890
Exp Date	02/01/2008
Reference Range or Result	250-300
Result	250 mg/dl
Person Performing Control	Fauna Stout, CMA

Help Box: Quality Control Logs

If the log you are working in has no prior entries, you can enter the data in Table 1 directly; however, if previous entries were made in the log, you need to click the Add Log icon before entering the information.

6. Once you have entered the requested information, compare your screen with Figure 4 to make certain it is correct.

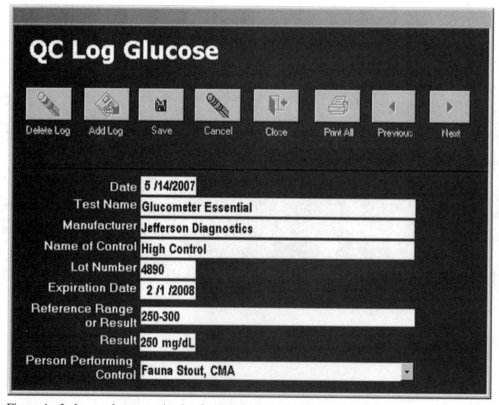

Figure 4   In-house glucose testing log for the glucose control

7. Click Save.

8. Next, click the Print All icon. Label your work as Task 1-1 and place it in your SYNAPSE folder.

9. Click Close. When you click Close, you should see the information you entered in the Glucose log. If the information does not match, delete the log by clicking the Update tab. This brings you back to the original screen in which you recorded the log entry. Make the appropriate changes and, once again, click Save. Click Print All, and click Close.

10. Close the Glucose log by clicking the Close tab next to Update.

11. Navigate out of the Open Selected Log screen by clicking Close, which is the little red box with the white X in the upper-right corner of the screen.

12. You should now be back in the Main Menu.

Task 1-2: Creating a New Chart and Progress Note for the Patient

The first patient of the day is Cindy Swaim. You greet the patient and take her back to the examination room. First, you will need to create a chart for Ms. Swaim. Information necessary to create the chart and progress note can be found in Table 2.

TABLE 2   CINDY SWAIM'S PATIENT DATA TABLE

Patient's Name	Cindy L. Swaim
Patient's DOB	04/14/1965
Patient's Chart Number	268506784
Patient's Address	429 Kingston Drive, Louis Center, NY, 01287-1111
Patient's Telephone Numbers	Home: 123-842-8421 Work: 123-652-9874
Patient's Employer Info	Lakeside Memorial Hospital Fostoria, NY, 01254-6543
Gender, Marital Status, Blood Type & Smoking Status	Gender: Female Marital Status: Single Blood Type: A+ Smoking Status: Smoker
Spouse Name, DOB, & Address	N/A
Responsible Party Info	Patient
Primary Payer Info	Signal HMO, 135 Carriagehill Lane, Douglasville, NY, 01268506784-00, Policy Holder: Self
Secondary Payer	None
Patient Drug Allergies	Tetracycline
Patient Other Allergy	Dust, Pollen
Current Mediation List	None
Preferred Pharmacy	Family Pharmacy Inc., 865 Livingston Ave, Fostoria NY, 01254
Lab Provider	National Diagnostics
Privacy Statement	Date the Privacy Statement was signed: 05/14/2007; note to be entered in the Notes box. April Patrick (mother of patient) can receive private information if unable to contact the patient directly. April Patrick's cell phone number is 123-328-9874.

Family Health History Info	Father: Age 62, Health: Fair Mother: Age 60, Health: Good Brother: Age 37, Health: Good Sister: Age at Death 6, Cause of Death: Leukemia Familial Diseases: Cancer: Enter the following note: Paternal grandfather died of liver cancer at age 72. Other: Father has emphysema.
Hospitalizations, Blood Transfusions, and Serious Injuries	Hospitalizations: 1984, Lakeside Memorial Hospital, emergency appendectomy (no complications) Blood Transfusions: The patient has not received any blood transfusions. Serious Injuries: None
Pregnancies	None
Medical History	Place checkmarks in the boxes for chicken pox, diabetes, and high cholesterol. Notes: Place the following in the Notes box: Chicken pox: 1970 (no complications). Diabetes: Diagnosed with borderline diabetes in 2003 (diet controlled) High cholesterol: Diagnosed in 2003 (diet controlled)
Health Habits	Check Caffeine: Two 12-ounce cups of coffee per day Check Tobacco: 1 to 1 1/2 packs of cigarettes per day × 22 years Check ETOH: Drink Type: Beer Drinks Week: Six 12-ounce cans per week Check the box for Heavy Lifting Occupation: Patient Care Associate
Subjective Information	Chief Complaint: Anxiety or stress Severity of symptoms is a 4 on a scale from 1 to 10. Duration of symptoms is 4 months. Associated symptoms: (Positives) Breathing irregularities, decrease in ability to concentrate, history of prior attacks, and increase in appetite or weight. (Negatives) Heart irregularities, and psychotic or delusional behavior Aggravating Factors: Crowded areas Relieving Factors: Eating and Sleeping
Objective Information	Vital Signs: Height: 64 inches Weight: 162 pounds Temperature: 99.8 Blood Pressure: 150/98 Pulse: 92 Respiration: 20 Pain: 0 Subjective Information and Vital Signs Entered By: Fauna Stout, CMA

CREATING A CHART

1. Begin by clicking the New Patients icon on the Main Menu.

2. The first tabbed screen under Patient Information is the Patient Main screen. Using the information provided in Table 2 fill in the requested fields. When you are finished, click Save. Check your work with Figure 5.

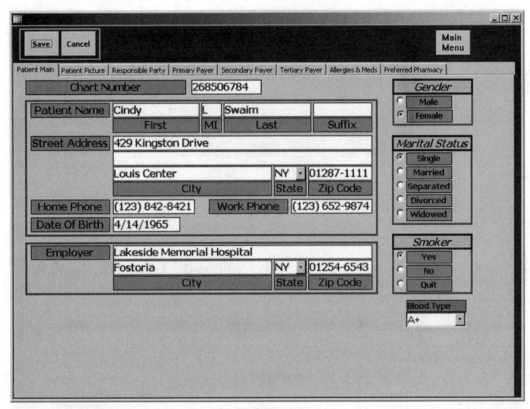

Figure 5   Patient Main screen completed for Cindy Swaim

Help Box: Navigating through Fields

Pressing the Tab key on your keyboard is an excellent way to move from one field to another. When you finish entering information in the field in which you are working, press the Tab key; this will move you to the next available field.

---

3. Next, click the Patient Picture tab. This is where you can attach a picture of a patient if you have a scanner or digital image. Check to make certain the patient's chart number is in the Patient Chart Number box. Under the Patient Picture box is another box labeled Patient Notes. This box serves as a reminder box. You will enter special facts about the patient in this box, such as how the patient wants to be addressed, special events in the patient's life (such as a wedding or graduation), or notes that remind you to take a certain action during the patient's next visit. These actions may include having the patient sign a specific form or making certain that the patient returned an X-ray that was borrowed from the office. You should look in this section of the record prior to rooming the patient to see if there are any specific notations directing you to take a specific action. Once the action has been applied, or the event has past, you should remove the note by deleting it and clicking Save. For this visit, enter the following information in the Patient Notes box: "The patient prefers to be addressed by her first name." Click Save.

4. Click the Responsible Party tab. The patient's chart number should have automatically populated in this screen, as well as the remainder of screens within the patient information section. Since Cindy is responsible

for her own bills, click Self. Note that all of Cindy's information automatically populates in this screen. Also notice that the numerals listed in the chart number is Cindy's Social Security number. Offices are currently moving away from using the patient's Social Security number as an identifier.

5. Click the Primary Payer tab. Click the drop-down menu arrow in the box next to the Name heading. Click Signal HMO. The address information for the insurance company should automatically appear after clicking Signal HMO. Next, enter the subscriber I.D. #, which is 268506784-00. There is no Policy/Group #, so leave that box empty. Under Policy Holder information, click Self. The remainder of the information should automatically populate within the Policy Holder section, except for Cindy's Social Security number. Enter 268-50-6784. Compare your work with Figure 6 and click Save.

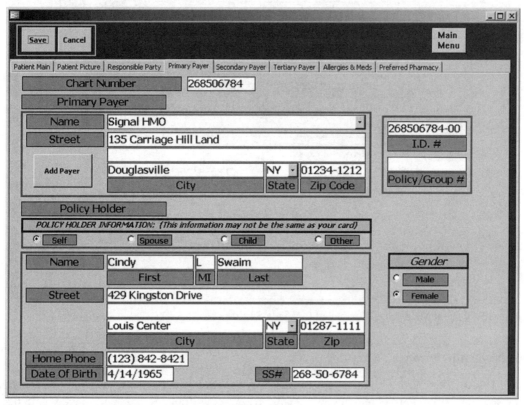

Figure 6   Primary Payer screen completed for Cindy Swaim

6. The patient does not have any secondary or tertiary insurance, so you can skip those tabs and go directly to the Allergy & Meds tab. The patient is allergic to Tetracycline. Begin this section by clicking the Click to Add tab within the Patient Drug Allergy List box. Another box will appear. Type Tetracycline in the Enter Patient Drug Allergy field. Next, click the Save button. Once you save your information, it should automatically appear in red in the Patient Drug Allergy List box. The patient is also allergic to dust and pollen, so click the Click to Add tab in the Patient Other Allergy List box. Type Dust in the Enter Patient Other Allergy field. Click Save. Repeat the same instructions for pollen. The patient is not taking any current medications, so click Save. Check your work with Figure 7.

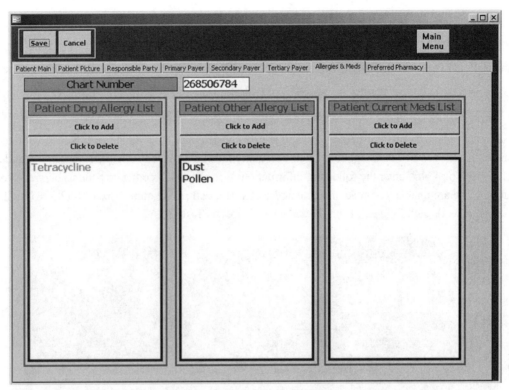

Figure 7   Allergies & Meds screen completed for Cindy Swaim

7. Next click the Preferred Pharmacy tab. Click Update Patient Preferred Pharmacies. The patient selected Family Pharmacy Inc., 865 Livingston Ave, Fostoria NY, 01254 as her preferred pharmacy. Click the Add/Remove button next to this pharmacy. A checkmark should appear in the box of the Add/Remove button. Click Close. The pharmacy you selected should now appear in the Patient Preferred Pharmacies box (see Figure 8). Click Save.

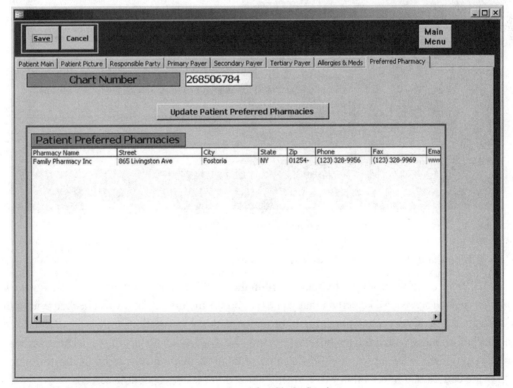

Figure 8   Preferred Pharmacy screen completed for Cindy Swaim

8. Review each tab and make certain that all of your information saved correctly.

9. Click the Main Menu icon.

10. Click the Patients icon. Cindy Swaim's name should now be listed within the alphabetical list of patients.

11. Highlight Cindy's name by clicking the patient selector column, which is the column just to the left of the patient's name. Click Open Patient Record. The Patient Information screen for Cindy Swaim appears.

12. Click the Legal Icon. You just finished reviewing the privacy statement with the patient. Now click the drop-down menu arrow in the Privacy Statement box. Click Yes. Enter today's date, May 14, 2007, in the box under the date column. In the Notes box, enter the following information: April Patrick (mother of patient) can receive private information if we are unable to contact the patient directly. Her cell phone number is 123-328-9874. Click Save, and check your work with Figure 9. Print the screen and label as Task 1-2A.

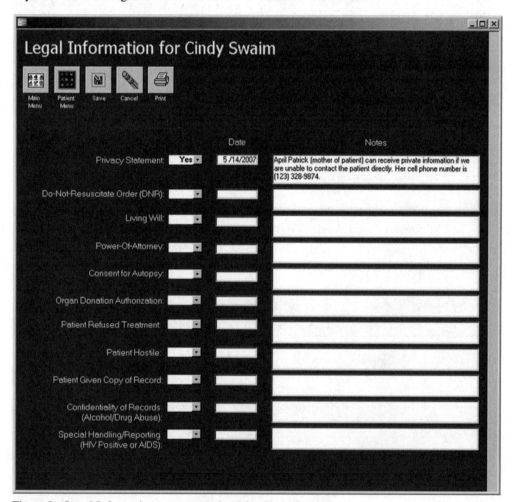

Figure 9   Legal Information screen completed for Cindy Swaim

13. Click Patient Menu and then click the Health History icon.

14. Using Table 2, enter all of the history information within the Health History sections. *Note: Save your information after completing each screen.* Make certain that you expound on any disease that was checked within the family history or past medical history tabs by entering information in the Notes sections of those particular screens. Do not enter any information within the lab history screen or the medication history screen. These screens will automatically populate when a prescription is written or a lab requisition is ordered. Refer to Figures 10, 11, and 12 to make certain that information was correctly entered in the corresponding screens.

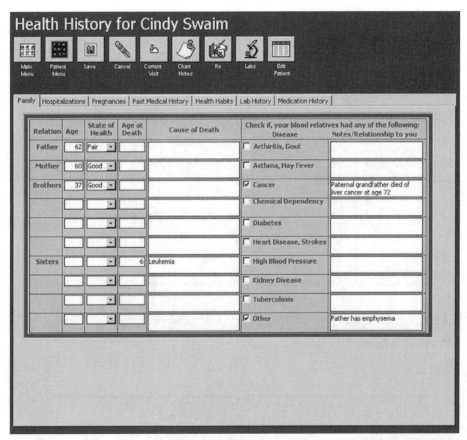

Figure 10   Family History screen completed for Cindy Swaim

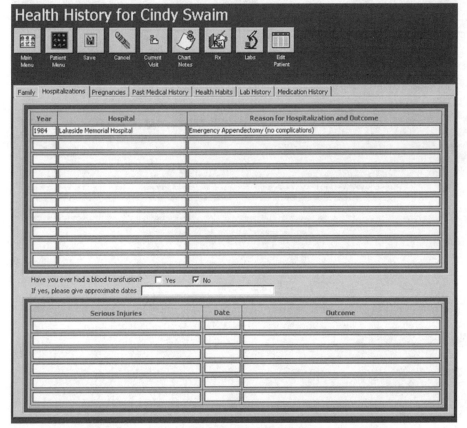

Figure 11   Hospitalization screen completed for Cindy Swaim

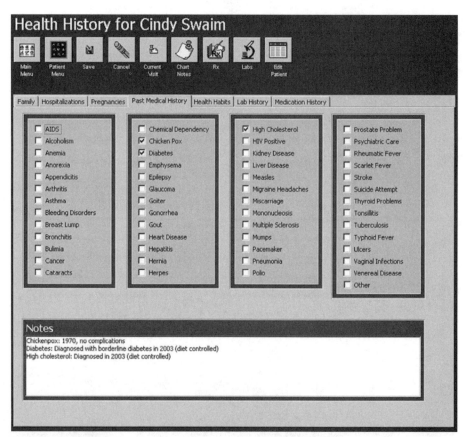

Figure 12   Past Medical History screen completed for Cindy Swaim

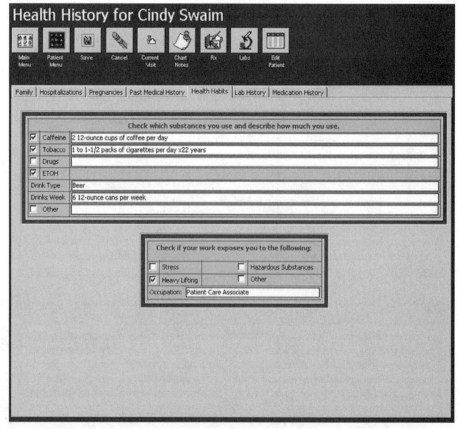

Figure 13   Health Habits screen completed for Cindy Swaim

Help Box: Entering Grandparent Information into the Family History Screen

When entering information about a grandparent, identify if it was the father's parents by placing the word "paternal" in front of the grandparent and by using the word "maternal" when referring to the mother's parents.

15. Click the Patient Menu icon. Next, click the Chart Notes icon.

a. You should see four icons at the top of the screen and two long boxes below the four icons (Figure 14).

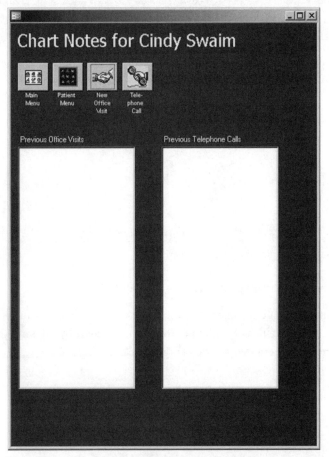

Figure 14   Chart Notes screen for Cindy Swaim

b. The two boxes below the icons will include a listing of all previous office visits and telephone calls that the patient has had in the past. Your boxes should be blank because the patient has not been seen in the past. When you want to read a previous note of an established patient, just click the date in question and the note from that visit will appear. Each time a patient comes in for a new office visit, you should click the New Office Visit icon. When the patient calls the office for medical results or advice, you should click the Telephone Call icon. Cindy is here for a new office visit, so click New Office Visit.

16. Once you see the New Office Visit Screen, enter the date of Cindy's visit, which is May 14, 2007. Next, enter the time of Cindy's visit, 9:00 a.m.

17. Click the Update Progress Note button at the top of the toolbar and then click Save.

18. Next, click the Subjective Tab.

19. Click the drop-down menu in the box under Chief Complaint.

20. Click the words "Anxiety or Stress" from the drop-down list (Figure 15).

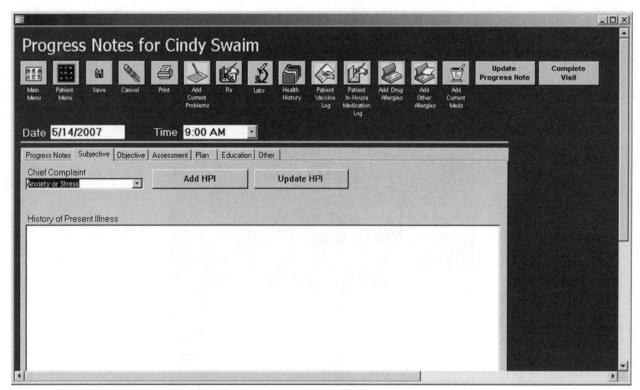

Figure 15   Chief Complaint screen completed for Cindy Swaim

21. Click Update Progress Notes and then click Save.

22. Most physicians will enter the patient's history of the present illness (HPI) information; however, you will enter it here to see how items populate within the progress note. Start by clicking the Add HPI button. The screen where HPI information is entered appears (Figure 16).

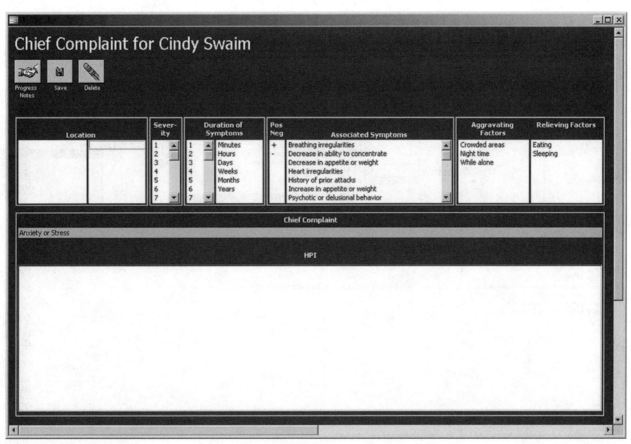

Figure 16 Chief Complaint screen that shows all of the HPI information for anxiety or stress

a. Since location is not a factor, the box is empty.

b. Under Severity of Symptoms, click 4. This signifies the severity of the patient's symptoms on a scale from 1 to 10.

c. In the row next to severity there is another set of numbers. Click 4 and then click Months. This signifies that the patient has had the symptoms for four months. All of this information should automatically populate within the white HPI box below the chief complaint.

d. Next is the Associated Symptoms box. Associated symptoms are symptoms that may be common with particular chief complaints. You will see a + symbol and – symbol. Click the + symbol first. Click all of the symptoms that are listed as positive in Cindy's patient data table. Positive symptoms included the following: *Breathing irregularities, Decrease in ability to concentrate, History of prior attacks, and Increase in appetite or weight.* Now click on the – symbol. Click the symptoms that do not apply, which include the following: *Heart irregularities and psychotic or delusional behavior.* You didn't click Decrease in appetite or weight because the patient already stated that she had an increase in appetite or weight.

e. Next is the Aggravating Factors box. Aggravating factors are factors that make the symptoms worse. Cindy stated that crowded areas make her symptoms worse, so click *Crowded areas.*

f. Next is the Relieving Factors box. Relieving factors are factors that seem to help the symptoms. Cindy stated that eating and sleeping seem to make her symptoms better, so click Eating and click Sleeping. Now that you are through entering the HPI information, click Save. Check your work with Figure 17.

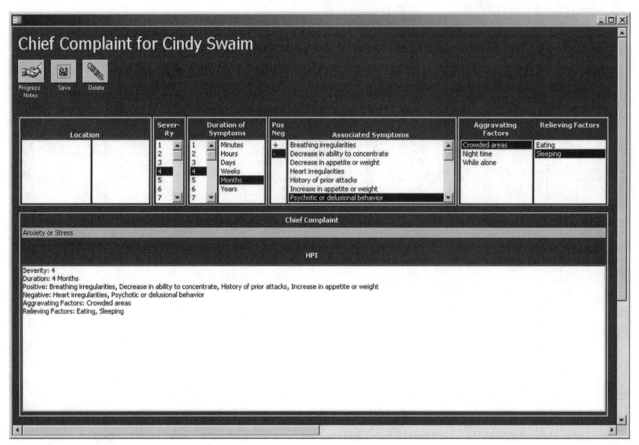

Figure 17   Cindy Swaim's completed HPI table

23. Next, click the Progress Notes icon. You should now be viewing the information within the Subjective Information tab. Click Update Progress Note and then click Save. Now click the Progress Notes tab. The subjective information should have automatically populated within the progress note. Refer to Figure 18 to make certain that your subjective information is correct.

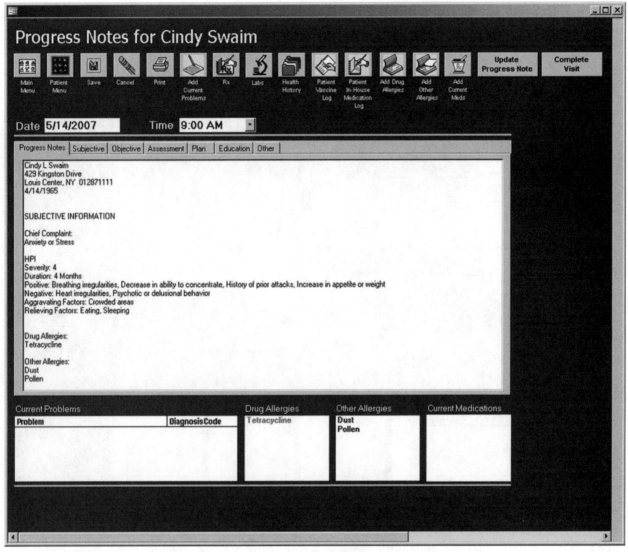

Figure 18   Progress Notes screen with the subjective information entered within the progress note

24. Click the Objective Tab. Enter the patient's vital signs in the requested fields:

   Vital Signs:

   Height: 64 inches

   Weight: 162 pounds

   Temperature: 99.8

   Blood Pressure: 150/98

   Pulse: 92

   Respiration: 20

   Pain: 0

25. Click the name of the medical assistant you are representing, which is Fauna Stout. This feature illustrates who entered the subjective findings and vital signs. Refer to Figure 19 to make certain that you entered the information correctly in the Objective screen.

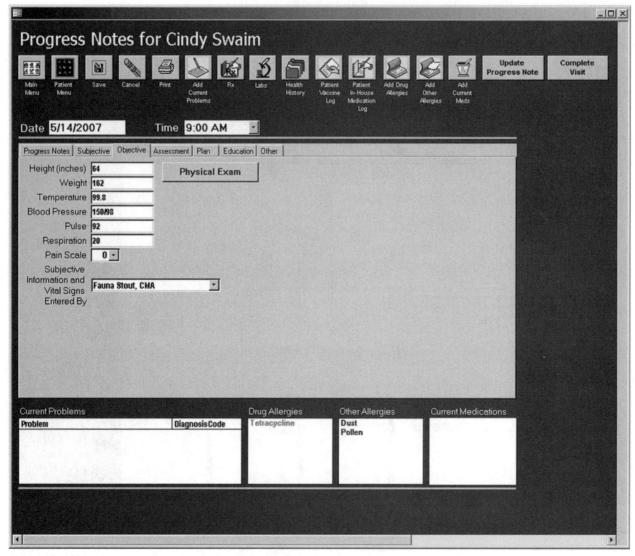

Figure 19   Objective screen completed with Cindy Swaim's vital sign information

26. Click the Update Progress Note icon at the top of the toolbar and then click Save.

27. Click the Progress Notes tab. Scroll down to view the objective information. You should see the information you entered within the Objective tab now populated within the progress note window. You should also see that the Patient's Drug Allergy Information and Other Allergy Information automatically populated within the note. You will also see the headings Physical Examination Findings, Assessment, and Plan. These headings illustrate the remainder of information to be added by the clinician. Check your work with Figure 20.

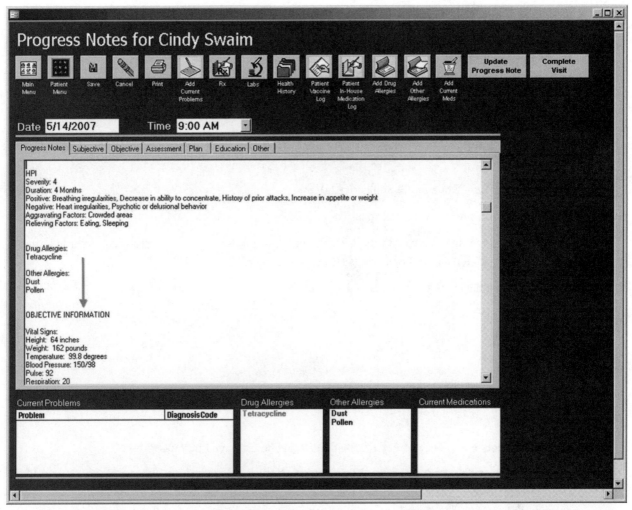

Figure 20   Completed progress notes for Cindy Swaim

28. Review the progress note and look for any errors. When you are satisfied the information is correct, click the Print icon. Print a copy of the progress note and label it Task 1-2B. Do not click the Complete Visit icon until the patient's visit is completed. Once you click this icon and leave the screen, you cannot enter any further information for this particular visit. The physician still has information to enter, so leave the screen for the physician.

Help Box: Progress Notes

If after viewing the progress note you notice any errors, take the following actions:

If the error occurs in the Subjective information:

1. You should return to the Subjective tab and make the appropriate corrections. Click Update Progress Note and then click Save. Make certain the information saved correctly.

2. If the updated subjective information does not save correctly after applying the above action, try the following:

   a. Click the Cancel icon while in the Subjective tab.

   b. Click Yes, you are sure you want to cancel.

   c. Click the drop-down menu arrow in the Chief Complaint box, even if the correct complaint is already displayed. (This should cause the previous HPI information to disappear.)

   d. Make certain that the correct complaint is displayed.

   e. Click Update Progress Note.

   f. Click Save.

   g. Click Add HPI.

   h. Click the appropriate symptoms.

   i. Click Save.

   j. Click the Subjective tab. The correct information should be displayed in the HPI box.

   k. Click the Progress Notes tab. You should be able to view the amended progress note. The information should now be correct. *Note: Remember, you will not click the Complete Visit tab until both you and the physician are completely finished with the patient. Once the note is completed, you will need to click the Complete Visit tab to complete the note; otherwise, the note will not save properly.*

If the error occurs in the Objective information:

1. Click the Objective tab.

2. Click Cancel.

3. Enter the corrected information in the appropriate boxes.

4. Click the Update Progress Note icon.

5. Click Save.

6. Click the Progress Notes tab.

7. You should be able to view the amended progress note now. The information should now be correct. *Note: Remember, you will not click the Complete Visit tab until both you and the physician are completely finished with the patient. Once the note is completed, you will need to click the Complete Visit icon to complete the note; otherwise, the note will not save properly.*

Now that the chart is created and all information is entered, you can alert the physician that the patient is ready to be seen.

When working in the field, the physician will typically exit the patient's room and instruct the medical assistant to read the Plan section of the progress note. Since this is not possible for these assignments, the plan will be provided in the instructions. The plan for Cindy Swaim states the following:

Plan: In-Office Glucose. Will send the patient's blood out for a Chem 12. Rx for Alprazolam, 0.5 mg, # 30, Take 1 tablet every day. One month prescription, no refills. Rx for Atenolol tabs, 50 mg, Take 1 tab each day before meals or at bedtime, One month prescription, no refills, Spoke to patient regarding hypertension, hypercholesterolemia, diabetes, and a smoking cessation program. Will give patient educational materials for hypertension, smoking cessation, heart disease, and diabetes. Re: Pt to follow up in one month for a thorough physical.

There are many things that you will need to do to finish with this patient. Time management will be very important. Let's start our tasks by creating all of the orders for the labs.

Task 1-3: Ordering Lab Tests

1. Since you should already be in the Progress Notes screen, click the Labs icon.

2. Click the drop-down menu arrow in the Laboratory box. A list of laboratories will appear. This box depicts which lab conducted the testing. Since the test will be performed in the office, select In-House Testing.

3. Next, click the drop-down menu arrow in the Ordering Provider box. Another drop-down list will appear. Click Dr. Heath.

4. Click the Payer drop-down menu arrow. Select Signal HMO.

5. Click the drop-down menu arrow in the General Lab Tests box. A drop-down list of tests will appear. Scroll and click Fasting Blood Sugar or FBS.

6. Leave the Number and Type of Specimens Sent box empty since we are not sending this test outside the office.

7. In the Today's Date box, enter the date of Cindy's appointment, which is 05/14/2007.

8. Next, click the Specimen Prepared By drop-down menu arrow. Click Fauna Stout, since she is the medical assistant taking care of the patient.

9. Click the drop-down menu arrow in the Was patient fasting? box. Click Yes. Check your work with Figure 21, and make the appropriate corrections before saving the information.

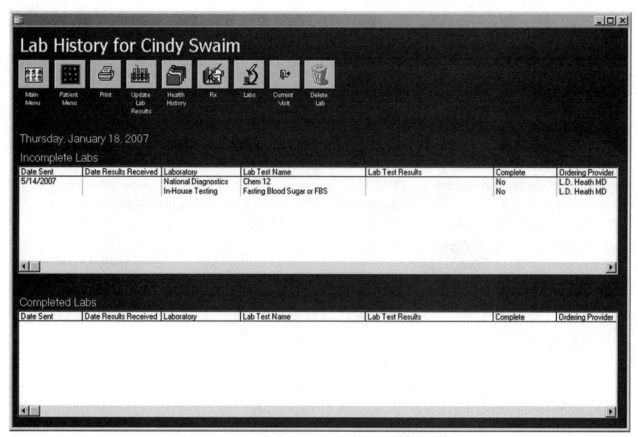

Figure 21   Completed Lab Requisition screen for Cindy Swaim illustrating the FBS order

10. Click Save.

11. Click the Preview Box to review the order. If you made an error, perform the steps in the Help Box: Correcting an Error in the Lab Preview Screen.

12. Once information is correct in the Preview box, click the Print icon in the upper-right corner of the lab requisition screen.

13. Label the requisition as Task 1-3A. Place it in your SYNAPSE folder. Close the screen by clicking the X in the upper-right corner.

14. Now click the Lab History icon. Your Fasting Blood Sugar order should be displayed in the Incomplete Labs table.

15. Since the doctor also ordered an outside test, which is the Chem 12, click the Labs icon. Since the patient is having an outside test as well, you should also create the requisition for that test. The patient's insurance company allows her to go to National Diagnostics, so select that name from the drop-down list.

16. Click Ordering Provider. Select Dr. Heath.

17. Click the Insurance box arrow. Select Signal HMO.

18. Click the General Lab Tests box arrow. Click Chem 12.

19. Type the following information within the Number of and Type of Specimens Sent box: One Red Top Tube.

20. Insert the date of the patient's appointment in the Today's Date box.

21. Next, click the Specimen Prepared By drop-down arrow. Select Fauna's name.

22. Click the drop-down arrow in the Was patient fasting? box. Click Yes. Click Save. Click the Preview Box to view the order.

23. Print a copy of this lab requisition by clicking the Print icon in the upper-right corner of the screen.

24. Label the form Task 1-3B and place it in your SYNAPSE folder. Close the screen by clicking the X in the upper-right corner.

25. Click the Lab History icon. Your order should be displayed in the Incomplete Labs table. Refer to Figure 22.

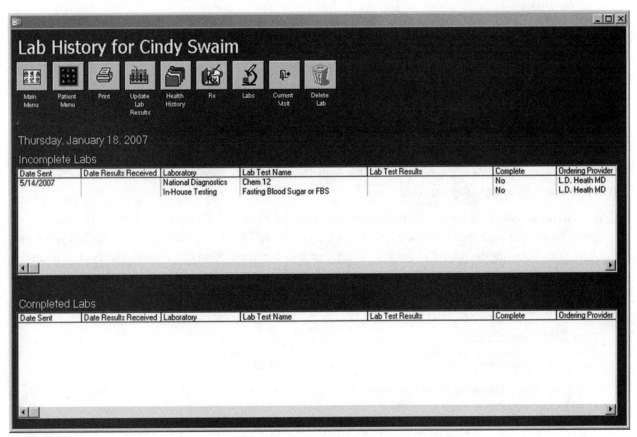

Figure 22 Lab History table showing the requests for both labs for Cindy Swaim

---

Help Box: Correcting an Error in the Lab Preview Screen

1. If you observe any errors during the lab preview, click out of the preview by clicking the Close box (the white X in the red box in the upper-right corner of the screen).

2. Click the Lab History icon.

3. Click the lab test that has the error.

4. Click the Delete Lab icon.

5. Click the small selector box next to the Click to Delete the Lab heading.

6. Close the screen. The information should no longer be listed in the table.

7. Go to the labs section by clicking the Labs icon, and start the whole lab requisition over.

Now that the lab requisitions are completed, you will need to create the prescriptions.

Task 1-4: Creating a Prescription

The first prescription listed is for the patient's anxiety: Rx for Alprazolam, 0.5 mg, # 30, Take 1 tablet every day. One month prescription, no refills.

1. Click Patient Menu.

2. Click Prescriptions.

3. Click the Pharmacy box drop-down arrow. Select Family Pharmacy Inc. 865 Livingston Ave, Fostoria NY, 01254.

4. Click the Common Drug Formulary drop-down arrow. Select Alpazolam. The instructions that autopopulate on the right side of the screen should match the order above.

5. Next, click the Payer box drop-down arrow. Select Signal HMO.

6. Next, click the drop-down arrow in the Clinician Ordering Medication box. Select Dr. Heath.

7. Next, click the drop-down arrow in the Prescription Created By box. Select Fauna's name.

8. On the bottom right side of the screen, enter the Start Date as today's appointment date. Select the End Date as a month from today's appointment.

9. You will notice two little boxes above the Start Date and End Date boxes. One box is labeled Do Not Substitute and the other box is labeled New Common Drug. The Do Not Substitute box is checked when the doctor does not want the patient to have the generic or less-expensive form of the drug. The New Common Drug box is checked when you create a prescription for a drug that is not listed in the Common Drug Formulary. The doctor did not give instructions that the drug could not be substituted, and the drug is already in the Common Drug Formulary, so uncheck both boxes if they are not already unchecked.

10. Under Refills, select None.

11. Double-check each box to make certain all information is correct.

12. Click Save. The information should automatically populate within the Prescription History table (Figure 23).

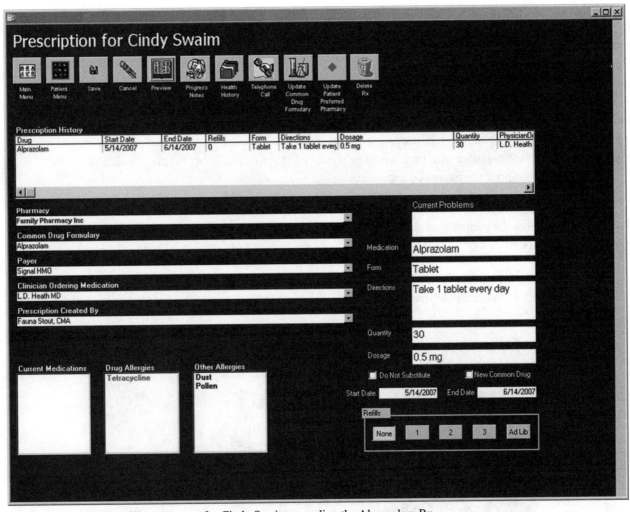

Figure 23   Prescription History screen for Cindy Swaim regarding the Alprazolam Rx

13. Click Preview. The Preview icon will allow you to view the prescription prior to printing it.

14. Click the Print icon in the Prescription Preview box and close the preview box.

15. In the medical office, the prescription would have been given to the physician to sign prior to giving it to the patient. Place the printed prescription in your folder and label it Task 1-4A.

Help Box: Correcting a Prescription Error after Saving

If you notice an error when previewing the information in the prescription screen after saving it, do the following:

1. Click the appropriate prescription within the Prescription History table.

2. Click the Delete Rx icon at the top of the toolbar.

3. Click in small empty box next to the Click to Delete the Prescription box.

4. Close the box.

5. Re-create the prescription and save.

The second prescription is for Atenolol, which is used to control the patient's blood pressure. The physician's order was for the following: Rx for Atenolol tabs, 50 mg, Take 1 tab each day before meals or at bedtime, One month prescription, no refills. This prescription should be easy to create because most of the necessary information was already entered for the first prescription. The only thing that needs to be changed is the name of the drug. Replace "Alprazolam" with "Atenolol." Make certain the information on the right matches the physician's order. The start date should be 05/14/2007 and the end date should be 06/14/2007. Be certain to click None under Refills. Take one final look at the information to make certain it matches the physician's order before clicking Save. Make certain the information saved in the Prescription History screen. Now click Preview, click out of the preview screen, and print the prescription. In the medical office, this form would be signed by the clinician. Label the prescription Task 1-4B.

Next, you should print the patient education materials.

Task 1-5: Printing Educational Handouts

The doctor stated that the patient should receive patient education materials for diabetes, smoking cessation, hypertension, and heart disease.

1. Click the Main Menu icon.

2. Next, click Patient Education Forms.

3. Next, click Education Letters.

4. Click the Diabetes box (Figure 24).

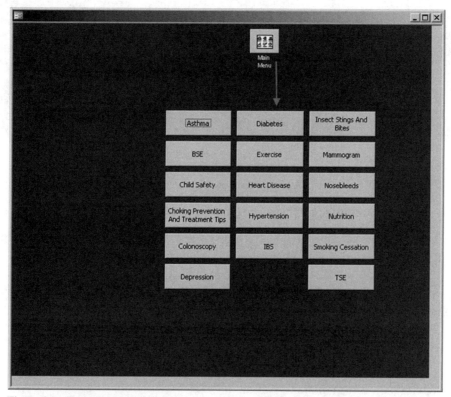

Figure 24   Education Letters screen

5. Choose Print from the File drop-down menu to print.

6. From the File drop-down menu, choose Close to return to the Education Letters screen.

7. Next, click Smoking Cessation tab.

8. Print the form and close the window, returning to the Education Letters screen.

9. Do the same for hypertension and heart disease.

10. Close the windows after printing.

11. After printing all of the handouts, label each handout as Task 1-5. Assign letters A through D for each individual handout. Place the educational handouts in your SYNAPSE folder.

Now you are ready to draw the patient's blood for outside testing and perform a finger stick for the in-house glucose testing. You finished the blood draw and blood glucose testing and are ready to log the information. The lab requisition forms have already been completed. Now you will need to record the glucose test in the In-House Test Log.

Task 1-6: Documenting an In-House Procedure within the In-House Test Log

1. Go to the Main Menu.

2. Click Logs.

3. Next, click the drop-down arrow in the In-House Log.

4. Select Glucose.

5. Click Open Selected Log.

6. Click Update.

7. Enter today's appointment date.

8. Choose the patient's name from the drop-down list in the Patient Name box.

9. Choose Dr. Heath's name from the drop-down list in the Ordering Provider box.

10. Enter the Manufacturer's Name, which is Jefferson Diagnostics.

11. Enter the Expiration Date from the test strips, which is 2/1/2008.

12. Enter the Lot Number, which is 4867.

13. Enter the results. Today's results are 204 mg/dl.

14. Click the drop-down arrow beside the Name of Person Performing the Test box. Click Fauna Stout's name.

15. Click Save. Refer to Figure 25 to make certain that you entered the information correctly.

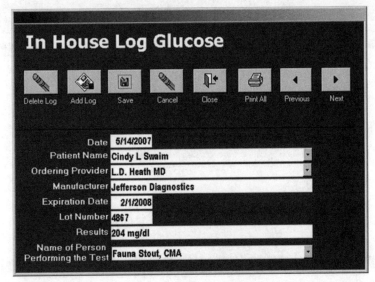

Figure 25   In-house log for Cindy Swaim's glucose

16. Print the glucose log by clicking the Print All icon. Label printout Task 1-6 and place it in your SYNAPSE folder.

17. Click Close.

18. The information should now appear on the In-House Glucose Test Log.

19. Click Close.

20. Close the Open Selected Log box by clicking the X in the upper-right corner of the window.

21. You should now be back in the Main Menu.

> **Help Box: In-House Logs**
>
> If the log you are working in has no prior entries, you can enter the information using the steps above; however, if other previous entries were made in the log prior to opening, you will need to click the Add Log icon before entering the information.

Task 1-7: Entering a Test Result in the Lab History Section

1. Select the Patients icon from the Main Menu.

2. Select Cindy Swaim's name.

3. Click Open Patient Record.

4. You should now be viewing Cindy's Patient Information Menu. Click the Lab Orders icon.

5. Click the Lab History icon.

6. Click the Fasting Blood Sugar test from the incomplete lab table.

7. Click the Update Lab Results icon (Figure 26).

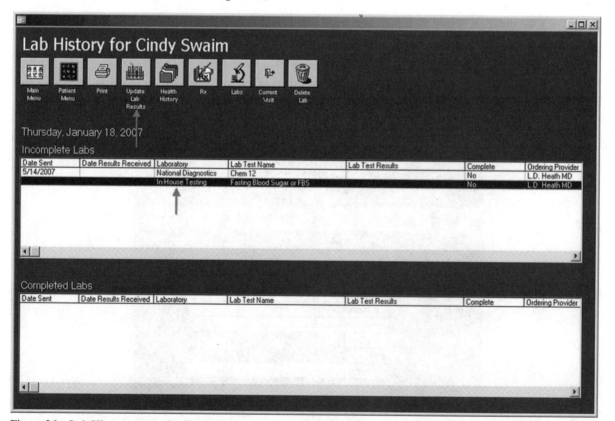

Figure 26   Lab History screen for Cindy Swaim

8. Type the lab result: 204 mg/dl.

9. Choose Fauna's name from the drop-down list in the Name of Person Who Recorded Results box.

10. Enter 5/14/2007 as the date the results were received. Check to make certain you entered the information correctly by comparing your information with Figure 27.

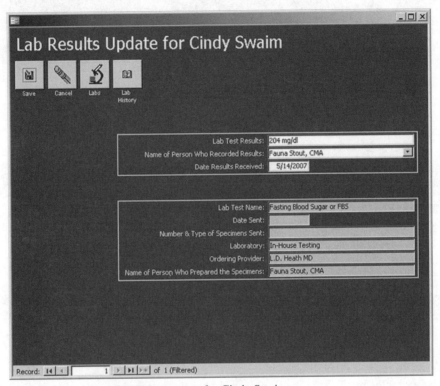

Figure 27   Lab Results Update screen for Cindy Swaim

11. Click Save.

12. Click Lab History.

13. The glucose results should have moved from the Incomplete Labs section to the Completed Labs section. (Figure 28).

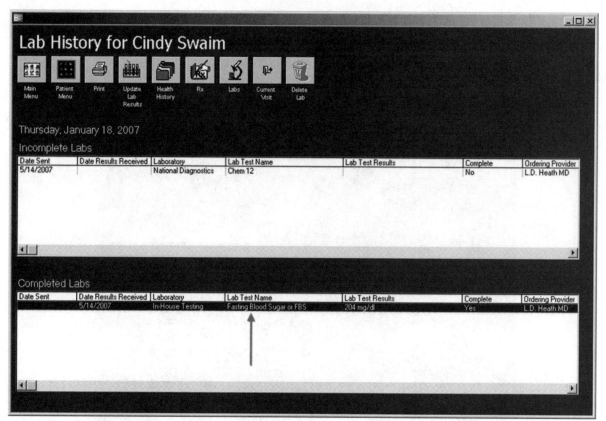

Figure 28   Lab History table for Cindy Swaim, illustrating how the glucose moved from the Incomplete Labs to the
Completed Labs

14. Print the lab history tables by clicking the Print icon. Label the Incomplete Lab table as Task 1-7A and the
Complete Lab table as Task 1-7B. Place both tables in your SYNAPSE folder.

Help Box: Printing Tables in the Lab History Screen

The Lab History Tables will not print unless there is data within the tables.

---

15. Click the Patient Menu icon.

Inform the physician of the patient's result and determine if he needs you to do anything else for the patient.
The physician tells you he wants to go in and discuss the results with the patient, and that he will let you know
when he is finished.

The physician re-enters the patient's examination room and discusses the findings. He notifies you that he is
finished and informs you that you can complete the visit. You have already gathered all of the patient's
prescriptions and educational handouts. You enter the patient's room and distribute and explain each prescription
and educational handout. You ask the patient if she has any further questions. She asks you for a proof of
appointment letter for her employer.

Task 1-8: Proof of Appointment Letter

1. Go to Cindy Swaim's Patient Information Menu, if you are not already there.

2. Click Patient Templates.

3. Click the Proof of Appointment button.

4. Insert the date of the appointment in the Date box.

5. Since Cindy's appointment was for 9:00, select 9:00 AM from the drop-down menu beside the appointment.

6. Click the Clinician drop-down list and select Dr. Heath. Refer to Figure 29 ensure you properly completed the template.

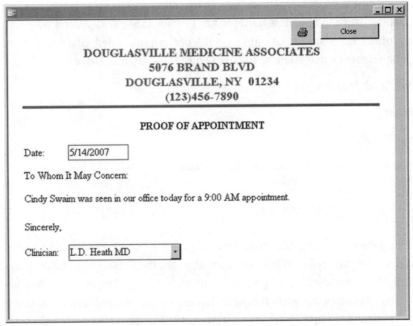

Figure 29   Proof of Appointment Letter template completed for Cindy Swaim

7. Print the letter and label it Task 1-8 and place it in your SYNAPSE folder.

8. Click Close.

9. Close the template letters by clicking the X in the upper-right corner of the window. You should now be in the Patient Information Menu for Cindy Swaim screen.

Task 1-9: Completing the Progress Note and Closing Out of the Patient's Record

Since the patient is gone and you are done working in the patient's personal EMR, you can now close the chart note.

1. Click the Chart Notes icon.

2. Click New Office Visit.

3. Click Save.

4. Click Update Progress Notes to make certain that all of the latest information was entered in the chart.

5. Click on the Complete Visit icon. *Note: When you leave this page, you will be unable to enter any additional data within the chart note.*

6. Click Patient Menu.

7. Click the Chart Notes icon.

8. Check to make certain that the date of your progress note saved to the Previous Office Visits box.

9. Click the visit and view the note.

10. Click Chart Notes.

11. Click Patient Menu.

12. Click the Main Menu.

Task 1-10: Phone Call from Blanche White

You will receive many phone calls, even while you are working in a clinical capacity. It is important that you document all encounters with the patient, including telephone calls.

Blanche White calls the office to request a refill for her Fosamax. She had several pills left from her previous prescription at the time of her last visit, so she didn't get the prescription filled. She lost the prescription and is now out of the drug. The pharmacy that Blanche uses is DanMart on Polaris Drive.

1. On the Main Menu, click Patients.

2. Select Blanche White.

3. Click Open Patient Record.

4. Now you should be in the Patient Information Menu screen.

5. Click Chart Notes.

6. Click the Telephone Call icon.

7. Notice there are four tabs in the center of this screen (Figure 30). The first tab is used when the patient is calling to request a prescription refill. When you click this tab, the Prescription History table will appear, which illustrates all of the medications the patient is currently taking. The second tab is labeled Follow-Up on Lab Test Results. You select this tab when the patient is requesting information regarding a lab test. This screen contains the patient's lab history for easy referencing. The third tab is labeled Symptoms. This tab is used when the patient has questions regarding symptoms he or she is currently experiencing, or when the patient has questions regarding his or her condition. The fourth tab is labeled Other Calls. This tab is used when the patient is calling about something other than the three previous tabs. Since the patient is calling regarding a prescription refill, keep the Prescription Refill tab current.

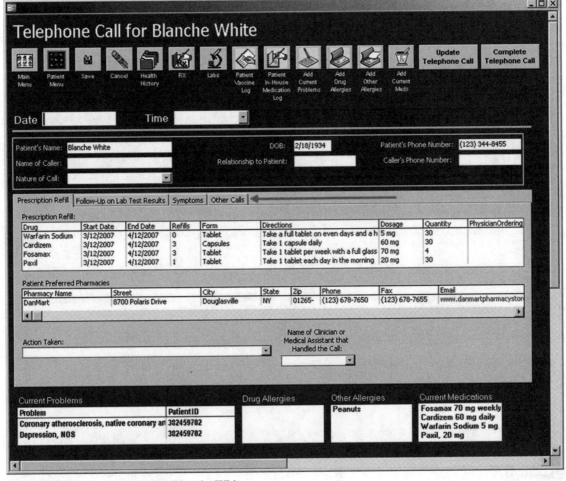

Figure 30   Telephone screen for Blanche White

8. Enter 05/14/2007 in the Date box.

9. Enter 9:45 AM in the Time box.

10. Enter Blanche White in the Name of Caller box.

11. Click the drop-down list arrow in the Nature of Call box, and select Prescription Refill.

12. The patient's birthday should have automatically populated in the DOB box.

13. In the Relationship to Patient box, enter Self.

14. The patient's home phone number should have automatically populated in the Patient's Phone Number box.

15. The caller's phone number is the same number as above, so type SAA in this box.

16. The patient's prescriptions will appear on the screen. Click Fosamax, since that is the prescription the patient is requesting.

17. Another box will appear. Place a checkmark in the box beside the Click to Indicate Telephone Inquiry box. Click out of the box by clicking the X on the upper-right corner of this window.

18. There is only one pharmacy, so you don't have to click in anything in that box.

19. Select the action you took from the drop-down list: Sent an Electronic Task to the Physician.

20. Select the person who handled the call (Fauna) from the drop-down list.

21. Double-check to make certain that you have all the information correct by comparing your screen with Figure 31.

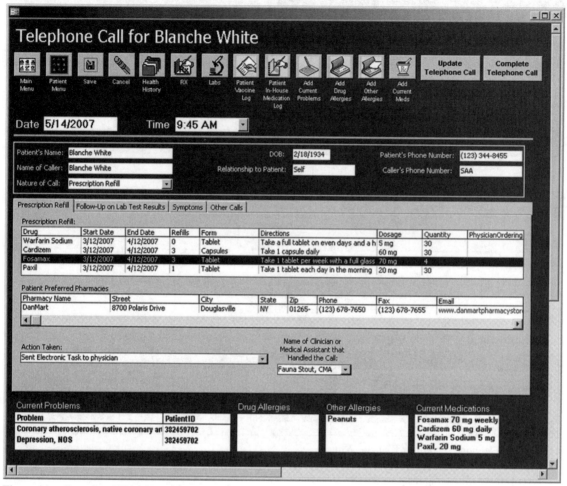

Figure 31   Completed Telephone Note for Blanche White

22. Click Update Telephone Call.

23. Click Save.

24. Click Complete Telephone Call. Once you click this icon and leave the screen, you will not be able to make any more adjustments, so make certain the information is correct before leaving the screen.

25. Click Patient Menu.

26. Click Chart Notes.

27. Click 5/14/2007 under Previous Telephone Calls.

28. Click the Print icon. Label your assignment as Task 1-10 and place in your SYNAPSE folder.

29. Click the Main Menu. The activities for Module I are now concluded.

Critical Thinking Questions for Module I

1. Cindy Swaim stated that she was a borderline diabetic and had high cholesterol during the health history portion of the interview. Her chief complaint was in regard to anxiety. Why shouldn't the medical assistant enter this information within the Current Problems screen? What information should be entered in the Current Problems screen? Whose responsibility would it be to enter such information?

2. Why is Cindy such a likely candidate for a heart attack?

3. What was the purpose of running a control on the glucometer? Why do you think that Fauna chose the High control?

4. Who may the office leave private information with when Cindy is not available?

5. What part of the chart should you check to find out how Cindy wants to be addressed for future visits? What other type of information may be entered in this section?

6. Cindy's complaint for today's visit was anxiety; however, after reading the history information and following her examination, Dr. Heath ordered patient education forms for diabetes, smoking cessation, hypetension, and heart disease. Explain the probable reason that each form was ordered. Dr. Heath did not order a patient education form for anxiety. This may be because there wasn't one stocked within the EMR. If Dr. Heath did order a patient education pamphlet that was not stocked in the EMR, what would be the next course of action?

MODULE II

Today's date: May 15, 2007
Appointments for May 15, 2007.

Patient's Name	Appointment Time	New Patient or Established Patient	Reason for Appointment	Clinician	MA
Morgan Penrose	9:00 AM	NP	UTI	Dr. Schwartz	Roger Wong, RMA

Work Assignments

You will be working as Roger Wong, RMA, for the next several tasks.

Task 2-1: Documenting in the Quality Control Log

After using the last rapid strep test in the rapid strep kit, Roger needs to open a new strep kit. He will need to run a control prior to using the new kit. Log information is found in Table 3.

TABLE 3 TASK 2-1 INFORMATION

Date	05/15/2007
Test Name	Two-Step Rapid Strep Test
Manufacturer's Name	Jefferson Diagnostics
Name of Control	+ Control
Lot #	6598
Exp Date	06/12/2008
Reference Range or Result	Positive
Result	Positive
Person Performing Control	Roger Wong, RMA

1. Go to the Main Menu and select Logs.

2. Go to the Quality Control Logs and click Rapid Strep Test. Open the selected log and click Update.

3. Enter the information from Table 3. **Do not forget to save the information.**

4. Print the log and label it Task 2-1.

5. Place the log in your SYNAPSE folder.

6. Close the log window. You should now see the information in the rapid strep log table. Close out of the log by clicking the Close box.

7. Close the Open Selected Log box by clicking the X in the upper-right corner of the window. You should now be back at the Main Menu screen.

Task 2-2: Creating a New Chart

Mrs. Morgan Penrose just arrived. You obtained her vitals and performed a medical history. You also obtained her chief complaint and reviewed the privacy statement with her. All responses to Mrs. Penrose's questions can be found in Table 4.

TABLE 4   MORGAN PENROSE'S PATIENT DATA TABLE

Patient's Name	Morgan A. Penrose
Patient's DOB	05/16/1960
Patient's Chart Number	257986523
Patient's Address	876 Honeycut Lane, Douglasville, NY 01234-1212
Patient's Telephone Numbers	Home: 123-457-9865 Work: None
Patient's Employer Info	None
Gender, Marital Status, Blood Type & Smoking Status	Gender: Female Marital Status: Married Blood Type: O– Smoking Status: Non-smoker
Patient Picture Screen: Patient Notes	Patient prefers to be addressed by her first name. Patient is getting ready to start nursing school (05/14/2007).
Spouse Name, DOB, & Address	Chad W. Penrose, DOB: 02/13/1955, Address: Same as patient
Responsible Party Info	Responsible Party: Spouse SS # or ID #: 365-84-9865 Address and Home: 876 Honeycut Lane, Douglasville, NY 01234-1212 Home Phone: 123-457-9865 Work Phone: 123-698-8888 Employer: Douglasville Textiles, 3658 City Park, N. Douglasville, NY 01236-1245
Primary Payer Info	Name: Flexihealth ID # 365849865-00 Policy/Group # 4ABDT DOB: 02/13/1955 Gender: Male SS # or ID #: 365-84-9865
Secondary Payer	None

Patient Drug Allergies	Codeine
Patient Other Allergy	Strawberries
Current Mediation List	Singulair, 10 mg/day, Albuterol Inhaler, and Clonazepam, 1 mg/day
Preferred Pharmacy	DanMart Pharmacy, 567 S. High Street, Douglasville, NY, 01234
Lab Provider	American Labs
Privacy Statement	Reviewed and signed May 15, 2007 Enter the following information in the Notes box: No one except the patient can receive private information. Do not leave any information on patient's answering machine.
Family Health History Info	Father: Age 69, Health: Good Mother: Age 68, Health: Fair Brother: Age 45, Health: Fair Brother: Age 41, Health: Good Sister: Age 39, Health: Good Heart disease: Mother has CAD. Had stent surgery in March 2001. High blood pressure: Mother, controlled with medication. Asthma: Brother has asthma. Controlled with steroids and breathing tx. Other: Stroke, maternal grandmother died of a stroke in 1992.
Hospitalizations, Blood Transfusions, and Serious Injuries	Hospitalizations: 　1982, Lakeside Memorial Hospital, birth of oldest daughter 　1986, Lakeside Memorial Hospital, birth of youngest daughter 　1987, Lakeside Memorial Hospital, birth of son Blood Transfusions: No blood transfusions Serious Injuries: None
Pregnancies	1982, female, C-section (baby's heart rated dropped) 1986, female, C-section (no complications) 1987, son, C-section (no complications)
Medical History	Click the following diseases: asthma, chicken pox, and other. In the Notes box, list the following: Asthma: Diagnosed in 1966. Treated with Singulair 10 mg/day and Albuterol Inhaler. Averages 1 attack every 1–2 months. Chicken pox: 1965 (no complications) Other: Seizure disorder, diagnosed in 1975. Clonazepam, 1 mg capsule/day. (Seizure-free for past 2 years)
Health Habits	Caffeine, 1 8-ounce cup of coffee/day. Does not smoke or drink alcohol. Occupation: Going to nursing school

Subjective Information	Urinary tract symptoms: Severity of Symptoms: 7 Duration: 3 days Associated Symptoms: + Abdominal pressure or pain, back pain, fever, nausea/vomiting, and urinary frequency. - Hx of UTI, mucus in urine, or vaginal symptoms Aggravating Symptoms: Not urinating Relieving Factors: OTC pain reliever
Objective Information	Vital Signs: Height: 67 inches Weight: 135 pounds Temperature: 101.4 Blood Pressure: 142/86 Pulse: 90 Respiration: 18 Pain: 7 Subjective Information and Vital Signs Entered By: Roger Wong, RMA

CREATING A CHART

1. In the Main Menu, click New Patients.

2. Complete all of the information within each tab of the Patient Information screen and save. Use Table 4 to complete each tab.

3. Save each screen as you complete each tab.

4. Go back through each tab and make certain your information is correct and saved.

5. Click Main Menu.

6. Click the Patients tab.

7. Highlight Morgan Penrose and click Open Patient Record.

8. You should now be in the Patient Information Menu for Morgan Penrose.

9. Click the Legal icon.

10. Click the drop-down arrow in the box next to Privacy Statement. Click Yes and enter the Date of today's visit in the date box. Enter the corresponding information in the Notes box from Table 4. Save your information.

11. Return to the Patient Menu and click the Health History icon.

12. Enter the corresponding information from Table 4 within each tab. Remember to save your information within each screen.

13. Click the Patient Menu, then Chart Notes.

14. Click New Office Visit. Enter the date and time of the patient's visit.

15. Click Update Progress Note and then Save.

16. You are now ready to enter the patient's subjective information. Start by clicking the Subjective tab.

17. Click the drop-down arrow in the Chief Complaint box.

18. Scroll and click Urinary Tract Symptoms.

19. Click Update Progress Note and then click Save.

20. Click Add HPI. Using the HPI information from Table 4, enter the appropriate information. Click Save after entering the HPI data.

21. Click Progress Note. You should now be on the Subjective tab.

22. Click the Objective tab.

23. Using the patient data table, enter the appropriate information.

24. List Roger Wong as the medical assistant who entered the subjective information and vital signs.

25. Click Update Progress Note, then click Save.

26. Click the Progress Notes tab. Make certain all of your information populated correctly within the progress note.

27. Print the progress note and label it Task 2-2. Place it in your SYNAPSE folder. Leave the screen for the physician. *Note: If you made an error in the progress note and do not recall how to correct it, refer to Help Box: Progress Notes.*

The doctor goes in to examine Mrs. Penrose. When he comes out of the patient's room, he instructs you to read the Plans section of the progress note. The plans state the following:

Plans: Complete UA and C&S. Rx for Septra DS Tab # 20, Take 1 tablet every 12 hours for 10 days, No refills. Rx for Singulair Tab, 10 mg, # 30. Take 1 tablet each day, 3 refills, Rx for Clonazepam Tablets, 1 mg, # 30. Take 1 tablet each day, 3 refills. Patient is getting ready to go to nursing school and needs the Hepatitis B series. Will give patient her first Hepatitis B shot today. Patient to return in 4 weeks for second Hepatitis B shot and a complete physical.

There are many tasks to perform, so time management is very important. Since the physician ordered a Complete UA and C&S, you will want to give the patient instructions for performing a clean-catch urine sample and hand the patient a labeled specimen container with cleansing towelettes. Inform the patient what to do with the sample once she collects it. While the patient is collecting the sample, you will create the electronic lab requisitions and prescriptions. Start by creating the lab requisition forms.

Task 2-3: Creating a Lab Requisition

1. You should still be in the Progress Note screen for the current visit.

2. Click the Labs icon.

3. Click the drop-down menu arrow in the Laboratory box and select American Labs. This is the lab that is listed as a provider for the patient's insurance company.

4. Click the Ordering Provider drop-down arrow. Click Dr. Schwartz, since he is the provider who saw Mrs. Penrose today.

5. Click the appropriate payer company.

6. Click the General Lab Tests arrow.

7. Scroll through the list and click UA Complete.

8. In the Number of and Type of Specimens Sent, type One Clean Catch Urine Sample (125 ml).

9. In the Today's Date box, enter the date of today's appointment.

10. In the Specimen Prepared By box, select Roger Wong.

11. Choose No in the Was patient fasting? drop-down list.

12. Click Save.

13. Preview the lab order. Make certain it is correct.

14. Click the Print icon. Label this Task 2-3A and place it in your SYNAPSE folder. Close the preview screen.

You now need to create a lab requisition form for the UA Culture & Sensitivity. The information for the last test should still be on the screen, so you will only need to change the name in the General Lab Test box to UA C&S, and change the Number of and Type of Specimens Sent to 1 UA Culture Swab in Liquid Media. Make certain all information is correct before saving. Click Preview. Click the Print icon. Label the requisition form as Task 2-3B and place it in your SYNAPSE folder. Close out of the print preview. Click Lab History and make certain that both tests populated within the Incomplete Labs table. Return to the Patient Menu.

Next, you will create the prescriptions.

Task 2-4: Creating Prescriptions

1. Start in the Patient Menu screen for Morgan Penrose.

2. Click Prescriptions.

3. Create prescriptions for all the prescriptions listed under the Plans section of the progress note. The patient's preferred pharmacy and payer information should automatically be loaded in the prescription screen. List the dosage for Septra as DS, which stands for double strength. Make certain you put today's date in the Start Date box and the end date for 30 days later on all the prescriptions. There shouldn't be any checks in the Start Date box or New Common Drug box.

4. Next click Save, Preview, and Print for each prescription. Label prescriptions as Task 2-4A through 2-4C and place in your SYNAPSE folder. *Note: If you made an error on one of the prescriptions and do not remember how to delete it, refer back to Help Box: Correcting a Prescription Error after Saving.*

Since the doctor also ordered a hepatitis B shot, you should print the vaccination information sheets form and consent form for that immunization.

Task 2-5: Printing Educational VIS Forms

1. Go to the Main Menu.

2. Click Patient Education Forms, and click Vaccination Information Sheets.

3. Click the Hepatitis B Form, and print it. Label it as Task 2-5 and place it in your SYNAPSE folder. Go to the File Menu and select Close.

4. Select Main Menu, then select Patients.

5. Select Morgan Penrose, and click Open Patient Record. You should now be in the Patient Information Menu for Morgan Penrose.

Task 2-6: Creating and Printing an Immunization Consent Form

1. Click the Authorization/Refusal Forms icon.

2. Click Immunization Consent Form.

3. Since the patient is only having one immunization today, click the drop-down arrow in the box beside 1. Click Hepatitis B. Do not do anything with the extra boxes.

4. Enter the name of the patient in the Typed Name box.

5. Enter the date of the visit in the Today's Date box. Refer to Figure 32 to make certain that the form is properly completed.

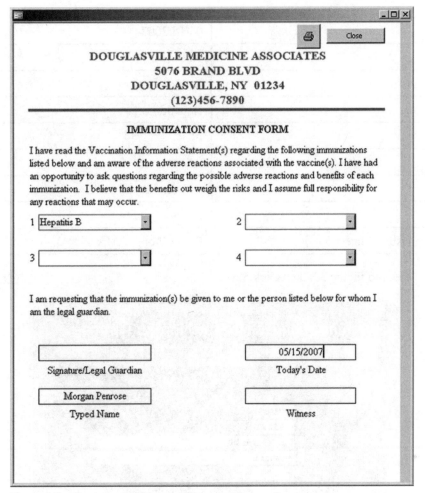

Figure 32   Immunization Consent Form for Morgan Penrose

6. Click Print.

7. In the medical office, both the patient and medical assistant would sign this form prior to scanning it back into the chart. This form must be signed. Label your work as Task 2-6 and place it in your SYNAPSE folder.

Once you have everything printed, take all of the paperwork into the patient's room. Give the patient all of her prescriptions and explain each one. Next, give the patient the VIS form for the hepatitis B immunization. Ask the patient to read the form thoroughly while you prepare the injection. After returning from preparing the injection, ask the patient if she has any questions. She states that she doesn't. Ask the patient to sign the consent form. Then, you give the patient the injection. Following the injection, you give the patient her prescriptions and tell her to schedule an appointment for a thorough physical. Dismiss the patient. You now need to enter the injection within the electronic chart.

Task 2-7: Entering Immunization Information in the Patient's Immunization Log

1. Go to the Patient Information Screen for Morgan Penrose.

2. Click Immunization Log.

3. Click the Update tab at the bottom of the screen. (If the patient had a previous vaccine, you will need to click Add Immunization before entering the information.)

4. Enter the information from Table 5.

TABLE 5   TASK 2-7 IMMUNIZATION INFORMATION

Date	05/15/2007
Time	9:30 AM
Ordering Physician	Dr. Schwartz
Immunization Name	Hepatitis B
Number in Series	#1
Amt. Given	0.5 ml
Location	R. Deltoid
Route	IM
Person Who Administered Injection	Roger Wong, RMA

5. Compare your screen to Figure 33, then click Save.

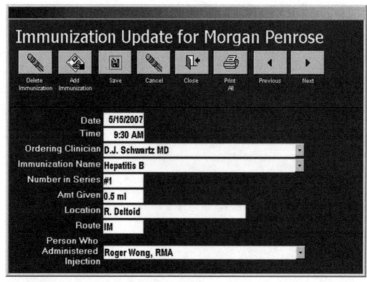

Figure 33   Immunization Update screen

6. Click Print All. Label the form Task 2-7 and place it in your SYNAPSE folder.

7. Click Close. You should now be in the Immunizations for Morgan Penrose log.

8. Close the screen. You should now be back in the Patient Information Menu screen.

Task 2-8: Closing the Chart Note for Morgan Penrose

Since the patient is finished and you are done working in the patient's personal EMR, you can now close the chart note.

1. Click Chart Notes.

2. Click New Office Visit.

3. Click Update Progress Note, and then click Save.

4. Click Complete Visit. After you leave this page, you will be unable to enter any additional data within this chart note.

5. Click Patient Menu.

6. Click the Chart Notes icon. Check to make certain that the date of your progress note saved to the Previous Office Visits box. Open the box and preview it.

7. Click Chart Notes. If the progress note is not listed in the Previous Office Visits box, you did not correctly exit the note. Return to the New Office Visit screen and review the information. If the information is correct, click the Update Progress Note button, click Save, and then click Complete Visit. Check to make certain that the information saved correctly this time. Click the Main Menu icon.

Task 2-9: Entering Immunizations on the Global Immunization Log

Now that you entered the information in the patient's personal information log, you will enter the information into the global immunization log. This log tracks all immunizations given in the office.

1. From the Main Menu, click Logs.

2. In the Global Immunization log drop-down list, choose Hepatitis B.

3. Click Open Selected Log, and then click Update.

4. Record the requested information. The only additional information you will need to complete this log is the Drug Form Injectable, Amt Given: 0.5 ml, Ordering Clinician: D.J. Scwartz MD, Manuf Name: CKD, Lot Number, 13698P, Exp Date: 06/15/2008, Who Administered: Roger Wong.

5. Click Save and then click Print All. Label the document Task 2-9. Click Close.

6. You should now see the Hepatitis B Immunization Log in the table.

7. Click the Close button at the bottom of the screen. Close the Open Selected Log screen. You should now be back at the Main Menu screen.

Critical Thinking Questions for Module II

1. Why do you think the physician ordered a culture and sensitivity in addition to the complete UA?

2. The patient arrived with urinary symptoms, so why do you think the physician ordered prescriptions for Clonazepam and Singulair in addition to the Septra DS? The patient also had Albuterol inhaler listed for her current meds. What might be a logical explanation as to why the physician didn't order a prescription for this medication?

3. What would you do if the patient refused to sign the immunization consent form?

4. Why did you have to record the immunization on two separate logs?

MODULE III

Today's date: May 16, 2007
Appointments for May 16, 2007

Patient's Name	Appointment Time	Reason for Appointment	Clinician	MA
Kevin Cook	1:00 PM	Sports physical	Megan Speck, NP	Roger Wong, RMA
Blanche White	1:15 PM	Complete physical	Dr. Schwartz	Roger Wong, RMA

TABLE 6   KEVIN COOK'S DATA TABLE

Patient's Name	Kevin R. Cook
Patient's DOB	03/12/1995
Patient's Chart Number	219365878
Patient's Address	1756 Edgeview Road, Douglasville, NY 01234-1212
Patient's Telephone Numbers	Home: 123-786-0098 No work number
Patient's Employer Info	None
Gender, Marital Status, Blood Type & Smoking Status	Gender: Male Marital Status: Single Blood Type: Leave blank (not known) Smoking Status: Non-smoker
Patient Picture Screen: Patient Notes	Patient prefers to be addressed by his middle name, which is Ryan.
Responsible Party Info	Responsible Party: Other (Father) Name: David M. Cook SS # or ID #: 356-98-5987 Address and Home: 1756 Edgeview Road, Douglasville, NY 01234-1212 Home Phone: 123-786-0098 Work Phone: 123-876-0987 Employer: Self-employed Douglasville, NY 01234-1212
Primary Payer Info	Name: Signal HMO ID # 356985987-00 Policy Holder Information: Other (father's information) Policy/Group: None Gender: Male DOB: 03/14/1967
Secondary Payer	None
Patient Drug Allergies	Aspirin
Patient Other Allergy	Dog and cat dander
Current Mediation List	None
Preferred Pharmacy	Douglasville Pharmacy, 7890 Cobblestone Place, Douglasville, NY
Lab Provider	Smith, Wright, & Kennedy
Privacy Statement	Reviewed and signed, May 16, 2007 Enter the following information in the Notes box: Father stated that private information may be left with him and the patient's mother.

Family Health History Info	Father: Age 40, Health: Good
	Mother: Age 39, Health: Good
	Brother: Age 16, Health: Good
	Sister: Age 9, Health: Good
	Heart disease: Maternal grandmother (heart attack at age 62).
	Other: Epilepsy, brother (onset at age 12, controlled with meds).
Hospitalizations, Blood Transfusions, and Serious Injuries	Hospitalizations: None
	Blood Transfusions: None
	Serious Injuries: None
Pregnancies	N/A
Medical History	Click the following disease: Chicken pox. In the Notes box, list the following: Chicken pox: 1998 (no complications)
Health Habits	Caffeine, 3 12-ounce cans of soda per day. Does not smoke or drink alcohol. Does not work.
Subjective Information	Patient here for sport's physical: Type "Sports Physical" in the Chief Complaint box.
Objective Information	Vital Signs:
	Height: 73 inches
	Weight: 165 pounds
	Temperature: 98.4
	Blood Pressure: 110/64
	Pulse: 64
	Respiration: 14
	Pain: 0
	Subjective Information and Vital Signs Entered By: Roger Wong, RMA

Task 3-1: Creating an Electronic Chart and Progress Note

You are acting as Roger Wong in these exercises.

1. Using Table 6, create an electronic chart and new progress note for Kevin Cook. Refer to Module I if you forget any of the specific components for creating a chart. The only difference in creating a progress note for this patient is that he is coming in for a sports physical instead of with symptoms.

2. Within the Subjective tab, type the words "Sports Physical" in the Chief Complaint box. You will not need to perform an HPI since the patient doesn't have any symptoms.

3. Click Update Progress Note, then click Save.

4. Next, click the Progress Notes tab. You should see the words "Sports Physical" under the Chief Complaint heading within the Subjective tab.

5. Click the Objective tab and enter the objective information.

6. Click Update Progress Note, then click Save.

7. Click the Progress Notes tab. Your subjective and objective information should populate in the progress note.

8. Click the Print icon and label the assignment Task 3-1.

You instruct Kevin on how to disrobe. Kevin's dad hands you a sports physical form from Kevin's school that needs to be completed. You give the form to Megan Speck, the nurse practitioner, before she examines the patient. Normally you would wait until the NP is finished with the patient to complete the record; however, you are finished recording this particular progress note, and you are ready to take a new patient to the room, so you complete and close the record at this time.

Task 3-2: Completing the Progress Note

1. Because you updated and saved the progress note information, you can now click the Complete Visit icon. *Note: Remember that once you leave the screen, you will be unable to make changes.*

2. Click the Patient Menu icon, and then click Chart Notes.

3. You should see the date of the visit in the Previous Office Visits box.

4. Click today's visit date to make certain the note saved properly.

5. Click the Chart Notes icon, and then click the Main Menu icon.

Task 3-3: Entering Information in a Previously Created Chart

While the nurse practitioner is in the room with Kevin Cook, Blanche White enters the reception area. She has an appointment with Dr. Schwartz. Since you are covering both Megan Speck and Dr. Schwartz, you will be taking care of Mrs. White.

1. Start by clicking the Main Menu icon, if you aren't already there.

2. Open Mrs. White's EMR by clicking the Patients icon, selecting her name, and then clicking Open Patient Record.

3. Click the Demographics icon. Read the information in the Patient Picture tab to see if Mrs. White has a preference on how she wants to be addressed, or to see if there are any other notes that may need attention before calling back the patient. You notice there is nothing entered in this section. When the patient enters the examination room, you ask her if she has a preference for the way she wants to be addressed. The patient states that she prefers to be addressed by her first name. The patient goes on to tell you that her granddaughter is getting married this weekend, on May 18. This is an important event in the patient's life, and you will want to ask her about the wedding on her next visit. Because of this, you should enter the information within the Patient Notes box as a reminder.

4. Enter the following notes in the Patient Notes box: Patient prefers to be addressed by her first name. Patient's granddaughter is getting married May 18, 2007. (The next time the patient comes in to the office, you may want to ask the patient about the wedding.) Click Save.

You ask Blanche if any demographic information has changed since her last visit. She states that it hasn't. Next, you ask if any legal information has changed since her last visit, such as privacy information, DNR information, etc. The patient once states it hasn't. Now you are ready to create a new progress note.

1. Click the Patient Main button at the top of your toolbar. You should now be in the Patient Information Menu for Blanche White.

2. Click the Chart Notes icon, and then New Office Visit.

3. Enter the date and time of the patient's appointment, and then click Update Progress Note. Click Save.

4. Click the Subjective tab. Enter "Complete Physical" in the Chief Complaint box. Click Update Progress Note, and then click Save.

5. Click the Objective Tab. Enter the following information:

   Height: 60 inches

   Weight: 164 pounds

   Temperature: 97.8

   Blood Pressure: 134/82

   Pulse: 88

   Respiration: 18

   Pain: 0

   Subjective information and vital signs entered by Roger Wong, RMA

6. Click the Update Progress Note button, then click Save.

7. Click the Progress Notes tab. Make certain that all of your information populated correctly in the progress note.

8. Click the Print icon at the top of the toolbar and label the assignment Task 3-3. Place the assignment in your SYNAPSE folder.

9. Do not click the Complete Visit icon until the clinician has finished entering the information. For now, click the Main Menu icon.

You are now finished entering the information within the patient's chart, and you instruct the patient how to disrobe. You leave the room and spot Megan, the nurse practitioner. Megan tells you Kevin Cook needs his second MMR shot because the parents cannot find records that prove he had the second immunization. The clinic in which he received the immunization is now closed. Mr. Cook and Kevin opted to have a second MMR instead of having a titer performed. Megan also tells you the patient needs a proof of appointment letter.

Task 3-4: Retrieving and Printing a VIS Form and a Consent Form

Since the patient needs an immunization, you will need to retrieve and print both a VIS form and an immunization consent form.

1. Click Patient Education Forms on the Main Menu screen.

2. Click Vaccination Information Sheets, then click MMR.

3. Print this form and label the assignment Task 3-4A.

4. Close the form and return to the Main Menu.

5. Click the Patients icon.

6. In the patient list, select Kevin Cook and click Open Patient Record.

7. Select the Authorization and Refusal Forms tab, and then click the Immunization Consent Form icon.

8. In box 1, choose MMR from the drop-down list.

9. Since the father is with the patient today, enter the father's name, David Cook, in the Typed Name box at the bottom of the form.

10. Enter the date of the appointment in the Today's Date box.

11. Print the form. Label the form Task 3-4B. In the medical office, the father would sign the form and the medical assistant would sign the witness box. Place Task 3-4A and Task 3-4B in your SYNAPSE folder.

12. Return to the Patient Information screen.

Now that you have printed the VIS and consent forms, you need to print a proof of appointment letter.

Task 3-5: Printing a Proof of Appointment Letter

1. Click the Patient Templates icon in the Patient Information screen. Choose Proof of Appointment.

2. Enter today's date, the time of the appointment, and the clinician's name.

3. Click the Print tab. Label the document Task 3-5 and place it in your SYNAPSE folder.

4. Return to the Main Menu.

You take the forms to the exam room, where the patient and his father are waiting. You ask the father to read over the VIS form and to sign the consent form while you go and prepare the immunization. You prepare the MMR immunization and re-enter the patient's room. You administer the injection in the subcutaneous tissue of the patient's left arm. The father of the patient asks if they can also have some kind of proof that the patient received his second MMR today. You tell the father that you can print him a copy of the immunization log from his electronic chart as soon as you enter the information.

Task 3-6 Documenting an Immunization in the EMR and Printing a Copy for the Patient

1. From the Patient Information Menu for Kevin Cook, click the Immunization Log icon.

2. Click the Update tab at the bottom of the box.

3. Complete the requested information by referring to Table 7.

TABLE 7   TASK 3-6 IMMUNIZATION TABLE

Date	May 16, 2007
Time	1:25 PM
Ordering Clinician	Megan Speck, NP
Immunization Name	MMR
Number in Series	2
Amt Given	0.5 ml
Location	Left Arm
Route	Sub Q
Person Who Administered Injection	Roger Wong, RMA

4. Save the information and print the form.

5. Label it Task 3-6 and place it in your SYNAPSE folder.

6. Click the Close icon. You should now see the immunization log for Kevin Cook. Close the immunization log for Kevin Cook.

You give the patient's father a copy of the immunization log so that they have verification that Kevin received the immunization. Kevin and his father leave after waiting the appropriate amount of time following the injection. You now need to enter the immunization information in the global immunization log within the Main Menu.

Task 3-7: Entering Immunization Information in the Global Immunization Log

1. From the Main Menu, click the Logs icon.

2. Click the Global Immunizations Log drop-down arrow, and select MMR.

3. Click Open Selected Log, and then select Update.

4. Enter the information found in the Table 8.

TABLE 8   TASK 3-7 GLOBAL IMMUNIZATION LOG TABLE

Date Administered	05/16/2007
Patient's Name	Kevin R. Cook
Drug Form	Injectable
Amt. Given	0.5 ml
Ordering Clinician	Megan Speck, NP
Manufacturer's Name	New York Pharmaceuticals
Lot Number	789451B
Exp Date	08/01/2008
Person Who Administered Injection	Roger Wong, RMA

6. Click Save and then print the form. Label the form Task 3-7.

7. Close the log and return to the Main Menu.

You just had a call sent back to you from the operator. It is Robert Green. He wants to know if he can have a prescription refill for his Cardizem.

Task 3-8: Documenting a Phone Call

You first need to bring up Robert Green's electronic chart. Follow the steps below.

1. Click the Patients icon on the Main Menu.

2. Select Robert Green, and then click Open Patient's Record.

3. Click Chart Note, and then click Telephone Call.

4. Enter 05/16/2007 in the Date box and 1:45 PM in the Time box.

5. Click Save.

6. Enter Robert Green's name in the Name of Caller box.

7. Enter "Self" in the Relationship to Patient box.

8. Enter abbreviation, SAA, in the Caller's Phone Number box.

9. In the Nature of the Call box, click Prescription Refill.

10. You should already be in the Prescription Refill tab, so check to see if the patient has any refills for Cardizem. The patient does not have any refills, so you will need to send an electronic task to the physician.

11. Click Cardizem in the Prescription Refill table.

12. A second box will appear. Put a check in the Click to Indicate Telephone Call Inquiry box. Close the box.

13. In the Action Taken box, click the drop-down arrow and select Sent Electronic Task to Physician.

14. Choose Roger Wong as the Name of Clinician or Medical Assistant that Handled the Call.

15. Double-check all of your information to make certain that the information is correct. Click Update Telephone Call, then Save.

16. Click Complete Telephone Call. Take one last look, because once you exit this screen, you will no longer be able to make any changes.

17. Click Patient Menu. Click Chart Notes.

18. Double-click the 05/16/2007 Previous Telephone Calls Entry to view the saved message. Click Print. Label the document Task 3-8 and file it in your SYNAPSE folder.

19. Return to the Main Menu.

Now that you have finished the call, you go to see if Dr. Schwartz is finished with Blanche. Dr. Schwartz is just exiting the patient's room when you arrive at the door. The doctor instructs you to read the Plans section of the progress note. The Plans section reads as follows:

Plans: In-Office PT and INR level today. After obtaining results, will adjust the patient's Wafarin Sodium medication if necessary. Depression much better; will continue to monitor over next couple of months. Patient to return in two weeks for another Pro-Time and INR.

You will need to perform a PT and INR level on the patient using your new CLIA-waived analyzer. Start by creating a lab requisition form for the patient.

Task 3-9: Creating a Lab Requisition Form

1. From the Main Menu, click the Patients icon.

2. Select Blanche White from the list of patients, and click Open Patient Record.

3. Click the Lab Orders icon.

4. Click In-House Testing in the Laboratory box, since we are performing this particular testing in the office.

5. Click D. J. Schwartz MD in the Ordering Provider box.

6. Click Medicare as the Payer, since Medicare is the primary payer.

7. Click Prothrombin Time in the General Lab Tests box.

8. Do not type anything in the Number of and Type of Specimens Sent box because we are performing the test in-house.

9. Enter today's date in the Today's Date box.

10. In the Specimen Prepared By box, select Roger Wong.

11. Select Yes in the Was patient fasting? box.

12. Click Save.

13. Click Preview, and then click the Print icon on the Preview screen. Label it Task 3-9A and place in your SYNAPSE folder. Close out of the preview.

14. Create a New Lab Requisition for the INR order. The only thing that will need to be changed is the name of the general lab test. Change the name of the general lab test to INR. Click Save.

15. Click Preview, and then click the Print icon. Label it Task 3-9B and place it in your SYNAPSE folder.

16. Next, click the Lab History icon. You should see both tests entered on the Incomplete Labs Log, as well as a previous test that was performed.

17. If you made an error, follow the instructions for deleting a log in Module I.

You enter the patient's room and perform the PT and INR via capillary stick. The results are as follows: PT 25.8 Seconds and INR 2.6. You will need to document this result in the Update Lab Results box.

Task 3-10: Entering Lab Results in the Electronic Medical Record

1. From the Lab Requisition for Blanche White screen, click Lab History.

2. Click the PT results, and then click Update Lab Results.

3. Enter 25.8 seconds in the Lab Test Results box.

4. Select Roger Wong as the Name of Person Who Recorded Results, enter the date of today's appointment, and click Save.

5. Click the Lab History icon.

6. You should notice that the result was sent from the Incomplete Labs box to the Completed Labs box.

7. Now repeat the same action for the INR results. There is no unit for INR, so you can enter 2.6 as the result.

8. Make certain that the test was sent to the Completed Labs box.

9. Print the screen and label the Incomplete Labs form Task 3-10A. Label the Complete Labs form Task 3-10B. File the forms in your SYNAPSE folder.

After completing the documentation, you immediately notify the physician of the result so that the physician can make any necessary adjustments in the patient's medication. If the physician was waiting on the result before finalizing the progress note, the physician would be responsible for closing the note. However, since you are finished with this project, you will complete the progress note.

Task 3-11: Finalizing the Progress Note

1. Click the Current Visit tab for Blanche White.

2. Click Update Progress Note, and then click Save.

3. Click Complete Visit. *(Note: Make certain that everything is correct before leaving this screen, because once you leave you will be unable to make changes.)*

4. Click the Patient Menu icon, then Chart Notes. Click the 05-16-2007 visit in the Previous Office Visits box to preview the note.

5. Return to the Main Menu.

Critical Thinking Questions for Module III

1. What was the purpose for writing down the date of Blanche's granddaughter's wedding?

2. Why do you think Kevin's father decided to have Kevin receive the second MMR instead of having a blood titer to determine Kevin's level of immunity?

3. In regard to the telephone call for Mr. Green, what information in the prescription history section caused you to send an electronic task to the physician instead of calling in a prescription for the Cardizem?

4. When you documented the labs in Blanche's electronic file, there was an outstanding blood test that was more than a month old? Which test was more than a month old. What would you do if you observed an outstanding test that was over a month old while working in the field?

5. What medication is Blanche taking that prompts the need to have Pro-Time and INR performed on a regular basis?

MODULE IV: CREATE AND MAINTAIN THE EMR

Module IV is an EMR competency, and it is designed to test your knowledge in performing tasks within the electronic chart. No step-by-step instructions are included; use the Competency Checklist on page 61 as documentation of your competency in this skill.

Today's date: May 17, 2007
Appointments for May 17, 2007

Patient's Name	Appointment Time	Reason for Appointment	Clinician	MA
Paul M. Myers	2:00 PM	Cold/flu symptoms	Dr. Heath	Fauna Stout, CMA

Task 4-1: Creating an Electronic Chart and Progress Note

1. Refer to Table 9 for patient information. Create an electronic chart and new progress note for Paul Myers.

TABLE 9   PAUL MYERS'S DATA TABLE

Patient's Name	Paul M. Myers
Patient's DOB	08/12/1945
Patient's Chart Number	985632998
Patient's Address	2487 Springdale Court, Douglasville, NY 01234-1212
Patient's Telephone Numbers	Home: 123-786-6890 Work: 123-879-9865
Patient's Employer Info	Douglasville Steel Douglasville, NY 01234-1215
Gender, Marital Status, Blood Type & Smoking Status	Gender: Male Marital Status: Married Blood Type: O+ Smoking Status: Smoker
Patient Notes	Patient is hard of hearing in the left ear.
Responsible Party Info	Responsible Party: Self SS #: 985-63-2998 Address: SAA Home Phone: SAA Work Phone: SAA Employer: Douglasville Steel, Douglasville, NY 01234-1215

Primary Payer Info	Name: Flexihealth ID # 985632998-00 Policy/Group: 6532001 Gender: Male Policy Holder: Self SS#: 985-63-2998
Secondary Payer	None
Patient Drug Allergies	Penicillin
Patient Other Allergy	None
Current Mediation List	Accupril capsules, 20 mg Glyburide tablets, 2.5 mg Viagra tablets, 50 mg
Preferred Pharmacy	DanMart Pharmacy 8700 Polaris Drive, Douglasville, NY 01234
Lab Provider	American Labs
Privacy Statement	Reviewed and Signed, May 17, 2007 Enter the following information in the Notes box: Can leave information on the patient's home answering machine and with wife, Carol.
Family Health History Info	Father: Age at death: 72, Cause of death: Heart failure Mother: Age 84, Health: Poor Brother: Age 66, Health: Fair Sister: Age 54, Health: Good Diabetes: Type II diabetes both father and mother Heart disease: CHF, father High blood pressure: Mother, father, and brother
Hospitalizations, Blood Transfusions, and Serious Injuries	Hospitalizations: 1976, Riverside Hospital, hernia repair Blood Transfusions: None Serious Injuries: None
Pregnancies	N/A
Medical History	Click the following diseases: Chicken pox, diabetes, high cholesterol, measles, mumps, other In the Notes box, list the following: Chicken pox: UCHD (no complications) Diabetes: Type II, diagnosed in 1995, controlled with diet and oral medication High cholesterol: Diagnosed in 2001, diet controlled Measles: UCHD (no complications) Mumps: UCHD (no complications) Other: Hypertension, diagnosed in 1992. Controlled by low-sodium diet and Accupril.

Health Habits	Caffeine, drinks 1 10–12-ounce cup of coffee per day.
	Tobacco: Smokes ½–1 pack of low-filter cigarettes per day. Has been a smoker for 32 years.
	ETOH:
	Drink type: Beer
	Drinks per week: 6 pack
	Occupation: Steel worker
	Heavy lifting
Progress Notes: Date, Time, Clinician, and MA	Date: May 17, 2007
	Time: 2:00 PM
	Clinician: Dr. Heath
	MA: Fauna Stout, CMA
Subjective Information	Chief Complaint: Cold, flu, sore throat
	HPI:
	Severity: 6
	Duration of symptoms: 7 days
	+: Ear pain, fever, head or facial pain, nasal drainage, productive cough.
	−: Light sensitivity, nausea or vomiting or other GI distubances, sore throat.
	Relieving factors: OTC: Sinus/flu medication
Objective Information	Vital Signs:
	Height: 70 inches
	Weight: 215 pounds
	Temperature: 99.7
	Blood Pressure: 146/92
	Pulse: 92
	Respiration: 20
	Pain: 6
	Subjective Information and Vital Signs Entered By: Fauna Stout

2. When finished, print the note.

3. Label it Task 4-1 and place it in your SYNAPSE folder.

4. You will not complete the progress note until later.

Task 4-2: Creating and Printing an Electronic Prescription

1. Accupril, 20 mg Cap. Quantity: 30, Take 1 capsule each day, 0 refills

2. Atenolol, 50 mg, Tab, Quantity: 30, Take 1 tab each day before meals or at bedtime, 0 refills

3. Glyburide, 2.5 mg Tab, Quantity: 60, Take 1 tab in the morning and one tab in the evening, 0 refills

4. Viagra, 50 mg, Quantity: 10, Take 1–2 tabs 30 minutes before sexual intercourse, 0 refills

5. All prescriptions are considered one-month prescriptions.

6. Print and label the documents Tasks 4-2A through 4-2D and place them in your SYNAPSE folder.

Task 4-3: Creating and Printing Lab Requisition Forms

1. HgbA1c (in-house), patient was fasting.

2. Print and label it Task 4-3A and place it in your SYNAPSE folder.

3. Chem 12: American Labs, Patient was fasting, sent 1 SST tube.

4. Print and label it Task 4-3B and place it in your SYNAPSE folder.

Task 4-4: Entering Lab Results in the Patient's Electronic Medical Record

1. Result: HgbA1c: 8.2% on 5/17/2007.

2. Print and label the Incomplete Lab table Task 4-4A.

3. Print and label the Complete Lab table Task 4-4B.

4. Place both forms in your SYNAPSE folder.

Task 4-5: Printing Educational Forms and VIS Forms for the Patient

1. Diabetes and hypertension educational forms.

2. Shingles VIS form.

3. Print and label the forms Task 4-5A through 4-5C and place them in your SYNAPSE folder.

Task 4-6: Creating a Consent Form to go with Immunization

1. Print the form, label it Task 4-6, and place it in your SYNAPSE folder.

Task 4-7: Entering an Immunization in the Personal EMR

Date	May 17, 2007
Time	2:45 PM
Ordering Physician	Dr. Heath
Immunization Name	Shingles
Number in Series	1
Amt Given	0.5 ml
Location	Left Arm
Route	Sub-Q
Person Who Administered Injection	Fauna Stout, CMA

1. Print and Label the form Task 4-7.

Task 4-8: Entering an Immunization in the Global Immunization Log

Date Administered	05/17/2007
Patient's Name	Paul Myers
Drug Form	Injectable
Amt Given	0.5 ml
Ordering Physician	Dr. Heath
Manuf Name	New York Pharmaceuticals
Lot Number	2365879 C
Exp	12/10/2008
Person Who Administered Injection	Fauna Stout, CMA

1. Print and label it Task 4-8 and place it in your SYNAPSE folder.

Task 4-9: Creating and Printing a Proof of Appointment Letter

1. Label it Task 4-9 and place it in your SYNAPSE folder.

Task 4-10: Properly completing Paul Myer's Progress Note from 05/17/2007

1. Label it Task 4-10 and place it in your SYNAPSE folder.

Task 4-11: Creating and Printing a Telephone Note

1. Date: May 27, 2007

2. Time: 4:15 PM

3. Patient is calling from home.

4. Prescription: Viagra refill.

5. Sent electronic task to the physician.

6. Medical Assistant: Fauna Stout.

7. Print and label it Task 4-11.

Student Name: _____   Date: _____   Score: _____

Competency Checklist
PROCEDURE   Create and Maintain the EMR

Task: Create an electronic medical record and perform various tasks within the EMR.

Condition: In a simulated medical office situation, students will be provided a computer, SYNAPSE, and Module IV text information to perform the procedure.

Standards: The student will accurately create a medical record and perform electronic tasks from the directions provided in Module IV. All documentation must be completed accurately. The student will have a total of 1 hour to complete all tasks listed below. A maximum of three attempts may be used to complete the competency.

STEPS START TIME: END TIME:	Points Possible	First Attempt	Second Attempt	Third Attempt
1. Task 4-1: Accurately create the chart by properly completing all of the tabs in the Patient Information screen within SYNAPSE.	15			
2. Task 4-1: Accurately create and print a progress note, closing it properly using the correct technique.	15			
3. Task 4-2: Accurately create and print the assigned prescriptions.	15			
4. Task 4-3: Accurately create and print the assigned lab requisition forms.	15			
5. Task 4-4: Accurately enter the assigned lab results in the patient's electronic medical record.	15			
6. Task 4-5: Accurately locate and print the assigned educational forms.	15			
7. Task 4-6: Accurately create and print an immunization consent form to go with Task 4-7.	15			
8. Task 4-7: Accurately enter an immunization into the patient's personal electronic medical record.	15			
9. Task 4-8: Accurately enter an immunization in the global immunization log.	15			
10. Task 4-9: Accurately create a proof of appointment letter for the patient.	15			
11. Task 4-10: Accurately complete the patient's progress note.	15			
12. Task 4-11: Accurately record a phone call in the patient's electronic medical record.	15			
Points Earned / Points Possible:	___ / 180			

Note: If grading on a 0–100 scale, when total possible points do not add up to 100, divide points earned by total points possible and multiply by 100 for equivalent score.

Key Competencies		
ABHES	VI.B.1.a.2.n	Application of electronic technology
	VI.B.1.a.3.b	Prepare and maintain medical records
	VI.B.1.a.3.d	Apply computer concepts for office procedures
	VI.B.1.a.3.e	Locate resources and information for patients and employers
	VI.B.1.a.5.b	Document accurately
CAAHEP	V.P.5	Execute data management using electronic healthcare records such as the EMR
	IX.P.7	Document accurately in the patient record

Student Name: _____   Date: _____   Score: _____

EVALUATION
Evaluator Signature: _____   Date: _____

Evaluator Comments:

DOCUMENTATION
Attach documentation for Tasks 4-1 through 4-11

Key Competencies		
ABHES	VI.B.1.a.2.n	Application of electronic technology
	VI.B.1.a.3.b	Prepare and maintain medical records
	VI.B.1.a.3.d	Apply computer concepts for office procedures
	VI.B.1.a.3.e	Locate resources and information for patients and employers
	VI.B.1.a.5.b	Document accurately
CAAHEP	V.P.5	Execute data management using electronic healthcare records such as the EMR
	IX.P.7	Document accurately in the patient record

CERTIFICATE OF COMPLETION

_____

has completed *SynapseEHR 1.1: An Electronic Charting Simulation Exercise Booklet*

_____
Evaluator Signature

_____
Date

System Requirements and Setup Instructions for
SynapseEHR 1.1

System Requirements for SynapseEHR 1.1

- Microsoft Windows 2000, Windows XP (Service Pack 3), or Vista (Service Pack 1), MS Office 2003, MS Office 2007
- Pentium or Celeron PC with 300 MHz or higher processor recommended; 233 MHz minimum required
- 128 megabytes of RAM or higher recommended
- 1.5 gigabytes of available hard disk space (if using a USB Flash Drive, must have at least 50 MB of free space available)
- Super VGA (800 x 600) or higher-resolution video adapter and monitor
- CD-ROM or DVD drive; USB port if using a USB Flash Drive
- Keyboard and mouse or compatible pointing device

Installation Instructions for SynapseEHR 1.1

1. Insert the CD in your computer's CD drive. It should automatically begin the setup process. If not, continue to step 3.
2. Follow the installation prompts on the screen. Continue to steps 7–10 if you would like to use Synapse with a USB Flash Drive. If you are not using a USB Flash Drive, the installation is complete.
3. Double click "My Computer."
4. Double click the Control Panel icon.
5. Double click Add/Remove Programs.
6. Click the Install button and follow the on-screen prompts from there. Follow steps 7–10 if you would like to use Synapse with a USB Flash Drive. If you are not using a USB Flash Drive, the installation is complete.

Note: Only follow steps 7–10 if you are using Synapse with a USB Flash Drive.

7. Insert a USB Flash Drive into your computer USB port. Your USB Flash Drive must have at least 50 MB of free space available.
8. Copy the SynapseEHR database, SynapseEHR.mdb, from C:\Program Files\SynapseEHR to your USB Flash Drive:
   - Open "My Computer."
   - Double click on C: (Drive).
   - Double click on Program Files.
   - Double click on the SynapseEHR folder.
   - Click one time on SynapseEHR.mdb to highlight the file.
   - Right click and select Copy.
   - Next, open "My Computer" again.
   - Double click to open your Flash Drive (if not already open).
   - Right click and select Paste.
   - SynapseEHR.mdb should now appear on your Flash Drive.
   - Close all open windows.
9. To open Synapse, select your Flash Drive and double click on SynapseEHR.mdb.
10. You can now begin working in the Synapse program. If you have questions regarding steps 7–10, please contact Delmar's Technical Support at 800-648-7450, Monday–Friday, 8:30 a.m. to 5:30 p.m. EST.

Signing into SynapseEHR 1.1

The default log-on is already populated (Student1, Student1), and the first-time user will only need to click "enter." Once in the program, the user may change the user name and/or password.

IMPORTANT! READ CAREFULLY: This End User License Agreement ("Agreement") sets forth the conditions by which Cengage Learning will make electronic access to the Cengage Learning-owned licensed content and associated media, software, documentation, printed materials, and electronic documentation contained in this package and/or made available to you via this product (the "Licensed Content"), available to you (the "End User"). BY CLICKING THE "I ACCEPT" BUTTON AND/OR OPENING THIS PACKAGE, YOU ACKNOWLEDGE THAT YOU HAVE READ ALL OF THE TERMS AND CONDITIONS, AND THAT YOU AGREE TO BE BOUND BY ITS TERMS, CONDITIONS, AND ALL APPLICABLE LAWS AND REGULATIONS GOVERNING THE USE OF THE LICENSED CONTENT.

1.0 SCOPE OF LICENSE

1.1 Licensed Content. The Licensed Content may contain portions of modifiable content ("Modifiable Content") and content which may not be modified or otherwise altered by the End User ("Non-Modifiable Content"). For purposes of this Agreement, Modifiable Content and Non-Modifiable Content may be collectively referred to herein as the "Licensed Content." All Licensed Content shall be considered Non-Modifiable Content, unless such Licensed Content is presented to the End User in a modifiable format and it is clearly indicated that modification of the Licensed Content is permitted.

1.2 Subject to the End User's compliance with the terms and conditions of this Agreement, Cengage Learning hereby grants the End User, a nontransferable, nonexclusive, limited right to access and view a single copy of the Licensed Content on a single personal computer system for noncommercial, internal, personal use only. The End User shall not (i) reproduce, copy, modify (except in the case of Modifiable Content), distribute, display, transfer, sublicense, prepare derivative work(s) based on, sell, exchange, barter or transfer, rent, lease, loan, resell, or in any other manner exploit the Licensed Content; (ii) remove, obscure, or alter any notice of Cengage Learning's intellectual property rights present on or in the Licensed Content, including, but not limited to, copyright, trademark, and/or patent notices; or (iii) disassemble, decompile, translate, reverse engineer, or otherwise reduce the Licensed Content.

2.0 TERMINATION

2.1 Cengage Learning may at any time (without prejudice to its other rights or remedies) immediately terminate this Agreement and/or suspend access to some or all of the Licensed Content, in the event that the End User does not comply with any of the terms and conditions of this Agreement. In the event of such termination by Cengage Learning, the End User shall immediately return any and all copies of the Licensed Content to Cengage Learning.

3.0 PROPRIETARY RIGHTS

3.1 The End User acknowledges that Cengage Learning owns all rights, title and interest, including, but not limited to all copyright rights therein, in and to the Licensed Content, and that the End User shall not take any action inconsistent with such ownership. The Licensed Content is protected by U.S., Canadian and other applicable copyright laws and by international treaties, including the Berne Convention and the Universal Copyright Convention. Nothing contained in this Agreement shall be construed as granting the End User any ownership rights in or to the Licensed Content.

3.2 Cengage Learning reserves the right at any time to withdraw from the Licensed Content any item or part of an item for which it no longer retains the right to publish, or which it has reasonable grounds to believe infringes copyright or is defamatory, unlawful, or otherwise objectionable.

4.0 PROTECTION AND SECURITY

4.1 The End User shall use its best efforts and take all reasonable steps to safeguard its copy of the Licensed Content to ensure that no unauthorized reproduction, publication, disclosure, modification, or distribution of the Licensed Content, in whole or in part, is made. To the extent that the End User becomes aware of any such unauthorized use of the Licensed Content, the End User shall immediately notify Cengage Learning. Notification of such violations may be made by sending an e-mail to infringement@cengage.com.

5.0 MISUSE OF THE LICENSED PRODUCT

5.1 In the event that the End User uses the Licensed Content in violation of this Agreement, Cengage Learning shall have the option of electing liquidated damages, which shall include all profits generated by the End User's use of the Licensed Content plus interest computed at the maximum rate permitted by law and all legal fees and other expenses incurred by Cengage Learning in enforcing its rights, plus penalties.

6.0 FEDERAL GOVERNMENT CLIENTS

6.1 Except as expressly authorized by Cengage Learning, Federal Government clients obtain only the rights specified in this Agreement and no other rights. The Government acknowledges that (i) all software and related documentation incorporated in the Licensed Content is existing commercial computer software within the meaning of FAR 27.405(b)(2); and (2) all other data delivered in whatever form, is limited rights data within the meaning of FAR 27.401. The restrictions in this section are acceptable as consistent with the Government's need for software and other data under this Agreement.

7.0 DISCLAIMER OF WARRANTIES AND LIABILITIES

7.1 Although Cengage Learning believes the Licensed Content to be reliable, Cengage Learning does not guarantee or warrant (i) any information or materials contained in or produced by the Licensed Content, (ii) the accuracy, completeness or reliability of the Licensed Content, or (iii) that the Licensed Content is free from errors or other material defects. THE LICENSED PRODUCT IS PROVIDED "AS IS," WITHOUT ANY WARRANTY OF ANY KIND AND CENGAGE LEARNING DISCLAIMS ANY AND ALL WARRANTIES, EXPRESSED OR IMPLIED, INCLUDING, WITHOUT LIMITATION, WARRANTIES OF MERCHANTABILITY OR FITNESS FOR A PARTICULAR PURPOSE. IN NO EVENT SHALL CENGAGE LEARNING BE LIABLE FOR: INDIRECT, SPECIAL, PUNITIVE OR CONSEQUENTIAL DAMAGES INCLUDING FOR LOST PROFITS, LOST DATA, OR OTHERWISE. IN NO EVENT SHALL CENGAGE LEARNING'S AGGREGATE LIABILITY HEREUNDER, WHETHER ARISING IN CONTRACT, TORT, STRICT LIABILITY OR OTHERWISE, EXCEED THE AMOUNT OF FEES PAID BY THE END USER HEREUNDER FOR THE LICENSE OF THE LICENSED CONTENT.

8.0 GENERAL

8.1 Entire Agreement. This Agreement shall constitute the entire Agreement between the Parties and supercedes all prior Agreements and understandings oral or written relating to the subject matter hereof.

8.2 Enhancements/Modifications of Licensed Content. From time to time, and in Cengage Learning's sole discretion, Cengage Learning may advise the End User of updates, upgrades, enhancements and/or improvements to the Licensed Content, and may permit the End User to access and use, subject to the terms and conditions of this Agreement, such modifications, upon payment of prices as may be established by Cengage Learning.

8.3 No Export. The End User shall use the Licensed Content solely in the United States and shall not transfer or export, directly or indirectly, the Licensed Content outside the United States.

8.4 Severability. If any provision of this Agreement is invalid, illegal, or unenforceable under any applicable statute or rule of law, the provision shall be deemed omitted to the extent that it is invalid, illegal, or unenforceable. In such a case, the remainder of the Agreement shall be construed in a manner as to give greatest effect to the original intention of the parties hereto.

8.5 Waiver. The waiver of any right or failure of either party to exercise in any respect any right provided in this Agreement in any instance shall not be deemed to be a waiver of such right in the future or a waiver of any other right under this Agreement.

8.6 Choice of Law/Venue. This Agreement shall be interpreted, construed, and governed by and in accordance with the laws of the State of New York, applicable to contracts executed and to be wholly performed therein, without regard to its principles governing conflicts of law. Each party agrees that any proceeding arising out of or relating to this Agreement or the breach or threatened breach of this Agreement may be commenced and prosecuted in a court in the State and County of New York. Each party consents and submits to the nonexclusive personal jurisdiction of any court in the State and County of New York in respect of any such proceeding.

8.7 Acknowledgment. By opening this package and/or by accessing the Licensed Content on this Web site, THE END USER ACKNOWLEDGES THAT IT HAS READ THIS AGREEMENT, UNDERSTANDS IT, AND AGREES TO BE BOUND BY ITS TERMS AND CONDITIONS. IF YOU DO NOT ACCEPT THESE TERMS AND CONDITIONS, YOU MUST NOT ACCESS THE LICENSED CONTENT AND RETURN THE LICENSED PRODUCT TO CENGAGE LEARNING (WITHIN 30 CALENDAR DAYS OF THE END USER'S PURCHASE) WITH PROOF OF PAYMENT ACCEPTABLE TO CENGAGE LEARNING, FOR A CREDIT OR A REFUND. Should the End User have any questions/comments regarding this Agreement, please contact Cengage Learning at delmar.help@cengage.com.

MOSS Procedures
from
Delmar's Comprehensive Medical Assisting:
Administrative and Clinical Competencies
4th Edition

Wilburta Q. Lindh
Marilyn S. Pooler
Carol D. Tamparo
Barbara M. Dahl

Patient Scheduling

Chapter 13

KEY TERMS

Encryption Technology
Matrix
Modified Wave Scheduling
Screening
Stream Scheduling
Wave Scheduling

OUTLINE

Tailoring the Scheduling System
Scheduling Styles
    Open Hours
    Double Booking
    Clustering
    Wave Scheduling
    Modified Wave Scheduling
    Stream Scheduling
    Practice-Based Scheduling
Analyzing Patient Flow
    Waiting Time
Legal Issues
Interpersonal Skills
Guidelines for Scheduling
  Appointments
    Screening Calls

Referral Appointments
Recording Information
Appointment Matrix
Telephone Appointments
Patient Check-In
Patient Cancellation and
  Appointment Changes
Reminder Systems
Scheduling Pharmaceutical
  Representatives
Scheduling Software and
  Materials
    Appointment Schedule
    Computer Scheduling Software
Inpatient and Outpatient Admissions Procedures

OBJECTIVES

The student should strive to meet the following performance objectives and demonstrate an understanding of the facts and principles presented in this chapter through written and oral communication.

1. Define the key terms as presented in the glossary.
2. Review six major scheduling systems.
3. Describe the six guidelines in scheduling appointments.
4. Explain the importance of screening in scheduling patient appointments.
5. Review proper cancellation procedures and explain the legal necessity of documenting cancellations.
6. Recall three types of reminder systems.
7. Choose an appropriate appointment scheduling tool and describe its advantages.
8. Establish a matrix for a new year and a new practice.
9. Check in patients using a daily appointment sheet.
10. Schedule appointments using a manual system and an electronic system.
11. Schedule outpatient procedures and inpatient admissions.

INTRODUCTION

Patient scheduling has undergone many changes. A medical appointment is most often scheduled over the telephone or in person. Information technology allows appointment scheduling through secure online access using the clinic's Web site. However the appointment is made, the medical staff will need the home telephone number and will want the cellular phone number that often accompanies the patient at all times or is used in place of a land-line telephone. In the case of online appointment requests, the patient's email address is necessary. If online appointment scheduling is new to the clinic, the medical assistant may ask if the patient has a computer and is willing to use the computer for online appointment scheduling.

Patient scheduling is an integral part of the daily workload for medical assistants, whether in large family practices, urgent care centers, or sole proprietor clinics. Scheduling becomes more complicated if providers are practicing in more than one location and traveling between them. Scheduling patients can be stressful, especially if the telephone rings constantly and the medical assistant is unable to provide patients a convenient appointment.

Although patient appointment scheduling may seem like a routine function, a smooth patient flow often determines the success of a day in the ambulatory care setting. A variety of administrative skills are used in the performance of this vital function. By effectively scheduling patients to fit a particular practice, it is possible to make profitable use of provider and staff time.

In addition, efficient patient flow pleases the patient. A common patient complaint is the time spent waiting in the reception area or the examination room. Most patients appreciate a clinic that recognizes the value of their time. Accordingly, these patients do not hesitate to advertise their experience (good or bad) to friends and families—a fact of great significance to any medical setting.

In addition to the required administrative skills, medical assistants involved in scheduling patients must put into practice their best interpersonal and communication skills. Scheduling an appointment may be the first contact patients have with the medical facility. They remember and value the treatment they receive from the time of first contact. The personality of the ambulatory care setting is always reflected in the treatment and respect given to patients.

Whether scheduling is done online, through a computerized system, or in the paper appointment book

Spotlight on Certification

RMA Content Outline
- Reception
- Appointment scheduling

CMA (AAMA) Content Outline
- Telephone techniques
- Equipment operation
- Computer applications
- Utilizing appointment schedules/types
- Appointment guidelines
- Appointment protocol
- Integrating meetings and travel with clinic schedule

CMAS Content Outline
- Medical office clerical assisting
- Appointment management and scheduling

(rare these days), practitioners and their staff must remember the importance of that first impression and make it satisfying for patients.

TAILORING THE SCHEDULING SYSTEM

The schedule of each medical facility will determine the best method for scheduling appointments. A surgeon's office will have a much different flow of patients than a pediatrician's office. The key is to customize the system to best accommodate the practice. Primary goals in determining this should include:

- A smooth flow of patients with a minimal amount of waiting time
- Flexibility to accommodate acutely ill, STAT (or emergency) appointments, work-ins, cancellations, and no-shows

Medical providers may feel uncomfortable if their days are not busy with patients or they experience idle time. It is also true that patients want access to their medical providers when needed and prefer not to wait several days to be seen. There is no one perfect scheduling style, and some facilities even may be unable to identify their style of scheduling by name. One thing is certain, however; patients, providers, and their staff will know when scheduling is not working successfully.

SCHEDULING STYLES

There are a number of methods for patient scheduling. The best method for a practice is the one that effects good patient flow and proper utilization of staff and physical facilities and meets the needs of the provider(s). Traditionally, all scheduling was done by writing appointments in a book by hand. Increasingly, however, scheduling is done using computer software designed specifically for that purpose or using scheduling programs that are part of total practice management software (Figure 13-1). Keep in mind that even the most sophisticated computerized system will fail if the scheduling style does not comfortably fit the predetermined and necessary patient flow.

HIPAA Some clinics ask patients to sign in as they arrive. Some legal authorities believe that the only infallible way to prove patients have kept a medical appointment is to have them sign their name upon arrival and give the time. The Health Insurance Portability and Account-

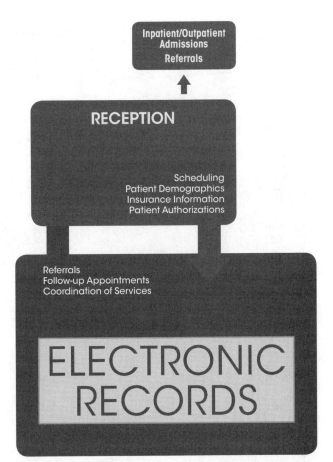

Figure 13-1   Total practice management software (TPMS) diagram showing the relationship of scheduling activities to a patient's medical record.

ability Act (HIPAA) has ruled that patients can be asked to sign their name upon arrival as long they are not asked to provide any other personal information, such as address, telephone number, Social Security number, or clinic identification number. HIPAA has also ruled that patients cannot be forced to sign if they feel uncomfortable in doing so. A word of caution is important here. The patient's right to privacy ensures that patients do not see confidential information (such as the reason for the visit) of other patients. HIPAA regulations have caused facilities to be more cognizant of patients' rights to privacy and confidentiality.

If the setting and circumstances indicate that a sign-in sheet for patients is the most efficient means of checking in patients, forms can be purchased that meet privacy and confidentiality expectations of patients.

Figure 13-2 illustrates a carbonized pack with perforations that allows a patient to sign in giving the necessary information. The patient is instructed to remove the top ticket, leaving the information on the bottom form only. The next

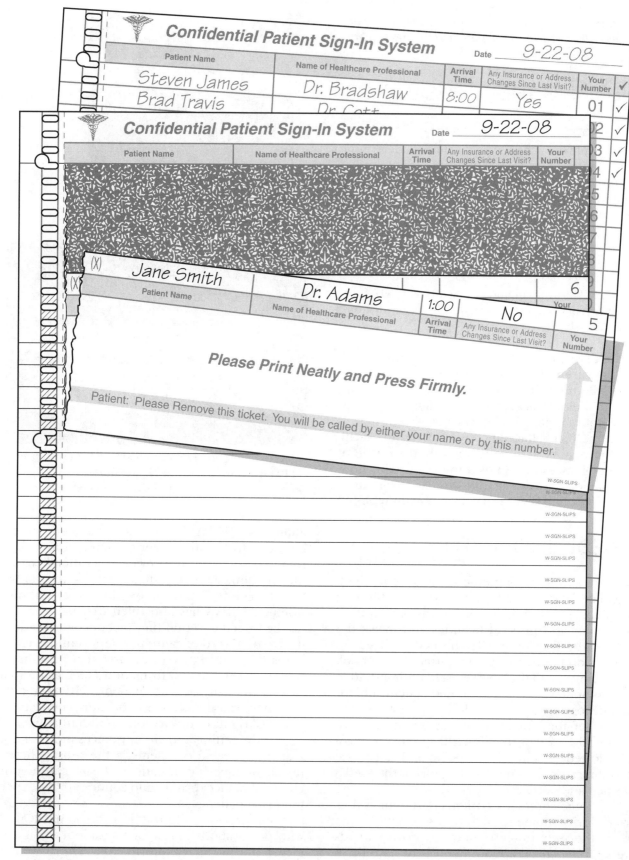

Figure 13-2 Confidential patient sign-in system that offers privacy. Patient can be called by the number of the ticket or by name.

person to sign in does not see the information of the previous patient. The ticket has a number in the upper right-hand corner that can be used by the medical assistant to call the patient if total confidentiality is preferred. However, many patients believe being called by a number is impersonal and unwelcoming.

Open Hours

In open hours scheduling, patients are seen throughout a particular time frame, for example, 9:00 AM to 11:00 AM or 1:00 PM to 3:00 PM. Patients are seen on a first-come, first-served basis. Many clinics frequently choose this method because they are able, by their nature, to maintain a steady flow of patients. Open hours scheduling is likely a place where a sign-in sheet is helpful, because patients are seen on a first-come, first-served basis. It is important to remember that a sign-in sheet can never replace a warm, welcoming greeting from the administrative medical assistant to set the tone for care given that day.

Double Booking

With the double-booking method, two or more patients are given a particular appointment time. This method is limited to a practice that can attend to more than one patient at a time. For instance, Maria Jover and Jim Marshal are both given a 9:30 AM appointment. Ms. Jover requires a complete checkup including lab tests, vitals, and provider visit. Mr. Marshal is being seen for suture removal. While the staff conducts the lab tests on Ms. Jover, the primary care provider can see Mr. Marshal. Obviously, this method requires a precise accounting for time, rooms, and adequate staff. A good rule to remember is that if patients are consistently having to wait for staff to attend to them, double booking is not a wise choice of method. Also, patients who do not understand the complex nature of patient scheduling may

Critical Thinking

When a sign-in sheet is used for patients but the administrative medical assistant is assisting the other staff members when patients arrive, what can be done to create an atmosphere that welcomes patients and puts them at ease?

mistakenly believe that their provider is trying to see two patients at the same time, forcing one of them to wait unnecessarily.

Clustering

The clustering method applies the concept used in production line work, namely, that performing only one step or process allows for efficient processing. In the ambulatory care setting, patients with similar problems are booked consecutively. Obstetricians and pediatricians commonly choose this method. A block of time, either hours or days of the week, is set aside for particular types of cases. For instance, an obstetrician might see only patients in their third trimester of pregnancy on Mondays and Fridays and gynecology patients on Tuesdays and Thursdays. A pediatrician's office might be organized for immunizations on Tuesday mornings and well-baby checkups on Monday and Friday afternoons.

Wave Scheduling

Wave scheduling is another method that can be used effectively in medical facilities that have several procedure rooms and adequate personnel to staff them. Using the wave scheduling system, patients are scheduled only in the first half hour of each hour. For example, three patients may be given the time of 11 AM. Generally, the first one to arrive is seen first. If they all arrive on time, the one who is most ill is usually seen first, and there will be a waiting time for the other two patients. Depending on the practice, some administrative medical assistants will be instructed to schedule three patients at the top of the hour and another two or three patients at the bottom of the hour (e.g., 11:30 AM). Patients who do not understand this system of scheduling may become irritated if they discover that another patient has the same appointed time with the same provider. This method takes into account that there will be no-shows and late arrivals. It can also accommodate work-in appointments. However, it does require personnel who are able to prioritize patient problems precisely when establishing the appointments.

Modified Wave Scheduling

Modified wave scheduling is a variation of the wave method where patients are scheduled in "waves." In this method, two or three patients are scheduled at the beginning of each hour, followed by single appointments every 10 to 20 minutes the rest of the hour.

A variation of this method assesses major and minor problems. Major time-consuming problems are seen at the beginning of the hour (e.g., new patients). Minor problems are seen from 20 minutes past the hour to half past the hour (e.g., follow-ups, bandage changes, and other minor procedures), and walk-ins (e.g., a child with a 103°F temperature) are accommodated at the end of the hour. Again, good screening will determine the success of this method.

With both the clustering and wave methods, empty or unscheduled periods can be used to catch up on other responsibilities.

Stream Scheduling

Stream scheduling is perhaps the best known and most widely used scheduling system. When this system works as it should, there is a steady stream of patients at set appointment times throughout the workday, for example, 30-minute appointment at 9:00 AM; 15-minute appointment at 9:30 AM; 15-minute appointment at 9:45 AM. Each patient is assigned a specific time. This can best be accomplished by establishing realistic time guidelines for particular types of appointments, such as 45 minutes for consultations, 15 minutes for immunizations, and 30 minutes for hearing tests.

Practice-Based Scheduling

As discussed earlier in this chapter, some ambulatory care settings find it necessary to develop a system unique to their patient load. In these customized systems (practice-based), the practice determines the schedule. An orthopedist might schedule cast removals on Mondays and Fridays using double booking and stream scheduling for new patients, with each patient having a 45-minute appointment. A group of vascular surgeons might use both a double-booking and a modified wave system. They might double book patients for short rechecks and quick procedures but use the modified wave for patients with preoperative and postoperative checks and long specialty procedures.

There are many variations of scheduling styles. An Oregon massage therapist who operates a private practice as a sole proprietor with no staff has found that an online welcome screen and appointment book is the best way for her patients to schedule a massage. Her online system also creates appointment reminder email messages. This massage therapist and her patients are pleased. They believe that the self-service scheduling gives their therapist more time to take care of their needs.

ANALYZING PATIENT FLOW

When reviewing the current scheduling practice, a simple analysis can maximize an office's scheduling practices. This entails looking at appointment times, patient arrival times, the actual time a patient is seen, and the time a visit is completed. A simple grid chart can be produced for a given period, for example, 1 to 2 weeks (Figure 13-3). In addition, chart the number of no-shows and cancellations. Electronic scheduling systems can automatically provide the detail necessary to analyze the effectiveness of patient scheduling. It has the capability of indicating the time for specific procedures, for each provider, and for each service given to the patient.

This analysis will provide a clear picture of patient flow and whether personnel are being used efficiently. The data will assist in estimating how many patients to schedule and realistic time frames for particular problems or procedures. If the staff is scheduling return patients every 15 minutes yet the analysis shows these visits average 24 minutes, the scheduling method needs adjustment. This may mean either allowing more minutes for follow-up visits or building in slack time when no appointments are made.

Develop a simple list of commonly scheduled visits with time estimates for each. This procedural sheet will be particularly useful when training new employees or when temporary help is used for scheduling (Figure 13-4).

PATIENT FLOW ANALYSIS

February 2, 20XX — Dr. King

Patient Name	Length of Appt.	Appt. Time	Time Seen	Time Out
Martin Gordon	15	10:20	10:22	10:45
Jason Jover	45	11:20	11:20	12:30
Nora Fowler	30	1:00	1:25	1:45
Jim Marshal	15	1:30	1:50	2:10
Herb Fowler	60	2:45	2:15	3:25

Figure 13-3   Patient flow analysis helps a practice determine realistic time frames for appointments.

TYPICAL SCHEDULING TIMES FOR INTERNAL MEDICINE PRACTICE	
New patients	30 minutes
Patients for consultation	45 minutes
Patients requiring complete physical examinations	45 minutes
All other patients (minor illnesses, routine checkups, etc.)	15 minutes

Figure 13-4 Most practices have a list of typical visits with time estimates.

Waiting Time

One of patients' frequently voiced frustrations with medical clinics is excessive waiting time. Obviously, emergencies and other unexpected interruptions cannot be anticipated. However, there are certain measures the medical assistant can take when attempting to keep the schedule on target. If patients are kept waiting, it is a good strategy to explain the reason for the delay and give patients an estimate of how long the delay will be. *Never* ignore the delay hoping patients will not notice; this, in fact, seems to increase perceived waiting time. Find ways to make patients comfortable while they wait; for example, provide an appropriate choice of reading materials (or in the case of children, activities). Refer to Case Study 10-3. If a delay can be anticipated, for example, the provider is called away for a baby delivery or surgery, attempt to contact patients before they leave home to reschedule the appointments.

If the delay is likely to be a half hour or longer, provide patients with options, for example:

1. Offer patients the opportunity to run an errand, having them return at a specified time.
2. Offer to reschedule appointments for another day, or later that day, or to see another provider in the practice if possible.

In any case, remember that good customer relations dictate your willingness to acknowledge the inconvenience to the patients and attempt to provide an acceptable solution. Remember also that some patients simply will not appreciate any efforts to apologize for a delay, in which case you must continue to act professionally toward them.

LEGAL ISSUES

  Information provided in any patient scheduling system may be used for legal purposes. A case of malpractice or questions regarding a provider's availability may require a copy of the daily schedule. It might become necessary to identify how many times a particular patient was a no-show or canceled an appointment, never calling to reschedule. The appointment schedule could verify that a patient was seen and treated on a particular day, thus affirming the information in the patient's record. A patient sign-in sheet may serve this purpose, also.

All computerized systems provide a permanent record of patients seen, and any alterations to that schedule are saved on the hard drive or disk and are shown when a printout is produced. If an appointment book is still used, the staff will have to make certain there is a permanent record or daily appointment sheet that indicates cancellations, work-ins, urgent care needs, and no-shows. Any changes to the daily appointment sheet are to be made in pen; therefore, there will be no question regarding accuracy.

Remember that anyone looking into a practice will be looking at the record of documentation. Taking the time to accurately and consistently document all aspects of patient care makes a statement about the providers in the practice and their staff and reflects positively on the presumed quality of patient care.

INTERPERSONAL SKILLS

Scheduling appointments requires interpersonal skills. Medical assistants convey a great deal to patients through attitude and actions as well as empathy. A hurried or disinterested manner communicates that the patient is not a priority. Because patients are often distraught or anxious when making appointments, it is extremely important to reduce rather than increase anxiety. Also, the medical assistant scheduling appointments may be the first contact a patient has with the clinic; patients do not easily forget rude or insensitive staff. A hurried, disinterested manner toward patients is just as often the basis for legal action as is a negligent act.

If any form of online scheduling is used, be certain that it is user friendly, has a rapid response time of no more than 24 hours, and provides patients an option if the online scheduling proves unsatisfactory for any reason. Make certain that staff are ready for online scheduling and that those responsible for assignments and backups are carefully prepared. It is important that patients not be made to feel inadequate if they choose not to use online scheduling.

The patient should always be made to feel worthy of attention. This validates his or her reason for calling. If you are scheduling a patient in the office and the phone rings, answer the call but excuse yourself first. Ask the caller to please hold for a moment. If you are on the telephone scheduling a patient and another patient walks in, acknowledge with a nod or signal that you will be right there—never let the person feel ignored (see Chapter 12). Today, patients have a variety of options for health care and tend to be much more consumer conscious of the treatment they receive.

GUIDELINES FOR SCHEDULING APPOINTMENTS

Whether completed by manual methods or computer technology, the process of scheduling appointments for patients and other visitors to the ambulatory care setting involves a number of variables, including (1) the urgency of the need for an appointment; (2) whether the patient is a referral from another provider; (3) recording methods for new and established patients; (4) implementation of check-in, cancellation, and rescheduling policies; (5) use of reminder systems; and (6) accommodating visits from medical supply and pharmaceutical company representatives.

Providers in some health maintenance organizations who are paid by a salary rather than by patient visit are experimenting with group scheduling. The group visits may be established around patients with specific chronic ailments such as diabetes, hypertension, or geriatric complaints. This is one method to provide patient education, support, and interaction while using time efficiently and keeping costs down. At the same time, patient-provider relationships are maintained in providing health care.

Screening Calls

Urgent calls will need to be **screened,** or assessed, before they can be scheduled. In other words, the person making the appointment will need to determine the actual urgency of that call and determine how the patient can best be scheduled. This requires both communication skills and medical knowledge.

Appropriate questions will be asked to determine the actual urgency. Is the patient in immediate need of medical assistance? Is there any bleeding? If so, where? How profuse is the bleeding? Are there chest pains? How intense is the pain? Is the in localized? How long have the symptoms been present? The medical assistant needs to determine whether this is a life-threatening matter, or whether the problem is urgent in the patient's eyes but not a medical emergency. Precise information will help to determine the critical or noncritical nature of the call.

In screening the patient's urgency of care, be tactful in questioning and avoid making the patient feel that the need is insignificant. If questioning indicates this is a medical emergency, follow the policy for having the patient seen (whether it be an emergency appointment or referral to the emergency department). If referral to the emergency department or a call to 911 is necessary, make the call for the patient, being certain you have the correct address and telephone number available. Such a referral minimizes disruption to patients being seen in the ambulatory care setting. If it is determined that the best method in handling this emergency is to see the patient in the office, let scheduled patients know of the emergency and offer them the opportunity of rescheduling or waiting until the emergency has been resolved. A built-in slack time of 30 minutes in the morning and 30 minutes in the afternoon can provide some flexibility in last-minute emergency scheduling. If it is determined that the situation is not an emergency, work the patient into the schedule as the situation warrants and time allows, and make certain the patient is comfortable with the scheduled time. Be sure to leave the patient with the understanding that you have done your best to address the situation. (See Chapters 9 and 12 for more information on screening.)

Referral Appointments

One of the primary sources for any provider is referrals from other providers. This is especially true in a managed care climate, where patients usually must have a referral from their primary care provider and where providers are part of an HMO network. It is important that these appointments be given special consideration and that referred patients be given an appointment as soon as possible.

Adequate information needs to be obtained to determine the urgency of scheduling. If the referring provider or clinic staff calls directly, the situation can be accessed at that time. However, if the referred patient calls, it is best to obtain necessary records and information from the referring provider's office to determine the urgency and appropriateness of an appointment. This can be done by obtaining general information from the patient and then scheduling an appointment after the provider's office is contacted for complete information regarding the patient's condition. Be polite and assure the patient of an appointment as soon as the referring provider's office is contacted.

Recording Information

Patients can be sensitive to the amount of information they are required to provide to make an initial appointment. Keep the information as simple as possible and obtain only essential information. It should be tailored to fit the practice; for example, an obstetrician and a pediatrician will have different questions for the first-time patient.

When patients schedule an appointment online via the clinic's Web site, they are directed to a patient preregistration and health history that can be completed online prior to coming to the facility. The information provided in this format is often more detailed than what is obtained over the telephone. Nevertheless, the following basic items should be obtained from a new patient:

1. The patient's full legal name (with the correct spelling)
2. A daytime telephone number
3. The chief complaint or reason for the visit
4. The referring provider, if relevant

In privacy, repeat this information back to the patient to ensure accuracy.

 Clinics with computerized scheduling and billing will require a few additional items, such as:

1. Date of birth
2. Type of insurance
3. Insurance number

The critical determination is whether the information is essential to the first contact or whether it can be obtained at the time of the visit.

An established patient, someone who has already been seen in the clinic, should be required to provide only the following information:

1. Full legal name
2. Chief complaint or reason for the visit
3. A daytime telephone number

When the information is recorded, print legibly and accurately in a manual system, and key in the information in a computer system. Check for accuracy in either system. Record the appointment as soon as it is made—never rely on memory.

When scheduling an appointment time, ask the patient what day and time is most convenient and then make the appointment for the first available time stated. If possible, provide the patient with a choice of appointment times. Finally, confirm that the patient clearly understands the date and time of the appointment; be sure to repeat the date and time to ensure that both of you have recorded the same information. If the patient is making the appointment in person, provide an appointment reminder.

Scheduling an appointment for the clinic's available times for anyone with an extremely busy schedule can require a great deal of patience. If the patient requests a particular appointment that is not possible, courteously offer an explanation.

Many ambulatory care settings, especially those specializing in family practice and pediatrics, provide alternative hours for scheduling appointments. Having evening appointments at least one day a week or Saturday morning appointments can be helpful for individuals whose work schedule does not permit weekday appointments.

Appointment Matrix

The appointment **matrix** must be established before patients can be scheduled. The matrix provides a current and accurate record of appointment times available for scheduling patient visits. Clinic hours are noted with times blocked when the facility is closed. Provider's schedules, vacations, holidays, hospital rounds, and any responsibilities that make providers unavailable for appointments, are recorded. The matrix of the scheduling plan might include slots for patients who need to see only staff members for their appointment; therefore, times when they are unavailable are important to the matrix. Any evening or weekend appointment slots available also are noted (see Procedure 13-1).

 Typically, when using an electronic system for scheduling, the program will search through a database of appointments, find an open appointment, and allocate an appointment time according to your instructions. These instructions can include finding an open appointment with a specific time length, on a specific day, or within a specified time frame. Once the appointment time is confirmed with the patient, patient data are keyed in, and the appointment is automatically scheduled (see Procedure 13-2).

Telephone Appointments

Appointments are made by telephone more than any other method. Remember the guidelines for appointment scheduling, appropriate screening of all calls to determine urgency and need, and to follow your provider–employer's instructions regarding patient referrals for appointments. Make certain that you get all the necessary information from the patient when the appointment is made. Procedures 13-3 and 13-4 provide practice for telephone appointments in both a manual system and an electronic system. The professional manner in which telephone appointments are made for patients sets the tone for their satisfaction with the clinic, its providers, and their care.

Patient Check-In

Records of patient appointments serve a legal purpose. Establishing a procedure for checking in appointments simplifies tracking of the arrival of patients (see Procedures 13-5 and 13-6). This is particularly true in multiprovider settings where patients are attended by a number of staff before, or instead of, seeing the primary care provider.

As mentioned earlier, more than one method can be used to check in patients. A sign-in sheet might be used, especially in a facility with open hours scheduling. The administrative medical assistant can place a check mark (usually in red) by the patient's name in the appointment book or make an indication electronically (usually an *X*) in scheduling software (Figure 13-5).

The check-in procedure serves the additional purpose of alerting the staff when a patient has arrived and is available to be seen. Communication among the administrative medical assistants and the clinical medical assistants is important for a smooth patient flow and to save time for both patients and providers (Figure 13-6).

Computer scheduling systems include a space to indicate when a patient arrives for an appointment. Some clinics use the printed activity schedule to check when patients arrive. Other clinics rely upon a copy of the day's schedule and the patient's chart indicating a consultation or visit to legally verify the patient's presence in the clinic.

Unfortunately, even the best of electronic systems may fail temporarily. In that case, the manual system is used as a backup. If the day's schedule has already been printed, it can be used to monitor the patient flow and to check in patients. It may also serve as adequate information for any work-in patients to be accommodated that day. However, for appointments

DAILY APPOINTMENT WORKSHEET

Thursday, August 21

8:00	Hospital Rounds		
9:15	Chris O'Keefe	30 minutes	Immunizations
9:30	Jim Marshal	15 minutes	Blood pressure check
10:00	Martin Gordon	60 minutes	PE/lab work
11:00	Nora Fowler	30 minutes	URI
11:30	Lunch break		
12:30	Dentist Appointment, Dr. Schleuter		
2:00	Maria Jover	30 minutes	Suspicious rash
2:45	Meet with drug rep regarding new beta-blocker agents		
4:00	Joseph Ortiz	30 minutes	Choking problems

Figure 13-5   Daily appointment worksheet.

to be made in the future, the administrative medical assistant may have to return a call to the patient when the computer is back up and running properly.

Patient Cancellation and Appointment Changes

A permanent record of no-shows should be designated on the appointment sheet with a red *X* or some other distinctive mark. Cancellations should be marked through on the appointment sheet with a single red line (Figure 13-7). Some facilities place a notation next to the patient's name. Computer scheduling will provide an area to indicate no-shows and cancellations also. No-shows and cancellations

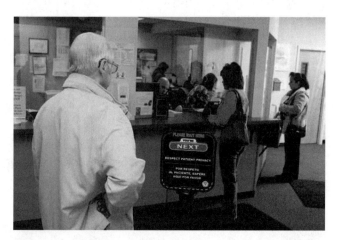

Figure 13-6   The administrative medical assistant checks in a patient and keeps the patient check-in list current.

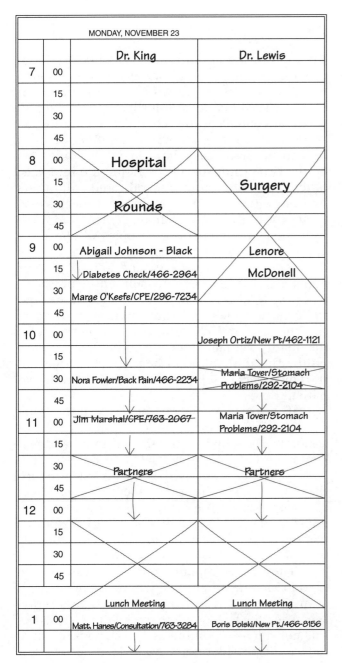

MONDAY, NOVEMBER 23		Dr. King	Dr. Lewis
7	00		
	15		
	30		
	45		
8	00	Hospital	
	15		Surgery
	30	Rounds	
	45		
9	00	Abigail Johnson - Black	Lenore
	15	Diabetes Check/466-2964	McDonell
	30	Marge O'Keefe/CPE/296-7234	
	45		
10	00		Joseph Ortiz/New Pt/462-1121
	15		
	30	Nora Fowler/Back Pain/466-2234	Maria Tover/Stomach Problems/292-2104
	45		
11	00	Jim Marshal/CPE/763-2067	Maria Tover/Stomach Problems/292-2104
	15		
	30	Partners	Partners
	45		
12	00		
	15		
	30		
	45		
		Lunch Meeting	Lunch Meeting
1	00	Matt. Hanes/Consultation/763-3284	Boris Bolski/New Pt./466-8156

Figure 13-7 Multiprovider clinic where providers' commitments and no-shows are marked with a red *X* and cancellations are marked with a single red line. Computer systems have slightly different tracking systems, but all no-shows and cancellations also should be marked in the patient's record.

should always be noted in the patient's individual chart. Again, it is imperative that the provider's care of the patient be thoroughly documented. Should a patient develop complications and claim a provider was unavailable, the daily appointment sheet and chart would document the patient's failure to show.

Occasionally, patients do not arrive for an appointment because they simply forgot, or sometimes they come on the wrong day or at the wrong time. That can happen simply by human error or miscommunication. However, if one patient begins a pattern of getting the dates and times mixed up or forgets the appointment entirely, the primary care provider should be made aware of the fact. Sometimes, a pattern of missed and mixed-up appointments is a first sign that the patient may be experiencing memory loss and mental confusion.

Many clinics have established firm policies for multiple no-shows and cancellations. The general rule is that after three no-shows or cancellations in a row, the provider will review the records. For the provider to adequately treat a patient, the patient's cooperation is necessary. A no-show pattern may indicate that the patient is not truly committed to assisting in treatment. If a patient routinely cancels or does not show, the provider may write a letter terminating services and explaining why the provider is discontinuing care. This should be sent by certified mail, return receipt requested, to ensure that the patient received the notice (see Chapter 7 for more information on termination of services). Procedure 13-7 outlines the proper cancellation procedures.

Although software programs differ, cancellations are typically performed by deleting the patient's name from the time slot; if the appointment is to be rescheduled, the name is then keyed in to the appropriate time, usually the first time open for other appointments (see Procedure 13-8).

When canceling appointments by computer, be certain that the program maintains a list of canceled appointments including patient name, date, and time. This documentation is necessary for legal purposes; also record canceled appointments in the patients' charts.

Reminder Systems

Studies show that the national average of missed appointments is more than 10%. Reminding patients of their scheduled appointments results in a greater rate of fulfilled appointments. Give patients appointment card reminders when appointments are made at the medical facility. Those cards may easily be tucked in a wallet and forgotten, however. Many clinics notify patients the day before the appointment with a reminder of their choice for the communication—telephone, pager, or email.

However, remember that this is confidential information and should not be left on a recording device without the

Patient Education

Encourage patients to participate in their health care by keeping appointments or by notifying the ambulatory care setting that they need to reschedule. Some cancellations are unavoidable, but gentle reminders and a two-way provider–patient relationship encourage responsible patient behavior.

patient's express permission to do so. (When initially seeing the patient, obtain a number where a personal message could be left.) Finally, reminders can be mailed. This would be most appropriate for patients who come on a regular basis (e.g., once every 6 months).

Scheduling Pharmaceutical Representatives

Some medical facilities schedule time with representatives of pharmaceutical and medical supply companies. There are medical clinics that refuse to see any pharmaceutical representatives. When representatives are seen, however, they can provide a valuable service to providers and staff, and with clear guidelines regarding when and how often representatives can visit, a working partnership can develop. Providers may set aside a specific time during the week to meet with these representatives; generally, a time allotment of 15 to 20 minutes is sufficient for these appointments. Some representatives try to establish a standard appointment once a month. If this is a representative your provider desires to see on a regular basis, that policy can be helpful to both the provider and the representative. However, this practice might not allow adequate time for other representatives; therefore, it is often discouraged.

SCHEDULING SOFTWARE AND MATERIALS

No matter what materials and which methods are used, the proper tools will enable patient scheduling to be a smoothly functioning, easily documented process. Materials needed for scheduling should be customized to the ambulatory care setting. For instance, a smaller practice may prefer a manual method involving appointment books; a large urgent care–type setting will use a computer program for patient scheduling that may be part of a practice management software program.

Appointment Schedule

An appropriate appointment schedule system is essential to any medical practice in the ambulatory care setting. Each clinic has unique needs in its physical facility and for its staff. The physical arrangement of the scheduler, including the various combinations of time allotments, must be determined. Some have major headings for hours with minor spaces for 15-minute intervals, others have 10-minute intervals, and still others only hour intervals. An appointment sheet is necessary for both legal risk management and quality management purposes. Copies of the daily appointment sheet are made available to the doctors, medical assistants, and any other staff members. Using the daily appointment sheet, it is easy to check in patients as they arrive and indicate no-shows and cancellations. Indicating the check-in and checkout times can be useful for quality management purposes. More importantly, the daily appointment sheet enables all staff members to see the total scheme of the day's patient flow.

If a provider works between two clinics or a hospital and office, it is helpful to have this appointment schedule transferred to a handheld computer device for immediate referral. If a handheld computer is not used by the provider, reduce the dimensions of the appointment schedule sheet to pocket-size for the provider's easy access. Generally, if the provider makes hospital visits before coming to the office in the morning, this schedule is printed the previous evening before closing.

These daily appointment sheets can also be used to include other provider commitments such as meetings and visits from pharmaceutical representatives. Such a complete record of time ensures that no patient appointments will be booked when, in fact, the provider is not available.

Computer Scheduling Software

Even the smallest of medical facilities today will benefit from the use of information technology. Numerous software programs for the ambulatory care setting require only basic computer hardware that can save time for providers and their staff members. Other programs are more sophisticated and may require on-site technical support.

Some scheduling software programs will schedule resources, equipment, examination rooms, and specialty staff, as well as patients and providers. Some will show copayments due, authorization expiration dates, and insurance expiration dates. They can select the next available appointment, search for appointments by provider, copy and paste appointments, and specify minimum time increments between appointments. The staff can view multiple schedules daily, weekly, monthly, or even yearly. Reminder notes can be created for both providers and patients.

EHR Computerized scheduling systems that are a component of a complete practice management facility, including medical records, are able to indicate no-shows and cancellations in the system and the patient's chart at the same time. Facilities that are partially computerized will still want to indicate patients who do not keep their appointments on the daily worksheet and in the patients' medical records.

Online systems can handle prescription refill requests, patient–provider email messages, and laboratory results. Some will allow patients to update insurance data and complete registration forms. All of the online systems are done within the provider's Web site, which includes security measures and sophisticated **encryption technology**. Therefore, security is less of a concern.

With America's goal of giving patients access to their electronic health record (EHR) by 2014 and with Congress pushing to have prescriptions transferred electronically by 2011, electronic scheduling becomes the "entry" to the entire field of computerized medical information. Employers in ambulatory care settings who make certain patients understand computerized scheduling, have put time and effort into determining the best program for their use, and have trained their staff well will not be disappointed with the outcome. Whatever system is chosen, keep in mind that the patient's time, the staff's time, and the provider's time are extremely valuable. The goal is to manage that time as efficiently as possible.

INPATIENT AND OUTPATIENT ADMISSIONS PROCEDURES

Often, patients are scheduled for either outpatient or inpatient hospital admissions or for special procedures performed in another facility. These appointments are most likely made while the patient is present in the ambulatory care center and has just been seen by the primary care provider. It will be especially helpful if the patient has an appointment book identifying current responsibilities. Have a calendar handy for visualization of the days discussed.

Outpatient procedures may include endoscopy examinations and specialized radiologic examina-tions such as mammography, bone scans, and ultra-sounds. Computerized tomography (CT) scans and magnetic resonance imaging (MRI) procedures will also require specialized admissions. If a patient prefers to make his or her own arrangements for a procedure, indicate that the following information is necessary:

- Name, address, and telephone number of patient
- Name of provider ordering the procedure
- Name of patient's insurance, ID number, and Social Security number

Follow up in a day or two to make certain the required procedure has been scheduled (see Procedure 13-9).

Generally, a real service is done for the patients and staff when the medical assistant schedules the procedure. With the patient present, place a telephone call to the facility where procedures are to be performed. Identify yourself, your provider, and the clinic from which you are calling. Identify any urgency to the request and ask for the next available appointment. As dates and times are discussed, your patient is able to give an immediate response. Consider travel time for your patient and whether there is apt to be any uncomfortable pre-examination procedures that might make travel difficult. Be certain to advise the patient if someone is needed to provide transportation home after the procedure. Often, there is a paperwork follow-up that indicates the nature of the illness and the reason for the specialty examination. Your employer will tell you if a phone response to the examination is required, or if it is acceptable to wait for the written test results.

Once a date has been established, make certain the patient knows the correct date and time, as well as how to get to the place where the examination is to be performed. Inform the patient how and when he or she will receive test results.

Scheduling inpatient admissions to the hospital is similar. However, the provider may want the patient in the hospital as quickly as possible. Call the preferred or designated hospital. Expect to provide pertinent patient and insurance information required by the hospital. Assist the patient in determining whether it is permissible to return home for some personal belongings and to make home arrangements or whether admission is immediate. Some large facilities have a surgery scheduler to make all these arrangements. In primary care, the medical assistant will do this kind of scheduling.

When a surgery is being scheduled, the medical assistant must sometimes coordinate several entities. Arrangement must be coordinated with an assistant in the surgeon's office, with the hospital or outpatient surgery center where the surgery will be performed, occasionally scheduling specialty equipment and personnel to be available, as well as with the patient's schedule. If any one of these entities is not available at the time requested, the process needs to begin again and can become quite convoluted. If the scheduling of the surgery is especially complex, the medical assistant should consider obtaining the patient's scheduling preferences and limitations and letting the patient go home to be contacted later when all the parts are in place.

Be sensitive to the patient's needs at this time. Scheduling a specialty examination or a hospital admission is rarely a convenience. More likely it is a great inconvenience to the patient, even when necessary. Anything that makes the scheduling more accommodating or pleasant for the patient will help in creating a beneficial atmosphere for all involved.

Procedure 13-1

Establishing the Appointment Matrix in a Paper System

PURPOSE:
To have a current and accurate record of appointment times available for scheduling patient visits.

EQUIPMENT/SUPPLIES:
Appointment scheduler
Clinic schedule and calender
Staff schedule

BLOCK CALENDAR EXERCISES:

1. Dr. Heath will be attending a Quality Care Committee meeting at New York County Hospital on the first of every month beginning June 1, 2009, through December 31, 2009, from 9:00 AM to 10:00 AM. *NOTE:* If the first of the month is on a weekend, the meeting will be held on the next business day.

2. Dr. Schwartz sees his patients who are residents in nursing homes every Thursday afternoon from 1:00 PM to 5:00 PM.

3. Staff meetings are held biweekly on Wednesday afternoons from 1:00 PM to 2:00 PM. This policy was put into place with an effective date of July 1, 2009, and will be in effect until June 30, 2010. All staff members are expected to attend.

PROCEDURE STEPS:

1. Block off times in the appointment scheduler when patients are not to be scheduled by marking a large *X* through these time slots. This establishes the matrix. Ideally, the whole year can be mapped out to avoid scheduling patients when the physician has other commitments or when the office is closed. RATIONALE: Identifies visually when patients cannot be scheduled for an appointment.

2. Indicate all vacations, holidays, and other office closures as soon as they are known. It may be helpful to indicate absences that might affect patient scheduling; for example, the vascular laboratory technician is gone April 20–23, so no Doppler procedures will be scheduled. RATIONALE: Informs all staff members of absences from the facility and indicates when these members are not available to see patients.

3. Note all provider meetings, hospital rounds, appointments, conferences, vacations, and other prescheduled provider commitments. If the provider has routine items, such as a Medical Society meeting that is always held on the first Thursday of the month at 7:00 PM or daily hospital rounds at 8:00 AM, write these in. RATIONALE: Informs all staff members of prescheduled commitments when a provider is unavailable to see patients.

4. If the clinic has a scheduling system for certain examinations or procedures (e.g., all cast removals are done in the morning before 10:30 AM), these can be color coded with highlighters. This way it is easily and quickly evident where particular types of appointments are available to be scheduled. RATIONALE: Allows all staff members to see at a glance where certain examinations or procedures can be scheduled. The color-coded highlighting helps prevent errors in establishing such specific times for certain procedures. *The completed matrix provides proof of the completed task.*

Procedure 13-2

Establishing the Appointment Matrix Using Medical Office Simulation Software (MOSS)

PURPOSE:
To have a current and accurate record of appointment times available for scheduling patient visits.

EQUIPMENT/SUPPLIES:
Computer with MOSS
Clinic schedule and calendar
Staff schedule

BLOCK CALENDAR EXERCISES:
1. Dr. Heath will be attending a Quality Care Committee meeting at New York County Hospital on the first of every month beginning June 1, 2009, through November 30, 2009, from 9:00 AM to 10:00 AM. *NOTE:* If the first of the month is on a weekend, the meeting will be held on the next business day.

2. Dr. Schwartz will see his patients at Retirement Inn Nursing Home every Thursday afternoon the month of January 2010, from 1:00 PM to 5:00 PM.

3. Dr. Heath's staff meetings are held biweekly on Thursday afternoons from 4:00 PM to 5:00 PM. This policy was put into place with an effective date of July 2, 2009, and will be in effect until December 31, 2009.

PROCEDURE STEPS:
1. Open MOSS and select File Maintenance from the main menu. View the practice settings by clicking on the "Practice Information" tab and then clicking "Practice Settings."

2. At the bottom of the dialog box, in Field 12, the practice hours are indicated. Make sure that the Start Time is set for 9:00 AM and the Stop Time is set to 5:00 PM (unless otherwise directed by your instructor). RATIONALE: Identifies when patients can be scheduled for appointments.

3. Verify that the Lunch Start Time is set for 12:00 PM and the Lunch End Time is set at 1:00 PM (unless otherwise directed by your instructor). RATIONALE: Identifies when patients cannot be seen for appointments.

4. Close the practice settings screen and return to the main menu. Select Appointment Scheduling.

5. Select June 1, 2009, by clicking on the date within the calendar in the upper right corner of the screen (Figure 13-8). Use the Y+/Y- and M+/M- buttons to navigate to the date.

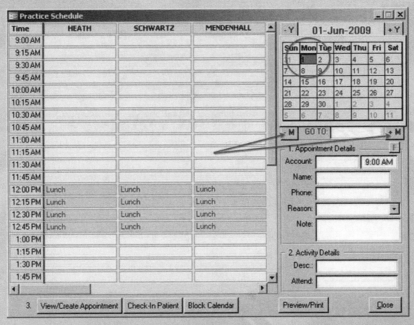

Figure 13-8   MOSS screenshot showing lunch hour schedule and present date.

continues

6. Once the date has been selected, click on the "Block Calendar" button at the bottom of the practice schedule screen.

7. You will receive a message "Do you want to create a NEW Calendar Block?" Select "Yes." The Block Calendar window will open.

8. In Field 1, type "Meeting." This field indicates the type of block you are creating (i.e., lunch, hospital rounds, committee meeting, etc.).

9. In Field 2, enter "06/01/2009," the date on which you wish to begin blocking a segment of the calendar.

10. In Field 3, enter "11/30/2009," the date on which you wish to end blocking the segment of the calendar. (This can be the same day or for an extended period of time.)

11. In Field 4, enter "09:00 AM," which indicates the start time.

12. In Field 5, use the drop-down menu to select "60," which indicates the duration of the block in minutes.

13. In Field 6, use the drop-down menu to select "monthly," which indicates the frequency of the block (i.e. daily, weekly, monthly, etc.).

14. Field 7 should automatically populate based on your selection in Field 6. This is the number of times the block will occur over the period of time selected.

15. In Field 8, select "Dr. Heath," the physician to whom this block applies.

16. In Field 9, indicate "Quality Care Committee, NY County Hospital." If the description in Field 1 needs no further explanation, leave Field 9 blank, as this would be used to enter any notes

applicable to the block that will provide additional information if necessary. Compare your work with Figure 13-9.

17. Click "SAVE" at the bottom of the screen. Review the calendar to make sure that the "BLOCK" has been appropriately applied and make any necessary changes. RATIONALE: This step ensures that your work will be maintained in the schedule.

18. Repeat the above steps, using the information provided in Block Calendar Exercises 2 and 3.

19. Take screenshots of the complete Block Calendar window (the window shown in Figure 13-9) for Exercises 2 and 3 to submit to your instructor either as a printout or in an email file.

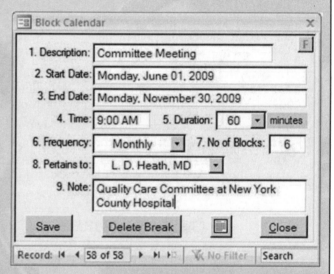

Figure 13-9   MOSS screenshot establishing a weekly

Procedure 13-3

Making an Appointment on the Telephone Using Paper Scheduling

PURPOSE:
To schedule an appointment, entering information in the appointment schedule according to clinic policy.

EQUIPMENT/SUPPLIES:
Telephone
Black ink pen
Appointment book or appointment worksheet
Calendar

APPOINTMENT SCHEDULING EXERCISES:

1. Jordan Connell calls the facility on June 3, 2009, because he has had a temperature of 101° F for 2 days. He also complains of a sore throat and ear pain. He is given a 15-minute appointment on the same day for 3:00 PM with Dr. Heath.

2. Ed Gormann calls the facility on June 1, 2009, to schedule his annual physical examination (60-minute visit) with Dr. Heath. He agrees to be seen on September 15, 2009, at 9:00 AM.

3. Elane Ybarra calls on June 2, 2009, because she has had persistent heartburn and indigestion along with intermittent bouts of diarrhea. She is given an appointment for June 4, 2009, at 10:15 AM (30-minute visit) with Dr. Schwartz.

4. Andrew Jefferson schedules an appointment on June 1, 2009 for June 5, 2009, because he has been bothered by a sore shoulder for the past 2 days. The 15-minute appointment is scheduled for 10:30 AM with Dr. Schwartz

5. Eric Gordon has been experiencing problems with urination for the past week. A 15-minute appointment is scheduled for Friday, June 5, 2009, at 9:00 AM with Dr. Schwartz.

PROCEDURE STEPS:

1. *In a private and quiet location,* answer the ringing telephone before the third ring. Identify the facility and yourself. RATIONALE: assures the patient calling that he or she has the correct number; sets the tone for the conversation. The private location ensures that others will not hear any information said during the telephone call.

2. As the patient begins to speak, make notes on your personal log sheet of the patient's name and reason for the call. RATIONALE: Makes certain you are focusing on the call and will not have to ask the patient to repeat something you missed.

3. Determine whether the patient is new or established, the provider to be seen, and the reason for the appointment. RATIONALE: Provides necessary information to determine when the patient should be seen and how much time will likely be necessary.

4. Discuss with the patient any special appointment needs, and search your appointment schedule (using appointment book or appointment worksheet) for an available time. RATIONALE: Tells the patient that his or her needs and the needs of the clinic are essential to this conversation.

5. Once that patient has agreed to an appropriate time, enter the patient's name in the schedule. Enter last name first, followed by the first name, telephone number (home, work, or cell), and the chief complaint (reason for the visit). Write or print legibly with a black pen in the appointment book or worksheet so that any staff member needing the information will be able to read it. RATIONALE: Provides necessary information for staff to pull a record or to make a chart; chief complaint helps identify the length of time to allot for the appointment. The telephone number provides immediate information should there be a need to change the appointment without having to pull the chart.

6. Repeat the date and time for the appointment, using the patient's name. Provide any necessary instructions about coming to the facility. RATIONALE: Confirms the appointment date and time with the patient and gives information about how to get to the facility.

7. End the call politely, perhaps saying, "Thank you for calling. We will see you at 3:45 PM Monday. Good-bye."

8. Make certain you transferred all necessary information from your telephone log to the appropriate appointment schedule. Draw a diagonal line through your notes on the log. This indicates you have completed the task.

Procedure 13-4

Making an Appointment on the Telephone Using Medical Office Simulation Software (MOSS)

PURPOSE:

To schedule telephone appointments using electronic software.

EQUIPMENT/SUPPLIES:

Computer and MOSS
Telephone
Calendar

APPOINTMENT SCHEDULING EXERCISES:

1. Jordan Connell calls the facility on June 3, 2009, because he has had a temperature of 101° F for 2 days. He also complains of a sore throat and ear pain. He is given a 15-minute appointment on the same day for 3:00 PM with Dr. Heath.

2. Ed Gormann calls the facility on June 1, 2009, to schedule his annual physical examination (60-minute visit) with Dr. Heath. He agrees to be seen on September 15, 2009, at 9:00 AM.

3. Elane Ybarra calls on June 2, 2009, because she has had persistent heartburn and indigestion along with intermittent bouts of diarrhea. She is given an appointment for June 4, 2009, at 10:15 AM (30-minute visit) with Dr. Schwartz.

4. Andrew Jefferson schedules an appointment on June 1, 2009, for June 5, 2009, because he has been bothered by a sore shoulder for the past 2 days. The 15-minute appointment is scheduled for 10:30 AM with Dr. Schwartz.

5. Vito Mangano calls the facility stating he has had a sore throat for the past 3 days. He is given a 15-minute appointment for June 10 at 9:00 AM with Dr. Heath.

6. Eric Gordon has been experiencing problems with urination for the past week. An appointment is scheduled for Friday, June 5, 2009, at 9:00 AM with Dr. Schwartz.

MOSS PROCEDURE STEPS:

1. Open MOSS and select the Appointment Scheduling module from the main menu.

2. From the calendar in the upper right corner of the screen, select June 3, 2009.

3. In the Appointment schedule, scroll down and click in the 3:00 PM time slot in the column for Dr. Heath. This will open an Appointment Scheduling dialog box with the list of patients in the practice.

4. Click in the search box and type "Con" and click on "Search." RATIONALE: This shows those patients whose last names begin with these letters.

5. Highlight the line with Jordan Connell's name and select "Add" at the bottom of the dialog box.

6. In the Patient Appointment Form, Field 1 will automatically populate with the patient name and account number.

7. In Field 2, use the drop-down menu to select Dr. Heath.

8. Fields 3 and 4 will automatically populate with the date, June 3, 2009, and the time, 3:00 PM.

9. In Field 5, use the drop-down menu to select 15 minutes for the amount of time to be set aside for the appointment.

10. In Field 6, using the drop-down menu, select Office Visit as the reason for the visit.

11. In Field 7, select the frequency of the visit as "Single" (i.e., single, daily, weekly, etc.) from the drop-down menu.

12. In Field 9, in the Note section, enter the reason for the patient visit, "Fever 101° F, sore throat, and ear pain." Compare your work with Figure 13-10.

13. Click on "Save Appointment." Click "OK" in the dialog box, which indicates "Appointment Information Posted." This will bring you back to the schedule for that day, and "Connell" should appear in the 3:00 PM time slot. Compare your work with Figure 13-11.

continues

Procedure 13-4 (continued)

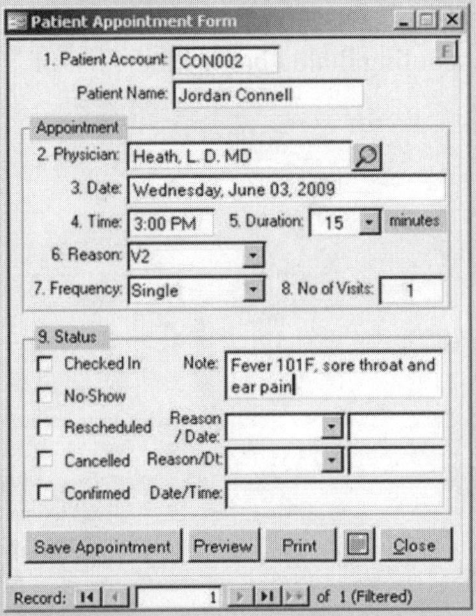

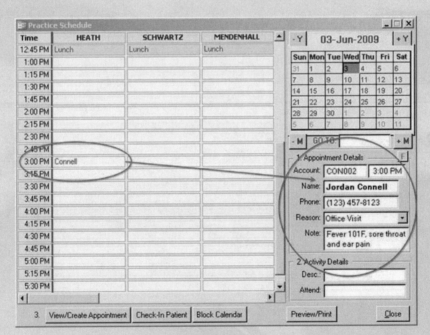

Figure 13-10   MOSS screenshot indicating patient's reason for visit.

14. Close the Practice Schedule dialog box by clicking on "Close" in the bottom right corner.

15. Repeat the above steps, using the information provided in Appointment Scheduling Exercises 2 through 6.

16. Print completed appointment forms and submit to your instructor either as a printout or in an email file.

Figure 13-11   MOSS screenshot showing completed appointment for Jordan Connell.

Procedure 13-4, Revised Step 3:

In the Appointment schedule, scroll down and **double-click** in the 3:00 PM time slot in the column for Dr. Heath. This will open an Appointment Scheduling dialog box with the list of patients in the practice.

Procedure 13-5

Checking in Patients in a Paper System

PURPOSE:
To ensure the patient is given prompt and proper care; to meet legal safeguards for documentation.

EQUIPMENT/SUPPLIES:
Patient chart
Black ink pen
Required forms
Check-in list or appointment book

CHECKING-IN PATIENT EXERCISES:
1. Jordan Connell arrives at the facility for his 3:00 PM appointment with Dr. Heath on June 3, 2009.

2. Elane Ybarra arrives at the facility on June 4, 2009, for her 10:15 AM appointment with Dr. Schwartz.

3. Ed Gormann arrives at 9 AM for his physical examination with Dr. Heath.

PROCEDURE STEPS:
1. The previous evening or before opening the ambulatory care setting, prepare a list of patients to be seen and assemble the charts. RATIONALE: Provides a patient list to use as a guide through the day's schedule; charts are ready before patient arrival. If the task is left to the last minute, it may not get done.

2. Check charts to see that everything is up to date. RATIONALE: Ensures that providers and staff have all the necessary data before seeing a patient.

3. When patients arrive, acknowledge their presence. If you cannot assist them immediately, gesture toward a chair; thank them for waiting as soon as you are available. RATIONALE: Patients feel welcomed, their time is valued, and their presence is noted.

4. Check in the patient and review vital information, such as address, telephone number, insurance, and reason for visit. *Be certain to protect the patient's privacy by reviewing this information where doing so cannot be overheard by others.* RATIONALE: Ensures that you have the latest personal information regarding your patient; provides patients with the privacy and confidentiality to which they are entitled.

5. Use a pen to check off the patient's name from the daily worksheet if one is used for the permanent record. RATIONALE: Ensures that there is a permanent record of the patient's arrival in the facility for an appointment. *Provides documentation for later referral if necessary.*

6. Politely ask the patient to be seated and indicate the appropriate wait time, if any. RATIONALE: Provides direction to the patient and indicates how long a wait might be.

7. Following clinic policy, place the chart where it can be picked up to route the patient to the appropriate location for the visit. RATIONALE: The patient's chart is in readiness when the clinical medical assistant, laboratory personnel, or provider is ready for the patient.

Procedure 13-6

Checking In Patients Using Medical Office Simulation Software (MOSS)

PURPOSE:

To check in patients when they arrive for their appointments using electronic software; to meet legal safeguards for documentation.

EQUIPMENT/SUPPLIES:

Computer and MOSS

CHECKING-IN PATIENT EXERCISES:

1. Jordan Connell arrives at the facility for his 3:00 PM appointment with Dr. Heath on June 3, 2009.

2. Elane Ybarra arrives at the facility on June 4, 2009, for her 10:15 AM appointment with Dr. Schwartz.

3. Ed Gormann arrives at 9 AM for his physical examination with Dr. Heath.

4. Vito Mangano did not keep his appointment with Dr. Heath on June 10, 2009. His appointment should be marked as "no-show" for record-keeping purposes.

MOSS PROCEDURE STEPS:

1. Open MOSS and select Appointment Scheduling from the main menu.

2. From the calendar in the upper right corner of the screen, select June 3, 2009.

3. Scroll down to the 3:00 PM time slot for Dr. Heath and double-click on "Connell."

4. This will open the Patient Appointment Form.

5. Go to Field 9 and click in the box next to "Checked-In." Compare your work with Figure 13-12.

6. Click "Save Appointment" and click "OK" when dialog box with "Appointment Information Posted" appears.

7. Select "Close" in the bottom right corner of the Patient Appointment Form.

8. Repeat the above steps, using the information provided in Checking-In Patient Exercises 2 and 3.

9. Take screenshots of the complete Patient Appointment Form (the window shown in Figure 13-12) for Exercises 2 and 3 to submit to your instructor either as a printout or in an email file.

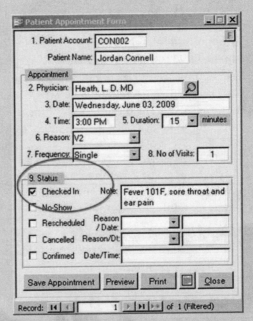

Figure 13-12   MOSS screenshot indicating Jordan Connell's check in.

Procedure 13-7

Cancellation and Rescheduling Procedures Using Paper Scheduling

PURPOSE:
To protect the provider from legal complications; to free up care time for other patients; to ensure quality patient care.

EQUIPMENT/SUPPLIES:
Appointment sheet
Red ink pen
Patient chart

CANCELLATION AND RESCHEDULING EXERCISES:

1. Eric Gordon contacts the facility today, June 4, 2009, because he is experiencing more acute symptoms related to his urinary problems: pain in the abdomen and burning when he urinates. His appointment for June 5 is rescheduled to today at 1:00 PM.

2. Andrew Jefferson calls on Thursday, June 4, 2009, to say that he cannot make the appointment tomorrow. His shoulder is no longer bothering him, so he does not want to reschedule.

PROCEDURE STEPS:
Develop a system so it is evident to staff making appointments that, because of cancellations, time is now open to schedule other appointments.

1. Indicate on the appointment sheet all appointments that were changed, canceled, or no-shows by:

   - *Changes:* Note rescheduling in the appointment sheet margin and directly in the patient's chart; indicate new appointment time. RATIONALE: Notifies all staff of a schedule change; *documents same information in patient's chart.*

   - *Cancellations:* Note on both the appointment sheet and the patient's chart. Draw a single red line through canceled appointments. Date and initial cancellation in the patient chart. RATIONALE: Notifies staff of a schedule change; *documents cancellation in patient's chart, thus identifying a change in the patient's plans.* A cancellation may initiate a follow-up call from a staff member to determine the reason for the cancellation.

   - *No-shows:* Note on both the appointment sheet and the patient's chart. Date and initial notations in the chart. No-shows can be indicated with a red *X* on the appointment sheet. RATIONALE: Notifies the staff of a schedule change; *documents the no-show in the patient's chart.* Provides a reminder to a staff member to follow up on the reason for the no-show.

Procedure 13-8

Cancellation and Rescheduling in Medical Office Simulation Software (MOSS)

PURPOSE:
To protect the provider from legal complications; to free care time for other patients; to ensure quality patient care.

EQUIPMENT/SUPPLIES:
Computer and MOSS

CANCELLATION EXERCISES:

1. Eric Gordon contacts the facility today, June 4, 2009, because he is experiencing more acute symptoms related to his urinary problems: pain in the abdomen and burning when he urinates. His appointment for June 5 is rescheduled to today at 1:00 PM.

2. Andrew Jefferson calls on Thursday, June 4, 2009, to say that he cannot make the appointment tomorrow. His shoulder is no longer bothering him, so he does not want to reschedule.

MOSS PROCEDURE STEPS:

1. Open MOSS and select the Appointment Scheduling module from the main menu.

continues

2. From the calendar in the upper right corner of the screen, select June 5, 2009.

3. Double click on "Gordon" in the 9:00 AM time slot for Dr. Schwartz. RATIONALE: This will open the Patient Appointment Form.

4. Go to Field 9 and click in the box next to "Rescheduled."

5. Click on the drop-down arrow in the field next to "Rescheduled" and select "Needs different date" tab to the field on the right. RATIONALE: This step indicates the need for a different date for the reschedule.

6. Now, click on the calendar button to the right of the reason/date line (see Figure 13-13). This brings up the practice calendar.

7. Select June 4, 2009 and then double click on the 1:00 PM slot for Dr. Schwartz. Click the Close button on the bottom right of the screen. *NOTE:* Double clicking on the slot will populate the original patient appointment form,

although nothing appears on the screen in the calendar.

8. Now you are back on the original Patient Appointment Form. In Field 9, in the Notes section, indicate the additional information regarding the patient's condition: "abdominal pain and burning sensation upon urination." RATIONALE: Indicates reason for appointment. Compare your work with Figure 13-14.

9. Click on "Save Appointment" and "OK" in the dialog box for "Appointment Information Posted."

10. Close the Patient Appointment Form and close the practice schedule.

11. Repeat the above steps, using the information provided in Cancellation Exercise 2.

12. Take a screenshot of the complete Patient Appointment Form window (the window shown in Figure 13-14) for Exercise 2 to submit to your instructor either as a printout or in an email file.

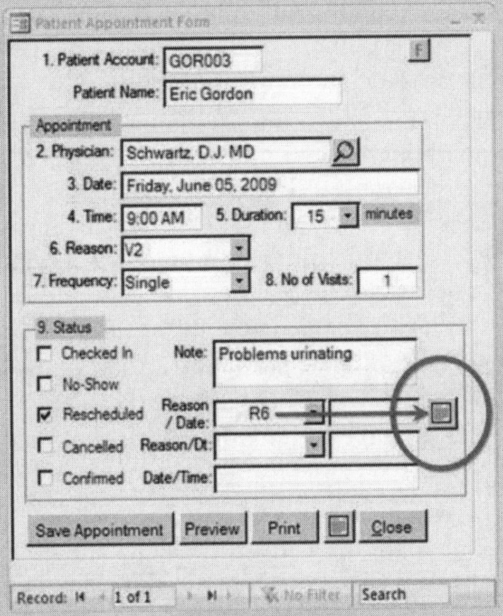

Figure 13-13   MOSS screenshot showing rescheduling for Eric Gordon.

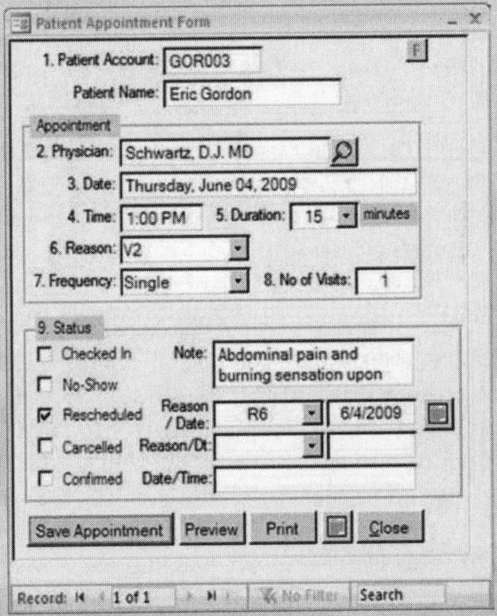

Figure 13-14   MOSS screenshot indicating additional information on reason for reschedule of Eric Gordon.

Procedure 13-9

Scheduling Inpatient and Outpatient Admissions and Procedures

PURPOSE:
To assist patients in scheduling inpatient and outpatient admissions and procedures ordered by the provider.

EQUIPMENT/SUPPLIES:
Calendar
Black ink pen
Telephones
Referral slip
Patient's calendar or schedule (helpful, but not critical)
Provider requests/orders regarding procedures/ admissions being scheduled

PROCEDURE STEPS:

1. In a private and quiet location, discuss with the patient the inpatient admission or outpatient procedure ordered by the provider. RATIONALE: Helps the patient identify the time necessary for this appointment and the reason for it.

2. If required, seek permission from the patient's insurance company for the procedure or admission. RATIONALE: Clearly identifies for the patient who is responsible for the bill and how it is to be paid.

3. Produce a large, easily read calendar and check to see if the patient has one also. RATIONALE: Visualization of the calendar is easier for determining available time for the appointment. Patient's calendar further identifies available days and times for the appointment(s).

4. Place telephone call to the facility where the appointment is to be scheduled. Identify yourself, your provider, the clinic from where you are calling, and the reason for the call. RATIONALE: Alerts the receiver of the call that a provider's office is calling to schedule an appointment. NOTE: *The more familiar the medical assistant is with the specific procedure to be scheduled or a hospital admission, the easier it is to make certain the patient has all the information necessary. It can be helpful for medical assistants to discuss such arrangements with specialty clinics and hospitals.*

5. Identify any urgency. Request the next available appointment for the particular appointment to be scheduled and provide the patient's diagnosis. Identify any time that is not possible for the patient. RATIONALE: Tells the receiver how quickly an appointment is to be made, for what reason, and if any dates or times are not possible.

6. As a time is suggested, confer with the patient for an immediate response.

7. Once the appointment has been scheduled, provide receiver pertinent information related to the patient (e.g., full name, insurance information, Social Security number, telephone number). RATIONALE: Provides essential information to secure the appointment for the proper patient.

8. Request any special instructions or advanced data necessary for the patient. RATIONALE: Helps to ensure that a smooth transition is made from the provider's office to the facility where the referral is made and provides the patient with any special instructions.

9. Complete the referral slip for the patient; send or fax a copy to the referral facility. RATIONALE: Ensures that the patient, the referral facility, and the patient's chart have a copy of the reason for the appointment, any specific instructions, and the date and time of the appointment.

10. If an immediate hospital admission is to be made, provide the patient time on the telephone to call family members to make arrangements to receive personal items and any other arrangements necessitated by the appointment. RATIONALE: Provides patients a little time to notify a family member and make necessary arrangements.

11. Place a reminder notice to yourself on the calendar or in a tickler file. RATIONALE: To check to make certain the appointment was completed and a report is received from the appointment facility.

12. Document the referral in the patient's chart. A copy of the referral slip and all pertinent data are to be included. Document in the chart when the appointment is completed and a report is received from the referral facility. Date and initial.

DOCUMENTATION

11/30/20XX— 10:45 am   Referral to Eastside Radiology for breast ultrasound made. C. Tamparo, CMA (AAMA)

12/01/20XX— 1 pm   Patient given instructions and copy of referral slip. Original referral slip sent to Eastside Radiology. C. Tamparo, CMA (AAMA)

Case Study 13-1

Review the scenario at the beginning of the chapter. It appears that this clinic has a smooth-flowing scheduling system and that Walter Seals has everything under control.

CASE STUDY REVIEW

1. What personal traits might Walter need to possess in order for this scenario to be true?
2. What factors, if any, might make the scheduling in Inner City Health Care work well?
3. If clients are seen on a first-come, first-served basis, how does the clustering system work if patients need to be referred to one of the specialty care clinics?

Case Study 13-2

Rhoda Au has persistently canceled her appointments at Inner City Health Care. Although she always reschedules, she has canceled her last four appointments. Today, she did not call to cancel nor did she arrive for her fifth appointment. Walter Seals, CMA (AAMA), who is responsible for scheduling and patient flow, is concerned that Rhoda is canceling because she is afraid to come in for some reason. Rhoda has been a patient for a few years now, and she was always responsible about keeping her appointments.

CASE STUDY REVIEW

1. From the point of view of the urgent care center, why should Walter be concerned that Rhoda is canceling appointments? What action might be taken?
2. From the patient's point of view, why should Walter be concerned?
3. How should Walter record these cancellations and no-shows?

Case Study 13-3

Audrey Jones, RMA, is a clinical medical assistant in Drs. Lewis and King's clinic. In the past 3 weeks, Audrey has been doing phone screening, primarily because the clinic has been so busy and the providers believe screening calls will help. In fact, Audrey discovered that the administrative medical assistant was screening quite well, but that there does not seem to be sufficient appointment slots to meet the patient demand.

CASE STUDY REVIEW

1. What might be done to determine whether there is a better scheduling style to fit the current demands?
2. What happens when professional staff, providers, and patients view this medical facility as "too busy"?
3. What are some solutions that you can identify?

SUMMARY

Today's ambulatory care setting needs to function efficiently to provide quality care, ensure adequate patient flow, and maintain positive patient relationships. Proper scheduling of patients and other visitors is key to an efficient operation, and the well-organized medical assistant will design a system that meets with both provider and patient satisfaction.

There are at least six common methods of scheduling; ambulatory care settings should use the one that is most appropriate to their patient population, practice areas, and provider preferences. Scheduling methods can and should be customized to the setting, for this usually provides the most adaptable, workable system.

Patient scheduling tools also vary and can be tailored to facility needs. All ambulatory care settings must carefully document appointments, cancellations, and no-shows. The goal is to use scheduling tools wisely and consistently in all scheduling activities while making the patient feel valued.

STUDY FOR SUCCESS

To reinforce your knowledge and skills of information presented in this chapter:

- Review the Key Terms
- Practice any Procedures
- Consider the Case Studies and discuss your conclusions
- Answer the Review Questions
  - Multiple Choice
  - Critical Thinking
- Navigate the Internet and complete the Web Activities
- Practice the StudyWARE activities on the textbook CD
- Apply your knowledge in the Student Workbook activities
- Complete the Web Tutor sections
- View and discuss the DVD situations

REVIEW QUESTIONS

Multiple Choice

1. Appointment scheduling should always be:
   a. recorded only in pencil
   b. current, accurate, and saved as documentation
   c. left on the front desk for patient viewing
   d. recorded only in red ink

2. Patient screening
   a. involves taking only emergencies
   b. is assessing the urgency of a call and need for appointment
   c. means sorting appointments by specialized procedure
   d. is only performed by providers

3. Representatives from medical supply and drug companies:
   a. should only be seen as a last resort
   b. should not be scheduled, but seen only if the provider has time
   c. can provide a valuable service and should be scheduled for short visits
   d. have complex information to communicate and need 1-hour appointments

4. The double-booking method:
   a. gives two or more patients the same appointment time
   b. keeps patients waiting unnecessarily
   c. is never the system of choice
   d. is purely for the provider's convenience

5. The stream method:
   a. gives patients appointments as they walk in
   b. schedules appointments at set times throughout the workday

   c. only works in sole-proprietor offices
   d. refers to streamlining paperwork for each appointment

6. Daily appointment sheets:
   a. indicate when providers and staff take lunch
   b. provide a permanent record for legal risk management and quality management
   c. are available only in computerized scheduling
   d. both a and b

7. Analyzing patient flow:
   a. can maximize a clinic's scheduling practice
   b. often reveals why patient flow is not efficient
   c. may indicate a change in pattern for patient scheduling
   d. all of the above

8. One principle above all else to be observed in scheduling is:
   a. always schedule in ink
   b. schedule for the patient's convenience
   c. be flexible and sensitive
   d. referral patients are first

9. If a patient must wait for an appointment:
   a. it is best to say nothing about the delay
   b. explain the delay and offer options when possible
   c. find ways to make the patient comfortable
   d. both b and c

10. Scheduling outpatient procedures is:
    a. best done by patients who understand their availability
    b. coordinated and completed by the clinic's staff
    c. an important way to enhance patient satisfaction
    d. both b and c

Critical Thinking

1. Why is there no one best system of scheduling?
2. Form small discussion groups and develop solutions to the following problems by (i) defining the problem, (ii) describing the appropriate steps if required, and (iii) developing a possible solution.
   a. Lenore McDonnell has called to cancel her appointment for the third consecutive time. (Background: Her last blood pressure reading in the office was 195/115, and there is a known history of stroke in her family.)
   b. Dr. Lewis is running an hour behind schedule. It is now 1:00 PM. He is now seeing a return patient. He has two new patients scheduled and has a surgery scheduled for 2:00 PM. (Background: Return patients require 30 minutes and new patients 60 minutes.)
   c. You are using the modified wave system. You have three appointments scheduled for 10:00 AM, one for 10:50 AM, and three for 11:00 AM. The office closes at 11:30 AM for lunch, so Dr. King can speak at a hospital luncheon. A patient calls and insists to be seen on an emergency basis. (Background: Dr. King's partner is unavailable to cover for her.)
   d. Two patients are scheduled to be seen at 11:30 AM. It is now 11:50 AM, and Dr. Whitney has indicated that he will not be through with his current patient for another 20 minutes. (Background: Both patients waiting to see Dr. Whitney have nonemergency problems.)
3. For the following situations, briefly explain which type of scheduling system you would choose and why.
   a. A four-provider practice has only two providers seeing patients at any one time. Three medical assistants share front- and back-office duties for all of the providers.
   b. An obstetrics practice specializes in problem pregnancies. There is one administrative and one clinical medical assistant.
4. With another person in your class, identify two or three public encounters where you feel ignored or rushed as a customer. How does it make you feel? What suggestions would you make to the business to change that feeling?

WEB ACTIVITIES

1. Go to http://www.physicianpractice.com for any information you can find regarding online patient scheduling. Identify advantages and disadvantages of online scheduling.
2. Go to your favorite search engine and key in "patient scheduling." Numerous sites will appear. Many offer a free download to examine components. What particular components seem most helpful? How many are separate software pieces as compared with software in connection with total practice management? How many require specialized training? Recommend two or three packages to examine more closely.

REFERENCE/BIBLIOGRAPHY

Lewis, M. A., & Tamparo, C. D. (2007). *Medical law, ethics, and bioethics for health professions* (6th ed.). Philadelphia: F.A. Davis.

Medical Records Management

KEY TERMS

Accession Record

Caption

Cross-Reference

Indexing

Key Unit

Out Guide

Problem-Oriented Medical Record (POMR)

Purging

SOAP/SOAPER

Source-Oriented Medical Record (SOMR)

Tickler File

Unit

OUTLINE

OBJECTIVES

The student should strive to meet the following performance objectives and demonstrate an understanding of the facts and principles presented in this chapter through written and oral communication.

1. Define the key terms as presented in the glossary.
2. List the purpose of medical records.

OBJECTIVES (continued)

3. Discuss the ownership of medical records.
4. State the reasons for accurately maintaining ambulatory care files.
5. Describe how and when information is released from the medical record.
6. State the pros and cons of the manual medical record and the electronic medical record.
7. Correct a medical record, manually and electronically.
8. Recall eight common supplies used in medical records management.
9. Identify the rules described under Basic Rules for Filing.
10. Describe the five steps commonly used when filing any documentation.
11. Name the two filing systems most often used in the ambulatory care setting.
12. State the purpose of cross-referencing.
13. Recall four common documents kept in the patient's medical record.
14. Discuss storage and purging of medical records.
15. Describe electronic medical records and their usefulness to the ambulatory care setting.
16. Discuss confidentiality and privacy as related to medical records.
17. Explain HIPAA security standards for electronic medical records.

Scenario

Consider a situation that might arise at the multiprovider Inner City Health Care. Patient Juanita Hansen was seen on Tuesday morning by Dr. Whitney for acute stomach pain. She was given a thorough examination and sent for appropriate testing that afternoon. She was then scheduled to return to Inner City on Friday to see Dr. Whitney.

After she was seen Tuesday morning, Juanita received an upper and lower gastrointestinal series; the results were then sent to Dr. Whitney's office. However, because Karen Ritter, RMA, the medical assistant, could not locate Juanita's chart to file the test results, she just set them aside. Friday arrived and Juanita came back to Inner City for her appointment, anxious to know the results of her tests. Dr. Whitney found Juanita's chart, which was inadvertently left on his stack of dictation, and realized the patient's test results had not been filed.

This left Dr. Whitney with an anxious patient. Karen Ritter is off today, so the provider checks with the other medical assistants on duty. They have no knowledge of the test results. Two acts—not replacing the file, and not promptly filing Juanita's test results—cause undue stress for the provider, medical assistants, and patient.

INTRODUCTION

Every medical facility generates a large amount of information. Business, insurance, personnel, and financial records must be maintained. Supplies and equipment records must be managed. Licensures and certifications must be current. Some records are kept for the life of the practice. The greatest bulk of information, however, comes from patient medical records. A vital function of any medical facility is the maintenance of patient records identifying the care given. Medi-cal assistants, both administrative and clinical, will spend a fair amount of time managing patients' records. Medical records potentially record all medical data about an individual from birth until death.

Even in medical facilities where patient records are managed electronically, there are ample paper records to be stored and retrieved manually. A number of functions essential to proper records management are discussed in this chapter. A clear understanding of the proper methods used to manage the records in a medical facility is an important and necessary skill for medical assistants.

Chapter 11 defined electronic medical records (EMRs) as those coming from a single medical practice, hospital, or pharmacy. When EMRs from multiple sources are combined into one database for a patient, the term electronic health record (EHR) is used (Figure 14-1).

THE PURPOSE OF MEDICAL RECORDS

The primary purposes of medical records in the ambulatory care setting are to:

1. Provide a base for managing patient care
2. Provide interoffice and intraoffice communication as necessary
3. Determine any patterns that surface to signal the provider of patient needs
4. Serve as a basis for legal information necessary to protect providers, staff, and patients
5. Provide clinical data for research

OWNERSHIP OF MEDICAL RECORDS

 State statutes have ruled that medical records are the property of those who create them. The information within the medical

Spotlight on Certification

RMA Content Outline
- Records management
- Protect, store, and retain medical records according to HIPAA regulations
- Release of protected health information in adherence to HIPAA regulations

CMA (AAMA) Content Outline
- Maintaining confidentiality
- Documentation/reporting
- Releasing medical information
- Records management

CMAS Content Outline
- Medical records management

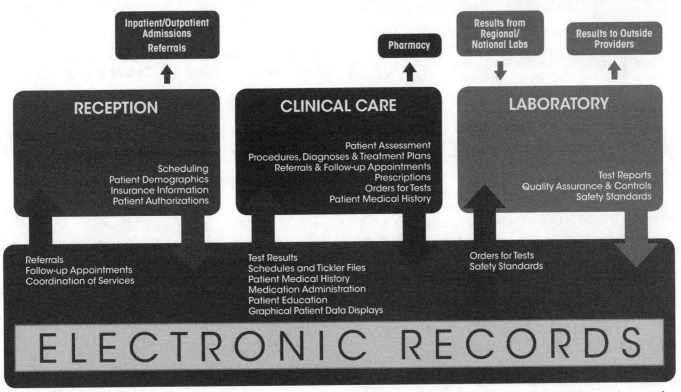

Figure 14-1   Medical records management relates to the laboratory, reception, and clinical care components in a total practice management system.

record, however, belongs to the patient, and that information is always to be protected with the utmost privacy and confidentiality. Patients can be allowed access to their medical records, ask for notes or information to be added to their files, and request certain information not be included in their files.

Providers who include their patients in their medical record keeping foster trust and respect with their patients. For example, a provider who enters patient data into the electronic patient record while sitting at a computer monitor in the examination room beside the patient has the opportunity to explain that the information is entered now so there is no room for error in reporting or in the provider not accurately recalling the patient information if entered at a later time. A patient who asks a primary care provider to put the pen aside while discussing possible depression symptoms is concerned about privacy, especially if the patient is the pediatrics department manager in the same large metropolitan medical center/hospital as the provider. The provider should realize that a discussion of how to keep this information confidential so that other employees are not aware of the patient's concern is in order.

AUTHORIZATION TO RELEASE INFORMATION

It is recommended that before any information is released from the medical record, even if it is subpoenaed, the patient be notified and written approval received. Medical facilities will have appropriate forms for such release of information. A sample release of information form is given in Chapter 23. The form should identify the reason for the release of information and what information is specifically requested. *Only* that information should be released. This does not include the release of information to a patient's chosen insurance carrier. A number of different methods exist to release that information. For some insurance carriers, the release is granted when the patient accepts the insurance coverage. For others, a yearly release form must be signed by the patient.

MANUAL OR ELECTRONIC MEDICAL RECORDS

Today's world has a mixture of manual, or paper, medical records and the electronic form of medical records. The world

is changing, however. In 2004, President George W. Bush announced his Health Information Technology Plan, which included the goal of ensuring that most Americans would have electronic health records by 2014. Planned projects include transmitting X-rays and laboratory results electronically to providers for immediate analysis and standardizing electronic prescriptions, hopefully decreasing errors in patient care. Medical clinics have scrambled to comply. Many have been successful; others have not and were hoping for federal funds to assist in the transition to electronic records. Although the complete transition to electronic health records by 2014 may not occur, it certainly will occur in the next decade. Frustrated by the slow response of medical providers, in 2007, lawmakers in the U.S. Senate and the House of Representatives introduced legislation to require electronic prescribing (e-prescribing) of medications for Medicare by 2011. EMRs are widely seen in large medical clinics, in metropolitan clinics with hospitals, and in hospital settings. Many ambulatory care settings, however, still have not fully computerized their medical records. This is in part because of providers' reluctance to let go of the paper medical record and the incredible expense of switching to computerized medical records. Also, there is the concern of how to transfer the current paper record to the computer record. Consider the following advantages and disadvantages of both records:

MANUAL MEDICAL RECORD

Advantages	Disadvantages
• Currently established and understood	• Can be used by only one person at a time
• Easier to protect confidentiality	• Easily misplaced or misfiled
• No worry of computer malfunction	• Equipment and storage space required
	• More susceptible to error

ELECTRONIC MEDICAL RECORD

Advantages	Disadvantages
• Multiple users are possible	• Needs protection to prevent loss of data
• Not easily misplaced or misfiled	• Expensive to establish and maintain
• Errors less likely	• May require on-site assistance
• Patterns and data more easily accessed	• Can require up to 12 weeks for staff to prove productive
• Quickly available in emergencies	

- Office storage space
  not required
- Legible, organized
  patient documentation
- Improved medication
  management
- Improved quality of care

Use of EMRs in ambulatory care is increasing in popularity every year. However, *Medical Economics* reported in a December 2006 survey that 65% of providers still had not adopted an EMR system. Solo practitioners are least likely to use EMRs; EMRs grow at faster rates in larger, multi-provider clinics. It is interesting to note that most patients believe they have greater access to and more control over their medical records when they are in electronic form and believe their primary care providers would be able to give more comprehensive patient care with EMRs. The medical record system must be one that fits the facility and satisfies the needs of the providers. Usually, medical record systems are adapted for a particular facility using certain common components. Whatever system is used, the management of the medical records must provide easy retrieval of information. All documentation must be complete and correct. Wording must be easily understood and grammatically correct. How corrections are made in the chart, how documents are removed or added to the chart, and the chart format must be predetermined and understood by all users of the information.

THE IMPORTANCE OF ACCURATE MEDICAL RECORDS

Accurate medical records are essential to patient care in any health care setting. One incorrect digit in a patient's Social Security number causes reimbursement problems. An incorrect address or telephone number or a misspelling of a name makes it difficult to contact patients about test results and prescription refills. Medical errors are even more disastrous and can cause serious medical problems for patients. Patient files are critical to the facility's smooth functioning and are important when referring the patient to outside specialists with whom the facility may need to coordinate care. Each treating primary care provider must be aware of tests, procedures, and diagnoses. Maintaining a conscientious record of patient care is also absolutely essential in controlling the costs of medical care.

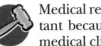 Medical records management is also important because of the legal issues that every medical clinic and health care professional must face today. The standard in court is that if there is no record of any piece of information related to a patient and that patient's care and treatment, then it did not happen. The question to ask yourself about any piece of information is: "Does this relate to the patient's care, and should it be in the chart?" To be prepared in the event of medical litigation, you must document all medical treatment. No matter how competently a provider has performed treatment, if a written record cannot prove how and what was done, there is no basis for a defense in a court of law.

Creating Paper and Electronic Charts

The patient's medical chart is prepared on or before the day of the patient's first visit in the medical facility. Paper medical records require the assembly of appropriate file folders, divider pages labeled with identifying tabs, and a number of essential forms to be completed by the patient. Included forms provide demographic information, social and family medical history, previous surgeries, HIPAA guidelines, and release of information details. Often, paper charts include adhesive twin prong fasteners to ensure that sheets of paper are securely held within the chart. Electronic patient medical charts are prepared in much the same manner with the exception being that all information is stored electronically. Patient information that is collected via the paper route will have to be scanned and entered into the record. The EMR will provide an orderly arrangement of patient information according to the particular software design or a predetermined plan selected by the providers and their staff. Procedures 14-1 and 14-2 allow creation of both a paper and an electronic chart.

Correcting Medical Records

The medical record must be readable and accurate; however, errors do occur and may not be discovered immediately. Any corrections necessary to a paper medical record should be corrected using the following method: draw a single line using a red ink pen through the error, make the correction, write "Corr." or "Correction" above the area corrected, and indicate your initials and the current date. The red line through the information indicates the "error" portion of the report. The words "Corr." or "Correction" by the correction indicates the change. The date and initials identify when the correction was made and by whom. Obliterations should never occur. When the medical record becomes the center of attention in malpractice litigation, forensic experts will be able to tell if a record has been tampered with or if information or pages have been added later. When not properly done, altered records become a detriment to any provider's defense in court (see Procedure 14-3).

Errors discovered immediately after the fact in an electronic medical record are corrected differently. Although it could be easy to do so, the error is *not corrected* by simple word processing. In a truly paperless clinic office, a notation is entered at the place of the error, a line is drawn through the error (using the tracking device in the word processing software), and the correction is made immediately after the information lined out. "Corr." or "Correction" is indicated and your initials and the date added. The finished product will look similar to a correction in a paper medical chart (see Procedure 14-4). To ensure accuracy and prevent tampering with the information in a patient's record, EMR software locks out any additions to a chart entry after a specific period of time. After the lockout has occurred and a correction is necessary, a new entry is created that identifies the error and the correction to be made. It is dated, signed, and inserted in the document. It will be clear to the reader the error that occurred, the correction made, who made the correction, and when.

If any correction is necessary of any information after either a paper chart or an electronic chart has been sent to another provider or facility, make a copy of the corrected information and send it to the provider or facility as quickly as possible.

TYPES OF MEDICAL RECORDS

Whether patient charts are kept manually or electronically, there are common threads that run throughout medical records. How material is stored within records is important. The choice of method must be in accordance with how the information needs to be accessed and used for each individual clinic. No one method is best. In the examples that follow, arrangement of materials is also discussed.

Problem-Oriented Medical Record

The **problem-oriented medical record (POMR)** places in a prominent location vital identification data, immunizations, allergies, medications, and problems. The problems are identified by a number that corresponds to the charting relevant to that problem number, that is, bronchitis #1, broken wrist #2, and so forth. If the patient returns in 9 months with recurring bronchitis, the same number (#1) is used.

The patient chart is then further built by adding a numbered and titled section for each problem the patient experiences, for example, bronchitis #1, broken wrist #2.

Each problem is then followed with the **SOAP** approach for all progress notes:

S Subjective impressions

O Objective clinical evidence

A Assessment or diagnosis

P Plans for further studies, treatment, or management

Some medical facilities have added two additional letters to the SOAP approach, creating **SOAPER**. This additional charting tool can be especially useful in large teaching hospitals with medical clinics:

E Education for patient

R Response of patient to education and care given

This process makes the chart easier to review and helps in follow-up of all the patient's medical needs. The SOAP/SOAPER approach also allows medical personnel to be aware of the patient's current medications. Starting and resolution dates for each problem also are noted on the tracking page.

Internists, family practitioners, and pediatricians use the POMR system more commonly than do specialists because they see their patients for a variety of problems over a long span of time. It is commonly used in manual medical records as well as EMRs.

A number of medical supply companies produce various formats for POMR manual charts. There are flip-up folder styles; book-style folders made of 125-1b manila or white stock with twin prong fasteners are the most popular. Divider pages may come with tabs that are preprinted to specific needs or have adhesive labels that can be printed on a printer exactly as you want them. Sometimes, the inside front and back covers are printed with information to be filled in. These areas are often used to provide essential personal information such as name, address, telephone numbers, insurance information, and responsible party. Over a period of time, however, when the information changes, entries on the inside cover are less desirable. A patient demographic form (see Chapter 23) can be attached to the inside cover. It can be updated annually and changed easily. In a prominent place, usually on the inside front cover, is the word **"ALLERGIES"** in big letters (often preprinted in red). Any allergies that patients have are listed here. Also prominently displayed should be any forms the patient has signed granting release of information, as well as any forms signed to comply with HIPAA regulations.

The problem list may be entered on a divider flap or on specially printed paper. Other dividers may be used for laboratory reports, progress notes, history and physicals, hospital admissions, and medications. Depending on the practice and the wishes of the provider, tab dividers are available for consultations, correspondence, insurance data, hospital notes, pathology reports, and electrocardiogram reports. The problem list is most likely the first divider used, followed by laboratory reports and progress notes, usually in the SOAP/SOAPER format.

SOAP/SOAPER is easily adapted to the EMR. There are a number of methods of indicating SOAP/SOAPER in the EMR. For a brief look at different models, use a computer search engine to key in "SOAP charting in EMRs." You will be able to compare a number of examples.

Source-Oriented Medical Record

The manual **source-oriented medical record (SOMR)** groups information according to its source; for example, from laboratories, examinations, provider notes, consulting providers, and other sources. Facilities use this method because it makes different types of information quickly accessible. A fastener folder is used that contains several partitions with their own fasteners. This allows for a separate section for laboratory reports, pathology, progress notes, physical examinations, and correspondence to be filed chronologically within each section. In the SOMR system, many providers use the SOAP/SOAPER method to record their chart notes.

The organization of the SOMR is quite similar to that of the POMR chart with the one exception that the SOMR does not have the problem list. Also, the SOMR may continually add sheets of identifying information with appropriate sections in the chart rather than transferring any data. Many EMR software packages use either the POMR or the SOMR format and are easily adapted to a particular provider's practice.

Strict Chronological Arrangement

Using strict chronology, data are filed strictly with the most recently charted materials to the top of the folder. For instance, a patient is treated from 2004 to the present. To locate information recorded in 2006, it is necessary to flip through the chart until the material for the year 2006 is located. This method makes it difficult for a provider or medical assistant to quickly assess a patient's clinical picture. This type of arrangement may seem confusing, but it may fit a specialty office such as a dietitian, radiologist, or physical therapist where patients are usually seen on a short-term basis.

EQUIPMENT AND SUPPLIES

Three primary types of file cabinets are used in medical clinics where manual files are stored: vertical, lateral, and movable.

Vertical Files

Vertical files are cabinets that have pullout drawers where files are stored (Figure 14-2). Files are retrieved by lifting the appropriate file up and out. These are likely used for business records and document, and should include a locking device.

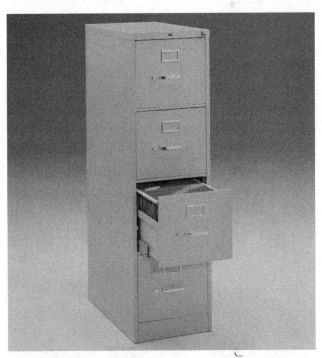

Figure 14-2   Vertical file cabinet. (Courtesy HON Company.)

The best vertical files have a center trough in the bottom of each drawer with a rod running through for holding divider guides. The rod and guides help keep file folders from slipping down underneath other file folders and getting misplaced or lost.

Open-Shelf Lateral Files

Open-shelf lateral file cabinets make quick retrieval of files possible (Figure 14-3). The records are retrieved by pulling them out laterally from the shelf. They are used most often with color-coded filing systems where visual inspection makes it possible to ensure files are kept in the proper order. Open-shelf lateral files are the most popular manual patient record system. It is necessary to be able to close and lock the open-shelf lateral files to protect confidentiality.

Movable File Units

Movable file units allow easy access to large record systems and require less space than vertical or lateral files. These units may be electrically powered to move on floor tracks or may be physically moved with an easy-to-turn handle mechanism. The movable shelving unit is electrically powered to open aisles for accessing files or to close aisles when those files do not need to be accessed. There are also movable file storage units that will automatically travel on a computer-controlled carousel track, moving files around until the required section reaches the operator.

File Folders

File folders are designed for different types of labels. Extending along the top edge (the edge that will be visible when filing) are tabs that are cut in varying sizes and positions to allow for different methods of labeling. Figure 14-4 shows the types of cuts, or tabs, found on file folders. File folders should be constructed of good-quality card stock. If they are too light in weight, they will soon be bent, torn, and battered from use. They need to be sturdy enough for years of use.

Identification Labels

A variety of labels are used to display the information required to select the correct name or number designation for a particular file. The identification label is adhered either along the top of the file folder (top tab) in vertical file cabinets or along the side of the file folder (side tab) in lateral file cabinets.

Guides and Positions

Guides are used to separate file folders. Guides are somewhat larger than file folders and are of heavier stock. Guides are described by the position of the tab, designated according to its location. For instance, a tab located at the far left would be in the first position, the next one to the right would be in the second position, and so forth. If using third-cut file folders, there are three positions of guides; if using fifth-cut file folders, there are five positions. Guides are used in vertical and lateral systems.

Captions. **Captions** are used to identify major sections of file folders by more manageable subunits (AA–AC, A, B, Office Supplies). Captions are marked on the tabs of the guides (Figure 14-5).

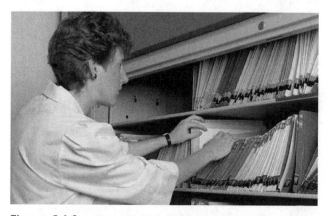

Figure 14-3   Open-shelf lateral file cabinet.

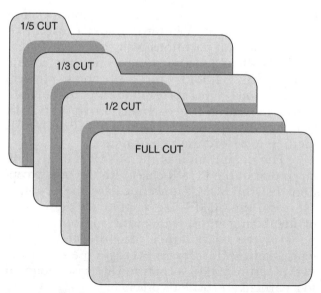

Figure 14-4   Types of cuts, or tabs, on file folders.

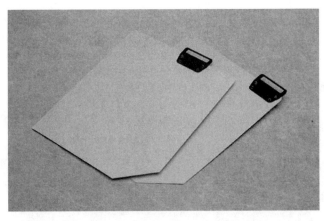

Figure 14-5   Guides separating file folders into subsections. Captions such as A, B, C (single captions) or Ab–Be, Co–Dy (double captions) are placed on the tabs of the guides to identify the sections.

These are denoted as single caption and double caption:

- *Single captions* contain just one letter, number, or unit:

  ○ A, B, C, D

- *Double captions* contain a double notation to denote a range of files:

  ○ Ab–Be, Co–Dy, Ho–Le

Out Guides

Out guides or out sheets are devices to help in tracking charts. An out guide is a piece of cardstock or plastic/paper sheet kept in place of the patient chart when charts are removed from the filing storage (Figure 14-6).

BASIC RULES FOR FILING

Regardless of the type of filing system used, alphabetizing is the key to organizing all files and charts. It is necessary to know more than just the alphabetic order of the letters *A* to *Z*. Thus, certain indexing rules have been developed by the Association of Medical Records Administrators (AMRA) to facilitate the alphabetic process in maintaining files in the medical office.

Indexing Units

There must be an organized method of identifying and separating items to be filed into small subunits. This is accomplished with the use of **indexing** units. A unit identifies each part of a name. In this process, each **unit** is identified according to unit 1 (the **key unit**), unit 2, unit 3, and so forth, with each segment of the filing label identified. This process can be applied to individual names, organizations, or clinics. Accepted filing rules describe how to assign unit numbers to each element.

Example.   Annette Barbara Samuels

Unit 1	Samuels
Unit 2	Annette
Unit 3	Barbara

 When working in a medical setting with patient charts, the patient's legal name is always used for the chart rather than a nickname or abbreviation. If the clinic has a practice of calling patients by preferred names, a note of name preferences and nicknames may be noted

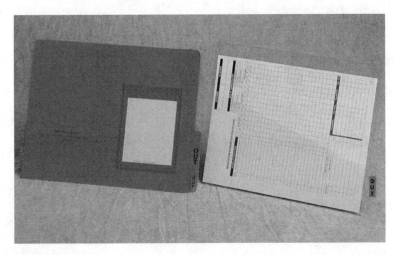

Figure 14-6   An out guide indicating the name of the person who has possession of the file should always be put in place of a patient's record when it is removed from the file.

on the chart. However, the filing label should use the proper name.

Example. The following items to be filed would be assigned units as illustrated:

	Units Assigned		
	1	**2**	**3**
Cole Blanche Little	Little	Cole	Blanche
Wayne Lee Elder	Elder	Wayne	Lee
Kelso Medical Supply	Kelso	Medical	Supply

Filing Patient Charts

Rule 1. The names of individuals are assigned indexing units, respectively: last name (surname), first name, middle, and succeeding names.

	Units Assigned		
	1	**2**	**3**
Jaime Renae Carrera	Carrera	Jaime	Renae
Lee Allen Au	Au	Lee	Allen
Bill Hugo Schwartz	Schwartz	Bill	Hugo

Rule 2. Names that include a single letter are indexed as the legal name and are placed before full names beginning with the same letter. "Nothing comes before something."

	Units Assigned		
	1	**2**	**3**
J. Larson	Larson	J	—
James R. Larson	Larson	James	R

Rule 3. Foreign language prefixes are indexed as one unit with the unit that follows. Spacing, punctuation, and capitalization are ignored. Such prefixes include *d, da, de, de la, del, des, di, du, el, fitz, l, la, las, le, les, lu, m, mac, mc, o, saint, sainte, san, santa, sao, st, te, ten, ter, van, van de, van der,* and *von der* (*st, sainte,* and *saint* are indexed as written).

	Units Assigned		
	1	**2**	**3**
Gerald Steven St. Simon	Stsimon	Gerald	Steven
Carol Louise del Rio	Delrio	Carol	Louise

Rule 4. When titles are used, they are considered as separate indexing units. If the title appears with first and last names, the title is considered to be the last indexing unit. When dealing with patient charts, the first name always accompanies the title and last name.

	Units Assigned			
	1	**2**	**3**	**4**
Dr. Marlene Elaine Smith	Smith	Marlene	Elaine	Dr
Prof. Marcia Tai Lewis	Lewis	Marcia	Tai	Prof

Rule 5. Names that are hyphenated are considered as one unit.

	Units Assigned		
	1	**2**	**3**
Adele Marie Johnson-Smith	Johnsonsmith	Adele	Marie
Ray Steven Reynolds-Martin	Reynoldsmartin	Ray	Steven

Rule 6. When indexing names of married women, the name is indexed by the legal name. Remember that patient charts are legal documents, making this practice necessary (use cross-referencing as necessary).

	Units Assigned			
	1	**2**	**3**	**4**
Amy Sue Sung (Mrs. John)	Sung	Amy	Sue	Mrs John
Tami Jo Strizver (Mrs. Todd)	Strizver	Tami	Jo	Mrs Todd

Rule 7. Seniority and professional or academic degrees are the last indexing unit and are used only to distinguish identical names.

	Units Assigned			
	1	**2**	**3**	**4**
James Edward Brown, Jr.	Brown	James	Edward	Jr
James Edward Brown, Sr.	Brown	James	Edward	Sr

Rule 8. Mac and Mc are filed in their regular place alphabetically. Some clinics will provide a special guide for both Mac and Mc for ease in filing.

Maasch
Mabbott
MacDonald
Mazziotti
McAffe

Rule 9. Numeric units are broken down such that numeric seniority terms are filed before alphabetic terms.

	Edward Lee Kletka, IV
BEFORE	Edward Lee Kletka, Jr.
	George Lee Curtis, II
BEFORE	George Lee Curtis, Sr.

Filing Identical Names

When names are identical, the address may be used to order files. The address is indexed by:

First:	City
SECOND	STATE
Third	Street Name
Fourth:.............	**Address #**

Therefore, the following Acme Drug Supply files would be arranged from first to last as follows:

1. Acme Drug Supply, **839** *Kentucky Boulevard,* <u>Crawford</u>, MISSOURI
2. Acme Drug Supply, **683** *Wildflower Avenue,* <u>Fairbanks</u>, ALASKA
3. Acme Drug Supply, **1539** *Wildflower Avenue,* <u>Fairbanks</u>, ALASKA
4. Acme Drug Supply, **742** *Terminal Street West,* <u>Fairbanks</u>, ARIZONA
5. Acme Drug Supply, **731** *Terminal Street East,* <u>New York</u>, NEW YORK

Although this is the official indexing rule, most medical facilities prefer alternative methods for filing identical charts. The primary consideration here is that patient addresses often change frequently. Therefore, preferred methods include date of birth or Social Security number.

STEPS FOR FILING MEDICAL DOCUMENTATION IN PATIENT FILES

Before a discussion of the common filing systems, it is helpful to review procedural steps that accurately and efficiently process data sheets, laboratory requests, dictation, and so forth from the time they are generated to the time the file is returned to the medical records section. Efficiently following these steps will save considerable time in the ambulatory care setting.

Inspect

Carefully inspect the report to identify the patient, subject, or file to whom the information belongs. Remove clips and staples. Make certain the information is complete.

Index

Use the indexing process to determine how the chart would be located, properly identifying indexing units and their order.

Code

Coding in medical records is the process of marking data to indicate how information is to be filed. If using a system other than a strict alphabetic system, determine the proper coding for the chart so it can be retrieved. Otherwise, identify the indexed units by underlining or highlighting. This makes refiling more effective and assures that the item will always be filed in the same place. If a cross-reference is required, identify the cross-reference by double underlining and placing an *X* nearby. This chapter includes detailed information on coding and cross-referencing.

Sort

If there are a number of reports/documents to be filed, sort them into units according to the captions on the charts. This will eliminate wasted time in working back and forth through the alphabet or numbers. Figure 14-7 shows a medical assistant using a desk sorter to put files and reports in alphabetic order.

File

The papers are placed in the proper charts and the charts returned to their proper place in the medical records section. Be alert to the labels and refile any information or charts that have been misfiled.

FILING TECHNIQUES AND COMMON FILING SYSTEMS

Three major filing systems are commonly used in the ambulatory care setting: alphabetic, numeric, and subject. The alphabet is intrinsic to all methods,

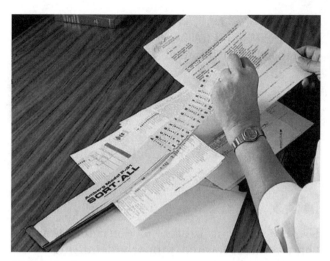

Figure 14-7   Medical assistant using a desk sorter to alphabetize reports to make filing easier.

and the basic rules for filing, covered previously, are used in all systems.

Color coding is used a high percentage of the time in all three systems to minimize filing errors. Another system, geographic, is seldom used in the ambulatory care setting unless there are multiple clinics. Even then, a form of color coding may be used.

Color Coding

Color coding is a technique often used in the three major filing systems. Numerous color-coding systems are available. Patient charts most often use an alphabetic system of color coding, although color coding can be used in numeric filing as well. Smead Manufacturing, Kardex, Bibbero, and American Corporate Services are companies widely known in medical and dental fields for their color systems and records management systems. Color coding may seem complicated at first, but once medical assistants understand the principles behind it and practice its application a number of times, the task becomes much easier, and there is immediate recognition if a chart is misfiled.

Color coding makes retrieval of files more efficient with the use of visible color differences that facilitate easier maintenance of the files. Color-coding filing systems also use an alphabetic system; after they are coded by color, that designation is used to order the files alphabetically.

Tab-Alpha System. The various forms of the Tab-Alpha system are designed primarily for filing systems in small offices that use vertical files where all individual charts are clearly visible in one unit.

Each alphabetic letter is assigned a different color. Each folder has a color-coded label. Only full-cut folders are used:

- Colored labels are applied over the edge of the full cut for the first two letters of the key indexing unit (Winston, Paul Lewis: WI).
- A third white label is placed over the tab edge, which contains all of the indexing units (Winston, Paul Lewis).
- In addition, some offices use a color-coded label to indicate the last year the patient was seen. This makes an efficient method for easily identifying active and inactive files.
- Any additional labels (e.g., allergies, last year seen, or industrial claim) are attached to the chart according to the office procedure.

Alpha-Z System. Forms of the Alpha-Z system are designed for use with either open lateral files or vertical drawer files (Figure 14-8A). Alphabetic letters are used as the primary guides. Breakdowns of alphabetic combinations are added as determined by the needs of a particular facility.

A combination of 13 colors is used in the Alpha-Z system with white letters on a solid colored background for the first half of the alphabet and white letters on a colored background with white stripes for the second half of the alphabet (Figure 14-8B).

The 13 colors used are shown in Table 14-1. Folders have three labels:

- The first label contains the typed name, a color block, and the letter of the alphabet for the first letter of the first indexing unit:

  Winston, Lewis Paul YELLOW "W"

- The second and third labels are color-coded to correspond to the second and third letters of the first unit:

  "I" on pink background and "N" on red-striped background

Customized Color-Coding Systems. Many offices use color systems to meet specific needs.

Colored File Folders by First Name. One method color codes the first letter of the first name. The folders then are filed alphabetically by last name.

Example.   A is assigned red folders; M is assigned green folders; S is assigned blue folders

Annette Samuels	Red Folder
Michael Taylor	Green Folder
Susan Boyer	Blue Folder

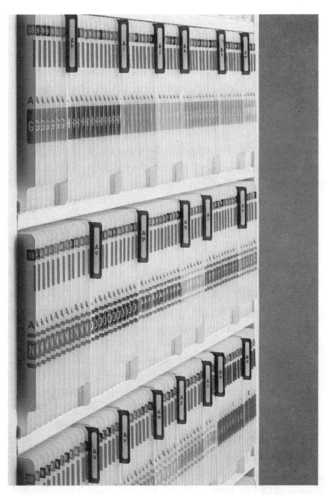

Figure 14-8A   Color-coding filing system uses open-lateral shelving unit with color-coded files. (Courtesy Smead Manufacturing Company.)

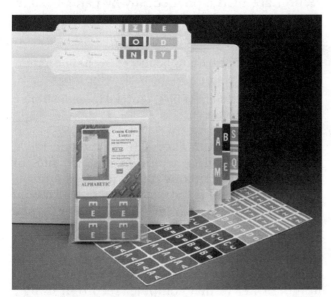

Figure 14-8B   Alpha-Z color-coded labels shown on top- and side-cut files. (Courtesy Smead Manufacturing Company.)

Table 14-1   Thirteen Colors Are Used in the Alpha-Z System

White Letter Colored Background	White Letter Striped Colored Background	Color
A	N	Red
B	O	Dark Blue
C	P	Dark Green
D	Q	Light Blue
E	R	Purple
F	S	Orange
G	T	Gray
H	U	Dark Brown
I	V	Pink
J	W	Yellow
K	X	Light Brown
L	Y	Lavender
M	Z	Light Green

Many small medical offices use this system and find it quite effective. In the multiprovider urgent care center, this would be quite time-consuming when locating files for patients of all providers.

Colored File Folders by Last Name. Another method using this system assigns colored folders according to the first letter of the last name. The folders are then filed alphabetically.

Example.   *S* is assigned pink folders; *B* is assigned gray folders.

Bill Schwartz	Pink Folder
Corey Boyer	Gray Folder

This system makes it easy to spot folders that have been misfiled under an incorrect first letter, but it does not break it down further for misfilings within the first-letter guides.

Color-Coded Numbers. The color-coded number system is used in a numeric filing system and operates in the same way as alphabetic systems. Numbers from 0 to 9 are color coded. The appropriate colored numbers are then placed on the tabs of the patient's folder.

Alphabetic Filing

Strict alphabetic filing is one of the simplest filing methods, as files are strictly maintained by assigning a label to each file. The first letter of that label (e.g., Jones, Invoices, or Pharmacies) is then used to alphabetize the files from A to Z. When a limited number of files is accessed, this is an acceptable method of maintaining records. Also note that every filing system will utilize the alphabet somewhere. Procedure 14-5 provides steps for manual filing with an alphabetic system.

Numeric Filing

Numeric filing is organized by number rather than by letter. A key benefit of numeric filing is that it preserves patient confidentiality because the individual's name is not obviously apparent on the file folder. The numeric filing systems most likely used in medical facilities are straight numeric and terminal digit.

Straight Numeric.

Straight numeric filing places charts in exact chronological order according to assigned number. For example, records numbered 45023, 45024, and 45025 will be in consecutive order on a shelf. This is an easy system to learn and use; however, there are some disadvantages. The greater number of digits to recall, the greater the chance for error. Numbers transposition is common. Chart number 45024 can be misfiled as chart number 54024. The use of color with straight numeric can decrease misfiling.

Terminal Digit.

In terminal digit filing, a six-digit number is most often used with a hyphen dividing three parts of two digits, for example, 85-32-07 and 86-32-07. Within these numbers, the primary units are the last two numbers; the middle digits are the secondary units; the first two numbers are the third and final units considered. In a terminal digit file, there are 100 primary sections from 00 to 99 to be considered. The medical assistant will consider the primary section first, match the record with the same group to the secondary set of digits next, and then file in numerical order by the third unit.

The advantage to this system is that files and numbers are equally distributed. Only every 100th new medical record will be filed in the same primary section. Filing using the straight numerical order of the first two numbers is simple to learn.

Middle Digit.

In middle digit systems, the staff still files according to pairs of digits, but the pairs of digits are in different positions. The middle pair of digits is primary, the pair of digits to the left is secondary, and the pair of digits on the right is third.

The terminal digit and middle digit systems are most likely seen in hospitals and large multi-provider clinics.

Components of Numeric Filing.

Four essential components are used with a numeric system, whether it is a manual or computerized system.

Serially Numbered Dividers with Guides. Consecutive numeric guides (5, 10, etc.; 50, 100, etc.) separate the individual file folders into smaller groups of files.

Miscellaneous (General) Numeric File Section. This is reserved for records that have not been assigned numbers. Patients should automatically be assigned a number on the first visit. However, on occasion patients cannot be assigned a number initially. The miscellaneous section is generally in front of all the numeric folders for ease of locating items. Files in the miscellaneous section are filed alphabetically by patient name. This is the best place for the miscellaneous file(s) for two reasons:

1. They do not have to be moved each time a numbered file is added to the back of the order.

2. In a large system of files, retrieval from the front is quick and easy.

Alphabetic Card File. This alphabetic file is necessary as a source to locate numeric files or records. A card contains name, address, and file number (or an *M* if located in the miscellaneous section); any **cross-reference** is here rather than in the numeric files.

The alphabetic card file in a manual system would be equivalent to the computerized record of the patient and whatever number is assigned to him or her in that computer record. If using a computerized system, the program generally will automatically cross-reference the number with the

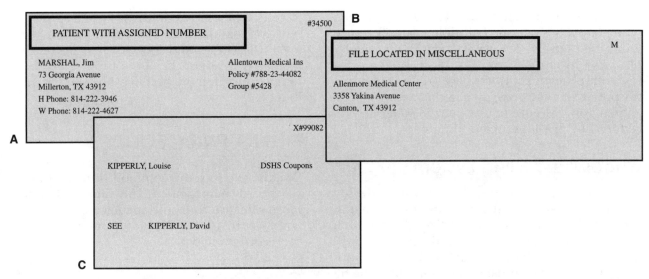

Figure 14-9   Card files used in numeric filing system: (A) Patient with an assigned number. (B) Patient record has not had a number assigned and is located in miscellaneous section. (C) Cross-reference card.

alphabetic list that was generated with the initial entry. If laboratory data come into the office on Leo M. McKay, there will need to be a method to know where to locate his chart to file the report, that is, the alphabetic listing.

With a manual system, the alphabetic file is kept in an index card fashion. This file will contain the complete name and address (and any other information denoted by the office policy, e.g., insurance and emergency numbers).

Noted with this information there needs to be either an *M* for miscellaneous (for those items not assigned a number) or an assigned number (Figure 14-9A and B).

If a cross-reference is required, prepare a cross-reference card and include an *X* next to the file number (or *M*) to indicate this is the cross-reference card and not the primary location (Figure 14-9C).

Accession Record. The **accession record** is a journal (or computer listing) where numbers are preassigned. Each new item to be assigned is written on the line next to the number (Figure 14-10). Each new entry for which a chart will be created must be assigned a number. A computerized system would have an accession record in its memory bank. Procedure 14-6 provides numeric filing steps.

Subject Filing

There are many reasons why material would be filed using a system of subjects in a medical clinic. If providers are doing research, they might wish to index

#	File Name
800	CARRERA, Jaime
801	AU, Rhoda
802	TREMONT Drug Supply
803	
804	
805	
806	
807	

ACCESSION LOGBOOK

Figure 14-10   Accession record or log sequentially lists predetermined numbers to be used to assign to numeric records. The next number available in this system is 803.

research according to diseases. Subject files are convenient for locating frequently used services or for filing reference materials for patient needs. Insurance company information also might be filed by subject.

When using a subject filing system, scan the material to determine the subject or theme. As with color-coding and numeric filing, an alphabetic file is necessary. This can be either a subject list or an index card file listing the subjects. Also, as with numeric filing, all cross-reference cards are done only with alphabetic file listings.

Within the folders, material can be arranged either alphabetically or chronologically; keep in mind the objective for maintaining the particular files. For instance, if using subject indexing for research projects providers have conducted, identify the subject category; then in the material, code an item for reference to that specific material. Procedure 14-7 provides subject filing steps.

Choosing a Filing System

To select a filing system, each facility must decide what the primary objectives are with respect to storage of patient files, business records, and research files. How will the charts be used primarily? Will information need to be tracked by others not familiar with the records? Often more than one filing system will be used, such as alphabetic filing for patient charts, a numeric system for research subjects, and a subject system for miscellaneous correspondence.

The number of documents to be filed is one primary determinant in selecting an alphabetic or numeric system. Alphabetic filing is quite manageable for many clinics. However, when the number of patients is quite large, a numeric system becomes practical because an infinite set of numbers is available. With the numeric system, there is only one of each assigned designation. However, with an alphabetic system, there are a number of common names (e.g., Smith, Jones, Adams, and Johnson) that can have many multiples requiring additional sorting to narrow the search for the correct chart. In addition, with multiple charts of the same last name, the chances for misfiling increases.

Confidentiality is another reason to select a numeric filing system. Confidentiality of charts is maintained more easily with numeric files because no name is visible on the outside of the chart. In addition, numerically referenced records can be used in research activities where random sampling and anonymity are required.

To make the medical facility HIPAA compliant when traditional paper-based or manual charts are used, you need to ensure that no patient-identifiable information is located on the outside of the chart. This includes the patient address or any other information that might be used to determine the identity of the patient, including Social Security number, birth date, or phone number. Any information that reveals a health condition or payment status also must be removed from the outside of the chart.

Recall earlier the example of locked storage cabinets for manual files. Note that all file cabinets are to be closed and locked when no one is immediately present in the office; that includes lunch time when the staff may be eating in the staff lounge.

FILING PROCEDURES

By adhering to some common principles in medical records management, any filing system will be more effective and will enable the medical assistant to store, identify, retrieve, and maintain medical records efficiently.

Cross-Referencing

In running an efficient medical facility, files must be stored for quick and accurate retrieval. If there is any doubt as to where a particular file would be located, cross-reference the file. Many offices fail to take the extra time it requires to do this. However, with the growing number of foreign names, hyphenated names, and stepfamilies, it is well worth the effort. When the office receives a letter and a release of information form inquiring about medical facts on Mr. David Kipperly's four stepchildren who were involved in an accident, how will these files be located? If they are cross-referenced under the stepfather's name, this will be a relatively easy procedure. However, if the medical assistant is unfamiliar with the family (as in a larger urgent care center with a large volume of patients), this may become a time-consuming job. Another scenario might involve insurance information on Janet Morgan. A search of the records does not produce a file for any Janet Morgan. The reason for this is that Janet Morgan is married, and her chart has been filed under Janet Hill-Morgan. Time spent cross-referencing contributes to a more efficient method of retrieving information.

A cross-referencing system does not need to be elaborate. It is quite sufficient to use inserts with labels attached that are inserted in the appropriate place in the storage units. For instance, a plain piece of cardstock, rather than a file or chart, could be inserted for "Janet Morgan." This insert would simply have a label directing one to the location of the primary file.

The proper steps for cross-referencing, together with several examples where cross-referencing might be used, are discussed in the next section.

Steps for Cross-Referencing.

1. Identify the primary filing label.

2. Make a proper file to be used as the primary location for all medical records.

3. Identify one (or more) alternatives where one might find the file.

4. For the alternative filings, make a cross-reference sheet, card, or dummy chart that lists the primary reference and refers back to the location of the primary file.

Example. The patient, Jaime Renae Carrera, has made it known to the office that most of his information received will refer to the name Renny Carrera, as this is his preference. The SEE reference will identify where the primary file is located.

PRIMARY FILE:	Carrera, Jaime Renae
X-REFERENCE FILE:	Carrera, Renny
	SEE Carrera, Jaime Renae

Rule 1.   Married Individuals. When taking a spouse's name, the primary file would be the patient's legal name with the cross-reference listed under the spouse's.

PRIMARY FILE:	Au, Rhoda A. (Mrs.)
	Lee Au
X-REFERENCE FILE:	Au, Mrs. Lee
	SEE Au, Rhoda A. (Mrs.)

Rule 2.   Foreign Names. The primary file would be located under the patient's legal name. It is important, therefore, that you identify the first, middle, and surname (last name) when the patient comes for the first visit. Unless people are familiar with a particular group of names, the first, middle, and surnames are often confused with one another. Again, your experience will teach you which cross-references should be set up.

PRIMARY FILE:	Sing, Yange Teah
X-REFERENCE FILE:	Yange, Sing Teah
	SEE Sing, Yange Teah
X-REFERENCE FILE:	Teah, Yange Sing
	SEE Sing, Yange Teah

Rule 3.   Hyphenated Names. With the proliferation of hyphenated names, it is common for materials to be listed under different combinations of the hyphenated name. For instance, a married woman may have records under her maiden name, her husband's surname, and her hyphenated name. Therefore, it is necessary to make two cross-references.

PRIMARY FILE:	Krenshaw-Skiple, Rose Marie
X-REFERENCE FILE:	Skiple, Rose Marie
	SEE Krenshaw-Skiple, Rose Marie
X-REFERENCE FILE:	Krenshaw, Rose Marie
	SEE Krenshaw-Skiple, Rose Marie

Rule 4.   Multiple Listings. A great deal of correspondence is received with multiple listings of names. At times, the medical office may receive correspondence from only one of the involved parties. Rather than keep a separate file for each, maintain a primary file as listed on the letter and then cross-reference file(s) for the individual names.

PRIMARY FILE:	Olsen, Piper, and Dillard Associates
X-REFERENCE FILE:	Piper, Richard C., M.D.
	SEE Olsen, Piper, and Dillard Associates
X-REFERENCE FILE:	Olsen, Francis William, M.D.
	SEE Olsen, Piper, and Dillard Associates
X-REFERENCE FILE:	Dillard, Thomas E., M.D.
	SEE Olsen, Piper, and Dillard Associates

Tickler Files

Sticky notes and writing notes on the calendar are popular methods of reminding office personnel to follow up with some required action. However, a well-organized, efficient office will maintain what is known as a **tickler file,** a method that serves as a reminder that some action needs to be taken at a date in the future.

 Some systems have a calendar that pops up to allow reminders to be placed on the calendar. The computer system reminds you of the note when that particular day arrives. Some EMR systems have built-in reminders that automatically give a reminder for such things as annual physical examinations, monthly blood pressure checks, medication checks, and anything else that might be beneficial to both patient and provider. Some systems automatically pick up these reminders from the progress notes that are a part of the electronic medical record.

Most computer systems today have provisions for establishing ticklers on files. However, a standard practice of using index cards for tickler files is easy to maintain (Figure 14-11).

The tickler card should contain the following information:

- Patient name
- Tickler date (when action should be taken)
- Required action (e.g., schedule surgery or mail reminder)
- Additional relevant information (telephone number)

If action is to be taken with a patient or on behalf of the patient (e.g., scheduling a hospital admittance or sending a reminder of a checkup visit), place the information on the tickler card as soon as possible so this task is not forgotten.

When filing records, be sure to look for words such as "on _____ date we will," "pending action," or "follow-up," indicating that some course of action needs to be taken.

It is important to remember that any tickler system, whether manual or computerized, is worthless if the reminder is not adhered to and appropriate action taken.

Release Marks

It is a good practice to use some type of release mark on every item that is filed (date stamp, initials, check mark). Ideally, the provider should initial the document after it has been read. Then, if action is required by the medical assistant, a release

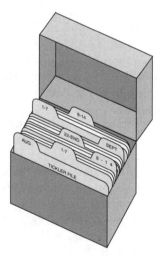

Figure 14-11   Tickler files should be reviewed daily or weekly to follow up on activities and actions that must be taken.

mark is in a consistently identified place on every document. If no action is required after the provider has signed or initialed, place a release mark on the document. A release mark on every piece of information serves as an excellent quality-control measure.

Checkout System

Many clinics have developed dummy charts or files labeled "out sheets" or "out guides" for use when the chart is removed. Most of these guides are identified by an OUT label or metal holder, but they could be assigned a particular color; the key is that they stand out as different from the primary folders (see Figure 14-6).

On the out guide, there should be a minimum of the following information:

- A record of when the chart was removed
- Where the chart can be located

Other information that is useful to note includes:

- Expected date of return
- Actual date the chart was returned
- Signature of the individual checking out the record
- Notation on what section of the chart file was borrowed, such as a laboratory report or specialty examination

Some clinics prefer to have *temporary folders* rather than just an out guide. There are also out guides with pockets to file data in the absence of a chart. This allows for data storage on a temporary basis until the primary file is returned. The data can then be filed permanently when the primary folder is returned. If these folders are of a different color or have a different type of tab/label, they can be spotted easily so the staff can track the temporary files to be sure they do not become permanent folders.

Locating Missing Files or Data

Misfiling can occur for a number of reasons. When this situation occurs, a specific procedure must be established to conduct a search for the missing information. By systematically searching, the missing data usually can be located. This systematic search can be aided by making a mental note of the particular items that commonly are misplaced, such as thin-paper laboratory reports, small laboratory slips, and look-alike names such as "Ward" filed under "Wart" or "Adam" filed under "Adams." Make a note of what was misfiled and where the information was located to more easily locate similar items in the future.

To locate missing pieces of information when the correct file is located but not the particular item within that file:

- Check all of the items within the file.
- Check other files with similar labels.

To locate missing files:

- Check the folders filed before and after the proper location of the misplaced file.
- Look at folders with similar labels.
- Check the provider's desk, the desk tray, and with other office personnel.
- If using a color-coding system, look for folders with the same coding as the misplaced file.
- If using a numeric system, look for possible transposition of combinations of numbers.
- Check for transposition of first and last names.
- Check for alternative spellings of names or look-alike names.

Misplaced files can be frustrating and time-consuming to locate. The best strategy is to check files for the proper filing order whenever returning or retrieving a file folder. When removing a file to answer a question, leave the file following it sticking out slightly to make its return easy and correct. Most importantly, when finished with a record, refile it immediately.

Filing Chart Data

Types of Reports. The patient's chart is the key source of information relating to treatment. A number of reports are kept in the chart, all serving to provide a total picture of patient care. Following are the most common documents that are part of the patient's medical record (see Chapter 16 for other documents).

Clinical Notes. Clinical notes include documentation such as the medical history, the physical examination, and the follow-up notes. They track the patient's course of treatment.

Correspondence. Filling of correspondence varies. Some file all types of correspondence together. Others file correspondence about the patient's treatment with the clinical notes.

Laboratory Reports. Included in laboratory reports are X-ray reports, CT scans, ultrasound reports, blood work, urinalysis, EEGs, ECGs, physical therapy–related reports, and pathology reports—information related to clinical data that assess the patient's condition.

Miscellaneous. The miscellaneous category includes insurance-related papers, requests for transfer of medical records, and personal notes from/to patients. In general, miscellaneous encompasses matters not related to direct treatment.

Retention and Purging

As information accumulates, it is necessary to maintain files by the process known as **purging.** Purging can involve several forms of action.

Record Purging. Record purging requires sorting through records and removing those not in active use. Each facility should establish a standard policy for control and processing of records.

States have different time requirements for retention of various types of records that will take into account the statute of limitations (see Chapter 7). Table 14-2 lists general guidelines. As a way of controlling risk and practicing responsible risk management, many facilities choose to maintain large numbers of inactive files rather than to destroy any records. Some keep them on computer disks or CDs (discussed later in this chapter). Check with the Medical Practice Act in your state to determine record-keeping requirements.

Active Files. Active files include records that need to be readily accessible for retrieval of information.

Inactive Files. Inactive files consist of records that need to be retained for possible retrieval of information. Files not currently being accessed for information would thus become inactive. Often, the type of practice dictates the relevant time period when files are determined to be inactive (generally 2 to 3 years).

Closed Files. Closed files are those that are no longer required. Again, patient files are retained for significantly longer periods of time because of litigation and research considerations, usually 3 to 6 years beyond the statute of limitations.

Table 14-2 Records for Retention

Patient Index Files

These include appointment books or daily appointment sheets. They are kept for an indefinite period. They may be required for litigation or research.

Case Histories

The length of storage depends on state requirements and individual practice requirements. Product liability cases have deemed long-term storage of these records necessary (20+ years). The records of minors must be retained at least until the age of majority. The statute of limitations is a deciding factor as well, usually 3 to 6 years.

If records are to be destroyed because of death of privider or closure of a practice, the following procedure is required: Each patient should be notified of the circumstances and given the opportunity to have his or her records forwarded to another provider. After notification, the records must be retained for a "reasonable" period (determined by state regulations). A period of 3 to 6 months is generally determined to be a "reasonable" period. The records must be destroyed by burning or shredding to protect confidentiality.

Laboratory and X-ray Data

Originals should be retained permanently with the patient's case history.

Personal/Professional Records

Professional licenses should be stored permanently in a secure location.

Office Equipment Records

These records are generally kept until the warranties and depreciation are no longer valid. They should be kept in an easily accessible location if under maintenance contract.

Insurance Records

Professional liability policies are kept permanently. Other policies are kept in active files while in force.

Financial Records

Bank records are kept in active files for up to 3 years and then placed in inactive storage. Tax records must be retained permanently.

CORRESPONDENCE

Most ambulatory care settings process a considerable amount of correspondence not directly related to patient care. Such items include employment applications, letters from/to pharmaceutical representatives, advertisements for medical supplies, magazine subscription information, and letters to/from other providers on a variety of subjects. This correspondence is processed using alphabetic filing rules. However, an additional step is necessary to determine whether the correspondence is incoming or outgoing. The correspondence must be filed under some aspect that will be distinctly identifiable; that is, what idea, subject, or name would most likely be thought of if someone wanted to retrieve that correspondence or file additional relevant correspondence.

Filing Procedures for Correspondence

Once it is determined whether correspondence is incoming or outgoing, follow the basic rules for filing. In addition:

- Remove paper clips and staple items together.
- Inspect to see if the item is ready to be filed; that is, if any appropriate action has been taken. If not, take care of copies and enclosures, and then place notes in the tickler file for future action before proceeding with the indexing.
- On incoming correspondence, be sure the letterhead is related to the letter.

Example:	A personal letter written by a patient on hotel stationery—index the signature on the letter.
Example:	When both the company name and the signature are important, index the company name. A letter from Preston Industries written by the company president—index Preston Industries, not the president's name, which may change.
Example:	If there is no letterhead and you have determined the material is not relevant to a patient, index the name on the signature line. A letter received from Carlton Fiske, RPT, advising your office of services his firm has to offer your patients—index Fiske.

- On outgoing correspondence, look at the inside address and the reference line.

Example:	A letter to the District Court regarding Karen Ritter, an employee who is summoned to jury duty—index Karen Ritter rather than District Court.

Example: If the correspondence is relevant to a patient, index the patient's name. A letter RE: Wayne Elder—index under Elder.

Example: If the correspondence is not relevant to a patient, look to the inside address for the indexing information. A letter inquiring about cost estimates for redecorating the clinic reception room—index the firm in the inside address.

Example: When the inside address is relevant and contains both a company name and a person's name, index the company name. (This avoids the problem of personnel changes.) Cross-referencing would be done under the individual name. A letter to Marvin Fairchild, President of Brandex Pharmaceuticals—index Brandex Pharmaceuticals with a cross-reference for Morgan Fairchild, President, SEE Brandex Pharmaceuticals.

Example: If the letter is personal, the name of the person to whom the letter is written would be used for indexing purposes. Dr. Whitney writes a letter to Dr. Lewis, one of his colleagues, asking if he plans to attend an upcoming conference—index Dr. Lewis.

- On incoming or outgoing correspondence, code the indexing units of the designated label. If the correspondence is being cross-referenced, be sure to note the cross-referencing unit and place the *X* in a visible place. You may find that the body of the letter contains an important name or subject.

- Create a miscellaneous folder for items that do not have enough in number to warrant an individual folder. Items in the miscellaneous folder are filed alphabetically first, and then identical items are filed with the most recent piece on top. An individual folder is then created when enough pieces accumulate on a particular item.

ELECTRONIC MEDICAL RECORDS

 Total electronic automation in any medical facility is a major undertaking. It can be both frightening and exhilarating. Careful study of systems available, impact on providers and staff, time necessary for moving from manual to electronic files, and cost involved are measured against the benefits incurred.

With the government's mandate to have EMRs for most patients by 2014 and Congress pushing to make all Medicare-covered prescriptions transferred electronically by 2011, EMRs are here to stay and one day will replace all paper/manual medical records. Evidence shows that fewer errors are created in EMRs because the "human element" is decreased. If all the data are entered correctly, the computer software "does all the thinking" to find the chart, store information appropriately, create reminder notices, check all medications for any contraindications, and flag any warning to providers, such as high cholesterol or blood pressure readings moving into the "alert" zone. The EMR will keep a record of all patient appointments and any missed appointments as well as any piece of information that might be found in a manual patient record. EMR software creates, stores, edits, and retrieves patient data. It has the added advantage of allowing more than one person to access a chart at the same time.

Electronic automation in the medical facility is discussed in several other chapters (in particular, see Unit 5: Managing Facility Finances). For purposes of this chapter and after reading about the fairly detailed "manual" records management tasks, consider the case for EMRs.

EMR software can be purchased as a single-computer application or as part of a larger "practice management" software package. Often, medical facilities start with one aspect of a practice management software package (usually not EMRs) and then gradually add the other pieces. EMRs are capable of the following:

- Create and print customized encounter forms and superbills

- View patient records of all provider encounters and laboratory results, transcription notes, radiologic images, and so forth

- Utilize predefined templates to make examination notes, procedures, review of systems, and postoperative checks quicker and more efficient

- Indicate or choose medications (from a predetermined list of those most prescribed), with specific instructions that can be electronically admitted into the chart and to the pharmacy

- Flag any drug interactions, contraindications, or allergies related to the patient

- Give providers pen units or small computers in which to enter data with a simple touch of the pen

- Provide immediate access of the patient record to providers and necessary staff members
- Be easily retrieved and never lost or misplaced
- Eliminate the manual coding and filing of medical charts
- Store medical charts for as long as necessary in a small space on computer disks or CDs
- Reduce the amount of phone tag retrieving necessary information from a paper file
- Create reminders for follow-up as necessary
- Provide more efficient method of signing charts
- Can be emailed to a referring provider or easily printed, whether part of or the whole chart

EMRs require that providers use computers to open and view charts and write prescriptions. Progress notes can be created using clinical templates and a point-and-click form of entry. Commonly used clinical phrases can be dropped into the progress note with a push of a button. If providers prefer to dictate and have their notes transcribed, that can also be done. The transcribed and entered note will automatically update relevant information such as problem lists, vital signs, laboratory results, and so on. As voice recognition improves, it will become possible for the provider to speak the entries normally keyed into the system (see Chapter 11).

Confidentiality is often mentioned as a concern in EMRs, but with network access limitations, system administrators can identify access and privileges according to the desired policy of the clinic. The EMR is fully recognized as a legal document, is able to track any changes made, and can be presented to a court of law. Because a standard part of any EMR installation is a system backup, you should never be without a medical chart even if the system goes down for a brief period.

Most medical assistants working in facilities that are fully computerized say they hardly remember how they could function any differently. They also report that moving from the manual to the electronic system can be frustrating at times, but it is worth the effort in the long run.

Archival Storage

Most providers preserve patient medical records for at least the life of their practice. This obviously is a space-consuming prospect, particularly in today's large practices. Computers help to solve this dilemma through EMRs. Records are copied onto optical disks or CDs. This method not only eliminates the bulky storage problems encountered with traditional

records, but records can be retrieved and viewed almost instantaneously on a computer screen.

 One of the advantages of the EMR is the small amount of storage needed for all the patient charts, but remember that computer files, including patient charts, should have a backup system that stores the information in a secure place should there be a computer problem. Some systems provide for automatic backup every 30 minutes or less. Some systems include a second hard drive that stores data as thay are being created or as often as determined by facility policy. With an effective and efficient backup system, no one on the clinic staff will ever be without a patient chart when it is needed.

Transfer of Data

 EMRs are easily emailed in whole or in part. Computers also streamline transfer of records from one medical facility to another. Faxing is an everyday part of the medical clinic. Gone are the days when it took a provider days to obtain information vital to treating a patient. Within minutes, a patient's entire medical record can be sent electronically from one clinic to another. Scanners (optical character recognition) are devices that allow information to be converted to an image on the computer screen. For instance, a patient's entire medical record can be scanned by the device and then recreated as a computer file exactly as it was in paper form.

Confidentiality

 Maintaining confidentiality is a major issue in using the computer and online devices for storage and transfer of medical information.

 Not enough emphasis can be placed on the confidentiality issue. Medical assistants employed in a medical facility will hear and see information that is completely private. It is never appropriate to discuss any of that information outside the clinic with any individual unless it is a person who needs that information for medical reasons. It is also unwise to discuss private information within the facility if it is not your concern, and especially if your voice might be overheard by someone waiting in an examination room, a patient using the restroom, or individuals in the reception area. An appropriate situation in which information can be shared is when giving the name, address, and Social Security number or clinic number to the radiology department that will be performing the X-rays ordered by the provider.

HIPAA

HIPAA compliance with EMRs is very specific in required security standards to protect the confidentiality of patients' health information. The standards include the following:

- Computers, servers, and network hubs must be secure from intrusion.
- Users who access medical information are to be identified and updated regularly.
- Firewalls and antivirus measures must block unauthorized access.
- Passwords are not to be easily guessed, must be securely stored, and should be changed no fewer than every 90 days.
- Passwords are to be hidden when entered and are not shared with anyone.

- The number of invalid entries to access information must be limited.
- Computer screens are to be out of view of unauthorized individuals.
- Screensavers are used for further protection when there is no computer activity.

It is recommended that users close any document prior to leaving a workstation for even a short period of time and that the password be required upon returning to the document.

Remember that HIPAA expressly gives patients the right to determine who has access to their protected health information (PHI). Any release of a medical record or PHI should be with the patient's permission.

Procedure 14-1

Establishing a Paper Medical Chart for a New Patient

PURPOSE:
To demonstrate an understanding of the principles for establishing a paper medical chart.

EQUIPMENT/SUPPLIES:
File folder used in the facility (flip-up or book-style)
Divider pages used in the facility (SOAP/SOAPER laboratory reports, HIPAA information sheets, and so forth)
Adhesive twin prong fasteners for divider pages
Twin hole punch for twin prong fasteners
Selected tabs to identify folder and divider pages
Demographic patient information completed before or at the first appointment

PROCEDURE STEPS:

1. Assemble all supplies at a desk or table. RATIONALE: Everything is in one place for efficient use.

2. Punch holes in the manila file folder and any necessary divider pages. RATIONALE: Creates holes for the twin prong fasteners.

3. Affix the adhesive twin prong fasteners. RATIONALE: Places fasteners as appropriate for material to be attached.

4. Assemble the divider pages dictated by the practice and the office policy in the proper location of the chart over the twin prong fasteners.

RATIONALE: Ensures that items are placed in the same place as all other charts in the facility.

5. Securely fasten twin prong fasteners over the divider pages. RATIONALE: Ensures that no pages will fall out of the chart.

6. Index and code the patient's name according to the filing system to be used (i.e., alphabetic, numeric, or color). RATIONALE: Determines where the chart will be placed.

7. Affix appropriately labeled tabs to the folder cut. RATIONALE: Prepares the chart for patient information.

8. Transfer demographic data in black ink pen or affix the demographic divider sheet to the inside front cover of the chart. RATIONALE: Identifying patient information is readily available inside the chart cover.

9. Affix HIPAA required information to the chart, after it has been read and signed by the patient, as determined by office policy. RATIONALE: Ensures that this task not omitted.

10. Place prepared chart in proper location for pickup by the provider or clinical medical assistant. RATIONALE: Signals to all staff that the chart is ready for the patient's visit.

Procedure 14-2

Establishing an Electronic Medical Record for a New Patient Using Medical Office Simulation Software (MOSS)

PURPOSE:
To demonstrate an understanding of the principles for establishing an electronic medical record.

EQUIPMENT/SUPPLIES:
Computer
MOSS

Electronic Medical Chart Exercises:

1. Jacalyn Dombrowski, DOB July 18, 1974, new patient of Dr. Schwartz. Home address: 936 East Jackman Drive, Douglasville, NY 12345. Telephone number: 123-862-9133. Social Security #: 999-82-1644; married. She is the subscriber to her insurance plan which is Consumer One HRA; Identification #: 463251178 and Group #: ADM246. Employer: Regent Medical Clinic, 847 Constitution Street, Kensington, NY 12355; telephone 123-928-5475, x2198.

2. Allen P. Boynton, DOB November 24, 1981, new patient of Dr. Schwartz. Home address: 18 Brick-yard Place, Unit #214, Douglasville, NY 12345. Telephone number: 123-862-8849. Social Security #: 999-33-1162; single. He is the subscriber to his insurance plan which is Flexi Health PPO In-Network; Identification #: 887912436 and Group #: 864BD. Employer: First Surety Invest-ments, 3175 Forest Grove Avenue, Ravensport, NY 12358; telephone 123-645-2189.

3. Jessica L. McFadden, DOB March 28, 1997, new patient of Dr. Heath. Home address: 97 Lindberg Street, Douglasville, NY 12345. Telephone num-ber: 123-862-4387. Social Security #: 999-76-0184; single. Jessica is a full-time student at Jefferson Middle School. She is a dependent on her father's insurance plan which is Signal HMO; Identifica-tion #: 012348756 and Group #: 9873. Her father is Patrick McFadden, Social Security #: 999-55-8374, DOB May 18, 1970, and he lives at the same address. Patrick's employer is Addison-Kemp Insurance Agency, 348 Main Street, Douglasville, NY 12345; telephone 123-323-6743.

MOSS PROCEDURES:

1. Open MOSS and select Patient Registration.

2. In the Patient Registration window select the "Add" button at the bottom of the screen. This will bring up the Patient Registration Form.

3. On the tab labeled "Patient Information" click in the Physician field and click on the magnify-ing glass to select Dr. Schwartz from the practice physician listing.

4. Tab to Field 1 and enter "Dombrowski", the patient's last name.

5. In Field 2, enter "Jacalyn", the patient's first name.

6. In Field 3, enter patient's middle initial, if known.

7. Enter "999-82-1644", patient's Social Security number, in Field 4.

8. In Field 5, enter "Female", the patient's gender.

9. In Field 6, enter "Married", the patient's marital status.

10. Field 7, enter "07/18/1974", patient's date of birth in MM/DD/YYYY format.

11. Field 8, enter "936 East Jackman Drive", the patient's street address (also enter apartment number or unit number if applicable).

12. In Field 9, enter "Douglasville", the patient's city of residence.

13. In Field 10, enter "NY", the state of residence.

14. In Field 11, enter "12345", the zip code.

15. In Field 12, enter "123-862-9133", the patient's home telephone number, including area code.

16. In Field 13, enter "123-928-5475 x2198", the patient's work telephone number, including area code and extension, if known.

17. In Field 14, use the drop-down menu to select "Employed", the patient's employment status.

continues

18. Field 15 should contain "Regent Medical Clinic", the name of the patient's employer (if known).

19. In Field 16, enter "847 Constitution Street", the patient's employer's street address.

20. In Field 17, enter "Kensington", the patient's employer's city.

21. In Field 18, enter "NY", the patient's employer's state.

22. In Field 19, enter "12355", the patient's employer's zip code.

23. In Field 20, click on the magnifying glass and select "Cynthia Brennen". This field would be used to indicate when another provider has referred the patient to the practice. Usually this is used when the provider is being seen on a consulting basis.

24. In Field 21, click on "Self" as the responsible party for this patient.

25. Check your work with Figure 14-12. Click Save.

26. A dialog box stating "Changes to Patient Registration Saved!" will open. Click "OK".

27. Click on the "Primary Insurance" tab at the top of the dialog box.

28. In Field 1, click on the magnifying glass and select "Consumer One HRA", the patient's insurance carrier.

29. Select "Self" in Field 2 to identify the patient's relationship to the policyholder of the health plan.

30. When selecting "Self", Fields 3, 4, 5, and 6 will populate automatically with the information from the Patient Information screen.

31. Click in Field 7 and enter "463251178" as the patient insurance identification number.

32. Leave Field 8 blank. This would only be populated if this information was available to you.

33. In Field 9, enter "ADM246" for the group number of the patient's insurance plan. (This also may not always be available to you.)

34. Field 10 will automatically populate with information entered on the Patient Information screen.

35. Field 11 will automatically populate with information from the Insurance Centers maintenance files based on how it was set up in the database.

36. In Fields 12 through 14, check "Yes".

37. In Field 15, click on the magnifying glass and select "Cynthia Brennen" as the patient's primary care provider (PCP). If a provider in this practice is the patient's PCP, no selection is made in this field. Check your work with Figure 14-13.

38. Click "Save". A dialog box stating "Changes to Primary Insurance Saved!" will Open. Click "OK".

39. Click on the HIPAA tab at the top of the screen.

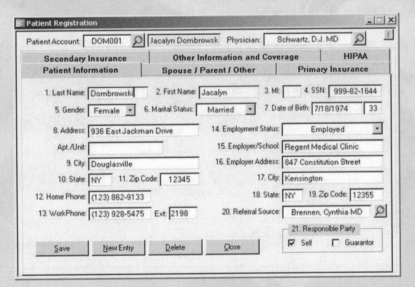

Figure 14-12   Completed Patient Information tab for Jacalyn Dombrowki in MOSS.

continues

Procedure 14-2 (continued)

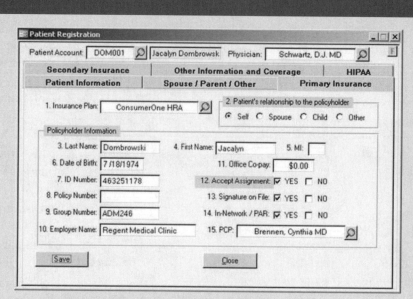

Figure 14-13   Completed Primary Insurance tab for Jacalyn Dombrowki in MOSS.

40. In Field 1, indicate "Yes" that the patient has been given the HIPAA form and enter today's date.

41. In Field 2, indicate "Yes" that the patient has signed the HIPAA form and enter today's date. Check your work with Figure 14-14.

42. Click on "Save". A dialog box "Do you want to save changes to Patient Registration" will come up. Select "Yes".

43. A new dialog box stating "Changes to Patient Registration Saved!" will open. Click on "OK".

44. Click "Close" at the bottom of the Patient Registration screen and "Close" at the bottom of the

Patient Registration list. Now you are back at the main menu.

45. Repeat the above steps, using the information provided in Establishing an Electronic Medical Chart Exercises 2 and 3.

46. Take screenshots of the complete Patient Registration window (the window shown in Figure 14-12), the Primary Insurance window (the window shown in Figure 14-13), and the HIPAA window (the window shown in Figure 14-14) for Exercises 2 and 3 and submit to your instructor either as a printout or in an email file.

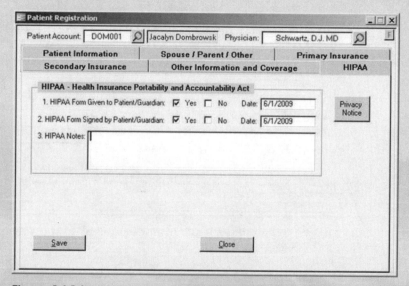

Figure 14-14   Completed HIPAA tab for Jacalyn Dombrowki in MOSS.

Procedure 14-2, Revised Steps 30-38:

30. When selecting "Self," several fields will populate automatically with the information from the Patient Information screen.

31. Click in Field 8 and enter "463251178" as the patient insurance identification number.

32. Leave Field 9 blank. This would only be populated if this information was available to you.

33. In Field 10, enter "ADM246" for the group number of the patient's insurance plan. (This also may not always be available to you.)

34. Field 11 will automatically populate with information entered on the Patient Information screen.

35. Field 12 will automatically populate with information from the Insurance Centers maintenance files based on how it was set up in the database.

36. In Fields 13 through 15, check "Yes."

37. Check your work with Figure 14-13. Click "Save."

38. A dialog box stating "Changes to Primary Insurance Saved!" will open. Click "OK."

Figure 14-13 Completed Primary Insurance tab for Jacalyn Dombrowski

Procedure 14-3

Correcting a Paper Medical Record

PURPOSE:
To demonstrate appropriate method of correcting an error in a paper medical chart.

EQUIPMENT/SUPPLIES:
Document containing error
Document containing correction
Red ink pen

PROCEDURE STEPS:

1. Review information on correcting medical records. RATIONALE: Ensures you know the rules for correcting paper records.

2. Draw a single line through the error using a red ink pen. RATIONALE: Identifies the portion of the record in error.

3. Write in the correction. RATIONALE: Corrects the noted error.

4. Write "Corr." or "Correction" above the corrected information. RATIONALE: Identifies the information as a correction of an error.

5. Initial and date the correction. RATIONALE: Identifies the person who made the correction and the date it was made.

Procedure 14-4

Correcting an Electronic Medical Record

PURPOSE:
To demonstrate appropriate method of correcting an error immediately discovered in an electronic medical record.

EQUIPMENT/SUPPLIES:
Computer with screen open to document containing error
Document containing correction

PROCEDURE STEPS:

1. Review information on correcting electronic medical records. RATIONALE: Ensures you know the rules for making corrections in electronic medical records.

2. Set the computer software to "track" the area to be corrected. RATIONALE: Ensures that any changes made in the document can be distinguished.

3. Using the dash key, line out the error. RATIONALE: Identifies the portion of the record in error. The line appears on the screen and will show when printed.

4. Key in the correction to be made right beside the error. RATIONALE: Corrects the noted error. The correction appears in a different color on the screen and when printed.

5. Key "Corr." or "Correction" after the corrected information. RATIONALE: Identifies the information as a correction of an error.

6. Initial and date the correction. RATIONALE: Identifies the person who made the correction and the date it was made.

7. If an error is discovered after the record has been finalized, create an addendum identifying the error and include the correction. This addendum must be signed and dated by the individual who is making the correction.

Procedure 14-5

Steps for Manual Filing with an Alphabetic System

PURPOSE:
To demonstrate an understanding of the principles of alphabetic filing.

EQUIPMENT/SUPPLIES:
Documents to be filed
Dividers with guides

PROCEDURE STEPS:

1. Inspect and index. RATIONALE: Ensures that the chart is ready for filing and determines the order in which the chart will be filed.

2. Sort the charts alphabetically. RATIONALE: Determines the order and placement of the record; allows for a second assessment for placement.

3. Create cross-reference files according to clinic policy.

4. File the charts appropriately.

5. Check the placement with the charts immediately before and after the chart being filed. RATIONALE: Makes certain the chart is filed in the correct location.

Procedure 14-6

Steps for Manual Filing with a Numeric System

PURPOSE:
To demonstrate an understanding of the principles of the numeric filing system.

EQUIPMENT/SUPPLIES:
Documents to be filed
Dividers with guides
Miscellaneous numeric file section
Alphabetic card file and cards
Accession journal if needed

PROCEDURE STEPS:

1. Inspect and index. RATIONALE: Ensures that the information is ready for filing and determines how the chart will be located.

2. Code for filing units. Check the alphabetic card file for each piece to see if the card has already been prepared. RATIONALE: Determines the number under which the chart will be filed.

3. Write the number in the upper right-hand corner if the piece has been assigned a number. RATIONALE: Tells you the number to be used in filing.

4. If no number is assigned (i.e., it has an *M* for miscellaneous), check the miscellaneous file. If a miscellaneous item is ready to be assigned a number, make a card and note the number in the right-hand corner of the card file, cross out the *M*, and make a chart file. RATIONALE: Tells you if a number should be prepared because of numerous items in miscellaneous, or if the piece to be filed should stay in miscellaneous.

5. If there is no card, make up an alphabetic card including a complete name and address, and then write either *M* or assign a number. RATIONALE: Ensures that there is always an alphabetic card with necessary demographic information and an assigned number or *M* for each piece of information and chart.

6. Cross-reference if necessary and file the card properly. You are then ready to file the document in the appropriate file folder/chart. RATIONALE: Ensures less likelihood of misfiling if necessary cross-references are prepared.

7. File in ascending order. RATIONALE: Establishes a pattern for filing.

Procedure 14-7

Steps for Manual Filing with a Subject Filing System

PURPOSE:
To demonstrate an understanding of the principles of the subject filing system.

EQUIPMENT/SUPPLIES:
Documents to be filed by subject
Subject index list or index card file listing subjects
Alphabetic card file and cards

PROCEDURE STEPS:

1. Review the item to find the subject. RATIONALE: Checks the item for the main topic of information to determine where piece will be filed.

2. Match the subject of the item with an appropriate category on the subject index list. RATIONALE: Saves you time so that you do not create an unnecessary subject index list.

3. If the item contains information that may pertain to more than one subject, decide on the proper cross-reference. RATIONALE: Ensures that any confusion will be checked with a cross-reference.

4. If the subject title is written on the material, underline it. RATIONALE: Readily identifies the subject used for filing.

5. If the subject title is not written on the item, write it clearly in the upper right-hand corner and underline (____) it. RATIONALE: Indicates the subject used for filing; consistently places the subject in the expected place.

6. Use a wavy (___) line for cross-referencing and an *X* as with alphabetic and numeric filing. RATIONALE: Clearly identifies any cross-referencing.

7. Underline the first indexing unit of the coded units. RATIONALE: Ensures the correct order for filing.

Case Study 14-1

Refer to the scenario at the beginning of the chapter.

CASE STUDY REVIEW

1. Juanita Hansen is waiting in the clinic. Dr. Whitney and the staff are scrambling for her medical record. They find the record on the provider's dictation stack, but they cannot find Juanita's test results. What can be done now to make certain Juanita has not made the trip unnecessarily?

2. Identify steps to be taken to prevent this situation from happening another time.

Case Study 14-2

Karen Ritter, administrative medical assistant at Inner City Health Care, has been chiefly responsible for managing this urgent care center's medical records. However, because Karen is only a part-time employee, the office manager feels she needs to delegate some of the responsibility of maintaining all office files to Liz Corbin, a medical assistant who also works part-time. Karen knows the system well and had a hand in designing an effective numeric filing method that both ensures patient confidentiality and satisfies the needs of Inner City and its large volume of patients. Now she is trying to orient Liz, who has little experience with the filing system, to the intricacies of medical records management.

CASE STUDY REVIEW

1. What is a good starting point for Liz Corbin's education in medical records management?
2. What are the basic procedures for filing any piece of documentation that Liz needs to learn?
3. Under the direction of the office manager, Inner City is gradually shifting to a computerized system for all operations. Eventually, patient files will be computerized. What can Karen and Liz do to prepare for this eventuality?

Case Study 14-3

Dr. King is notorious for misplacing files. Often, Dr. King, who does not want to bother busy staff, walks to the lateral file shelves and removes a file or two. Likewise, he may decide to refile a chart that he has had on his desk. He has been known to take charts home when he wants to do some research.

CASE STUDY REVIEW

1. What might the staff do to ensure that Dr. King does not remove charts or refile them without proper use of out guides?
2. Devise a plan to give Dr. King the comfort he desires in the medical clinic where he is a founding partner, yet still protect the patients' charts and ensure the staff knows of the charts' locations.

SUMMARY

Records management plays an ever-increasing role in the ambulatory care setting today. With the need for thorough and proper documentation, a majority of interaction on the patient's behalf is concerned with proper information processing. It is imperative that medical records be managed efficiently, and that the medical assistant possess the skills required for sorting, filing, retrieving, and maintaining information effectively.

A key aspect of managing patient records is selecting a filing system that achieves the goals of information access and storage. Once an alphabetic, numeric, or subject filing system is chosen, patient charts must be assembled and maintained accurately. Increasingly technology and computer applications play a prominent and varied role in the organization and utilization of charts in the medical facility as electronic medical records are more widely used. The medical assistant who is knowledgeable of procedures/rules related to the management of manual/paper medical records will find the transition to electronic medical records exciting and much easier to organize and control.

STUDY FOR SUCCESS

To reinforce your knowledge and skills of information presented in this chapter:

- Review the Key Terms
- Practice any Procedures
- Consider the Case Studies and discuss your conclusions
- Answer the Review Questions
  - Multiple Choice
  - Critical Thinking
- Navigate the Internet and complete Web Activities
- Practice the StudyWARE activities on the textbook CD
- Apply your knowledge in the Student Workbook activities
- Complete the Web Tutor sections
- View and discuss the DVD situations

REVIEW QUESTIONS

Multiple Choice

1. Maintaining order in files by separating active from inactive files is:
   a. indexing
   b. coding
   c. purging
   d. alphabetizing
2. A system used as a reminder of action to be taken on a certain date is called:
   a. accession log
   b. tickler file or reminder note
   c. release mark
   d. purging system
3. To maintain an accurate filing system, select from the following list the tool used to ensure that records are tracked when borrowed:
   a. release mark
   b. out guide
   c. alphabetic card file
   d. cross-reference file
4. The correct indexing from first to last for assigning units to the name John Porter O'Keefe II would be:
   a. O'Keefe John Porter II
   b. John Porter O'Keefe II
   c. II O'Keefe John Porter
   d. the "II" would be disregarded
5. Of the four systems of filing, the best for every ambulatory care setting is:
   a. the numeric system
   b. the color-coding system
   c. one customized to the needs of the clinic
   d. the alphabetic system

6. Medical records are the property of:
   a. the patients for whom the record is about
   b. insurance carriers who help to pay medical costs
   c. the providers who create the record
   d. a and c
7. Corrections to medical records:
   a. are made by erasing the error and replacing it with the correction
   b. are made by placing a single line through the error and replacing it with the correction
   c. are never made to charts because of the legal nature of the information
   d. are made only by the provider
8. The following statements about EMRs are all true except one:
   a. are initially more expensive than paper medical records
   b. should be available to most Americans by 2011
   c. eliminate coding and filing of medical charts
   d. create reminders for follow-up as necessary
9. When identical names are being indexed, the system most preferred in a medical clinic to index is:
   a. the address
   b. the telephone number
   c. the birth date or Social Security number
   d. a preassigned clinic number
10. The preferred order for steps in filing medical documentation is:
    a. code, index, sort, inspect, file
    b. inspect, code, index, sort, file
    c. sort, inspect, index, code, file
    d. inspect, index, code, sort, file

Critical Thinking

1. A patient's chart has been subpoenaed for pending malpractice litigation. In preparing the chart, you discover an error that was made when the results of the laboratory report were incorrectly documented in the chart. You have the original laboratory report. What should you do?
2. Identify how you would index and cross-reference the following medical chart:

Patient:	John Bryan Houk	
Mother:	Sara (Houk) Judson	(Assumed her maiden name following divorce)
Father:	Brett J. Houk	(Covers son on his medical insurance)

3. Research the statute of limitations in your state for medical records to determine how long a medical record should be kept. The statute will also tell you what triggers activity on a medical file that might dictate it be kept longer than normally indicated.
4. Identify the steps you might take in "inspecting" the charts before filing. What would you do if you found something missing or an unsigned report?
5. It has been said that filing records is the easiest task the medical assistant will perform, yet it is often the most difficult. What reasons can you give for this statement?

WEB ACTIVITIES

1. Using your favorite search engine, key in "medical record authorization for release of information." Are you able to find a site that has a sample blank form to be completed? Are there any surprises? For how long is the authorization valid?
2. Go to http://www.smead.com to view their many color-coded filing systems. Can color be used in both alphabetic and numeric filing? Now go to http://www.kardex.com to review their systems. Select a system and identify why it would be your choice for a medical clinic. What problems might occur with the self-adhesive products shown on these Web sites?
3. Search for information on electronic medical records. Identify the number of sites that come up. Select two or three sites that allow you to view or download a sample of the product software. Identify your likes and dislikes and give your rationale. What would influence you if you were helping to select electronic medical record software for a medical facility where you are employed?

REFERENCES/BIBLIOGRAPHY

Burt, C. W., Hing, E. & Woodwell, D. (2005). *Electronic medical record use by office-based physicians: United States,* 2005. Hyattsville, MD: U.S. Department of Health and Human Services, Centers for Disease Control and Prevention.

Fordney, M. T., French, L., & Follis, J. J. (2004). *Administrative medical assisting* (5th ed.). Clifton Park, NY: Delmar Cengage Learning.

Hansen, D. (2008). *"Congress considers mandate for medicare e-prescribing.* Retrieved February 2008, from http://ww.ama-assn.org/amednews/2008/01/07/gvsb0107.htm.

Johnson, J. (1994). *Basic filing procedures for health information management.* Clifton Park, NY: Delmar Cengage Learning.

Lewis, M. A., & Tamparo, C. D. (2007). *Medical law ethics & bioethics for health professionals* (6th ed.). Philadelphia: F. A. Davis.

Chapter 17

Medical Insurance

OUTLINE

Understanding the Role of
Health Insurance

Medical Insurance Terminology

Terminology Specific to
Insurance Policies

Terminology Specific to Billing
Insurance Carriers

Types of Medical Insurance
Coverage

Traditional Insurance

Managed Care Insurance

The Impact of Managed
Care

Medicare Insurance

Medicare Supplemental
Insurance

Medicaid Insurance

TRICARE

Civilian Health and Medical
Program of the Veterans
Administration

Workers' Compensation
Insurance

Self-Insurance

Medical Tourism Insurance

Screening for Insurance

Referrals and Authorizations

Determining Fee Schedules

Usual, Customary, and
Reasonable Fees

Resource-Based Relative Value
Scale (RBRVS)

Hospital Inpatient Prospective
Payment System (IPPS)

Hospital Outpatient Prospective Payment System (OPPS)

Capitation

Legal and Ethical Issues

HIPAA Implications

Insurance Fraud and Abuse

Professional Careers in
Insurance

KEY TERMS

Abuse

Adjustment

Assignment of Benefits

Beneficiary

Benefit Period

Birthday Rule

Capitation

Centers for Medicare and
Medicaid Services (CMS)

Coinsurance

Coordination of
Benefits (COB)

Co-payment

Deductible

Defense Enrollment
Eligible Reporting
System (DEERS)

Donut Hole

Exclusion

Exclusive Provider
Organization (EPO)

Explanation of Benefits
(EOB)

Fiscal Intermediary

Fraud

Health Maintenance
Organization (HMO)

Integrated Delivery
System (IDS)

Managed Care
Organization (MCO)

Medicare Part A

Medicare Part B

Medicare Part C

Medicare Part D

Medigap Policy

OBJECTIVES

The student should strive to meet the following performance objectives and demonstrate an understanding of the facts and principles presented in this chapter through written and oral communication.

1. Define the key terms as presented in the glossary.

2. Define the terminology necessary to understand and submit medical insurance claims.

3. Recall at least five examples of medical insurance coverage and discuss their differences.

4. Describe six primary managed care organization models.

5. Recall the steps involved when screening patients for insurance.

6. Discuss the importance of obtaining referrals and preauthorizations.

OBJECTIVES (continued)

7. Discuss legal and ethical issues related to medical insurance and the provider's office.

8. Discuss the impacts of HIPAA requirements related to insurance and the release of patient information.

9. Explore career opportunities in the insurance profession.

Scenario

At Inner City Health Care, a multiprovider urgent care center in a large city, medical assistant Jane O'Hara, CMA (AAMA), is responsible for all patient billing procedures. Inner City participates in a number of insurance plans, so Jane must stay abreast of policy changes regarding reimbursement, preauthorizations, and claims filing. She also tries to become acquainted with the conditions of each patient's insurance coverage and helps patients understand their responsibility, if any, for payment. Finally, Jane holds periodic meetings with her assistants to update them; she continually stresses to them the importance of timeliness in filing claims and the need for absolute accuracy in diagnosis and procedure codes, which must always reflect services actually performed.

INTRODUCTION

An understanding of medical insurance and proper coding techniques is absolutely critical to the survival of the ambulatory care setting. In recent years, much has changed in medical insurance coverage: more patients are choosing health maintenance organizations (HMOs) and other managed care options, and even traditional insurance carriers such as Blue Cross and Blue Shield are modifying their insurance plans to include some aspect of managed benefits.

In some ways, managed care coverage has simplified the patient's responsibility for payment, but it is more important than ever for the medical assistant to be accurate, timely, and conscientious in both filing insurance claim forms and understanding—and helping the patient to understand—the conditions of individual insurance policies.

The increasing complexity of health insurance today means that medical assistants must continually update their base of information. This chapter provides the groundwork for understanding the role of insurance, its terminology, and its various forms, and it gives the medical assistant the confidence to take responsibility for claim filing in the ambulatory care setting.

Spotlight on Certification

RMA Content Outline
- Insurance
- Computer applications

CMA (AAMA) Content Outline
- Maintain confidentiality
- Legislation
- Provider–patient relationship
- Computer applications
- Coding systems
- Third-party billing

CMAS Content Outline
- Confidentiality
- Insurance processing
- Coding
- Insurance billing and finances
- Fundamentals of computing

UNDERSTANDING THE ROLE OF HEALTH INSURANCE

Health insurance was designed to help individuals and families compensate for the high costs of medical care. Medical care consists of the diagnosis of diseases/disorders and the care and treatment provided by the health care team of professionals to individuals who are ill or injured. Medical care, which also includes preventive services, is designed to help individuals avoid health or injury problems and is termed *health care.*

Health care insurance is a contract between an individual policyholder and a third-party or government program that reimburses the medical provider or the policyholder for medically necessary treatment or preventive care covered by that specific health care provider.

There is much discussion today about changes in the health care insurance industry. Foremost is the idea that health care insurance should be available to all citizens of the United States. At this time, health insurance is usually tied to the employment package that covers the employee, and possibly the spouse and dependent children. One problem with work-related coverage is that some part-time employees are not eligible for health insurance and thus often go uninsured. Another problem is if an employee takes a position elsewhere, medical benefits may not transfer equally. If a family member is ill with a preexisting condition such as cancer or diabetes mellitus, the new insurance policy may not cover that disease or condition for a fixed time period. This time-dependent limitation of coverage is known as an **exclusion**. If health insurance has previously been in effect for at least 18 months and any lapse in coverage between policies did not exceed 63 days, a preexisting condition cannot be given as a reason for exclusion. Some states have laws limiting the length of an exclusion period; otherwise it is at the discretion of the carrier. An exclusion also may include illnesses or conditions for injury specifically not covered by the policy.

Another controversial aspect of health insurance is refusal to provide coverage for certain procedures because they are not sufficiently proven to be effective. In the early 1990s, bone marrow transplants were being performed on patients with breast cancer, at that time an experimental treatment for breast cancer. Because most insurance carriers will not extend coverage to experimental treatment, family and friends of patients often gathered for fund-raising drives to ensure that medical costs would be covered.

Not all insurance carriers cover the same exposures equally, and few carriers pay at the same rate. Similarly, not many carriers charge the same premiums to policyholders. Some insurance companies cover individuals, families, or employee groups through work or through groups such as the American Association of Retired Persons (AARP). Some premiums reflect the insured person's past medical history and the company's exposure in covering the person. Premiums may be less if the insured person selects a higher annual deductible. Other premiums represent the rate that a group is able to obtain based on the group's claim history.

MEDICAL INSURANCE TERMINOLOGY

 Before discussing the types of insurance coverage, one must understand the language used by the insurance industry. The terminology is specific in meaning and has been tested in courts of law to further define its meanings.

Terminology Specific to Insurance Policies

A policy is an agreement between an insurance company or government program and the insured, or **beneficiary**, that is, the person covered under the terms of the policy. The insured person may include as beneficiaries a spouse and dependent minor children; others may be included if related by blood and dependent on the insured for more than 50% of their support. The insurance carrier pays a percentage (**coinsurance**) of the cost of the services covered under the policy in exchange for a monthly premium or charge. This premium is paid by the insured or the employer, or it is shared by both.

At the inception or beginning of the policy, the insured is given an identification card, which must be presented before receiving medical treatment. This card contains the insured person's name, identification number, group number, and any co-payment amount or restrictions for treatment. The back of the insurance card contains an address where claims should be submitted and telephone numbers needed to receive prior authorization for treatment when required.

Deductible.

The language of the policy spells out the terms of the coverage. Usually there is an annual **deductible,** or an amount of money that the insured must incur for medical services before the policy begins to pay. This deductible can range from $100 to $1,000, or an even greater amount depending on the language of the policy. The deductible must be met each year by medical charges that are incurred after the inception or anniversary date of the policy.

For instance, if Boris Bolski went to the provider on January 22 and incurred $258 in charges but his policy did not go into effect until February 1, none of these charges would apply toward his deductible. If, however, he returned to the doctor on February 3 and incurred another $85 charge, this amount could be applied against his deductible.

Coinsurance.

After application of the deductible to the submitted bills, the insurance policy pays a percentage of the remaining amount. This percentage or coinsurance can vary from 50% to 100% depending on the language in a specific policy. Most traditional plans pay 80%.

Co-payment.

Some insurance policies, especially **health maintenance organizations (HMOs)** and other managed care policies, require the patient to make a payment of a specified amount, for instance $5 or $10, at the time of treatment. This payment must be collected at the time of the office visit. Some policies have both a **co-payment** and a coinsurance clause.

Preexisting Condition.

The earlier example of Boris Bolski presents another problem. If a person had an illness, disease, or injury before the inception of the insurance regardless of whether treatment was received, there is a good chance that most insurance policies will not cover any charges related to that specific illness, injury, or disease because it is considered a preexisting condition. Most policies have a specific waiting period before coverage is extended to those preexisting conditions. This waiting period can be a matter of months, years, or the lifetime of the policy. If the person had a previous insurance policy that was not as inclusive as the new policy, often the new policy would still consider this a preexisting condition and will deny payment until the waiting period is met. However, if the new policy has similar benefits and the person had no lapse in coverage, legally, the company must cover those conditions without applying a preexisting condition or waiting period to the policy.

Exclusions.

Exclusions are noncovered services and are an important part of a policy. Some policies exclude elective procedures (procedures that are not medically necessary) such as cosmetic surgery, whereas other policies may allow some elective procedures. Other examples of exclusions or noncovered services might be preexisting conditions, dental services, chiropractic services, or routine eye examinations. Not every policy has the same exclusions.

Coordination of Benefits.

When more than one policy covers an individual, the policy language provides for **coordination of benefits (COB).** This is determined by the policy language and coordinates payments between the policies so that the final total benefit is not greater than the original charge. Policy language again determines which of the two policies is primary or will pay first.

The employee's policy will pay first for the employee. For instance, if John O'Keefe is covered by an insurance policy where he works and is also covered by his wife's medical coverage, the policy Mr. O'Keefe gets from his employer will pay benefits first for him. The coverage under his spouse's policy will pay second because John is considered a dependent under that policy.

Whichever insurance is primary pays for their covered services up to the maximum allowed under the plan, less deductible and co-pay. The secondary insurance will coordinate the benefits and pay as appropriate, but never to exceed the total amount of the services. If the secondary insurance offers a COB, they will only consider the percentage paid as if they were primary; that is, Boris's $258 claim was allowed at 80% by both his primary and his secondary insurances. His primary insurance would pay $206.40, and if his secondary plan offered

COB, they would pay 80% as well. Because $206.40 and $206.40 total $412.80, which is more than the total bill of $258, Boris's secondary insurance will pay the balance left by the primary insurance, in this case, $51.60 (which may cover the co-pay, too). If Boris's secondary insurance does not offer COB, they would cover the same 80% the primary covered, and therefore would pay nothing. This is assuming that his deductibles have been satisfied.

The issue of which insurance is primary and which is secondary only applies when there are dependents covered under two policies. In this case, the **birthday rule** usually applies. When children of married parents are covered under both parents' policies, often the birthday rule is used to determine which policy is primary. This rule simply states that the policy of the parent with the birthday falling earlier in the year is primary. Thus, if the father's birthday is October 17 and the mother's birthday is May 12, the mother's policy is primary. The year of the birth date is not relevant.

If the parents share the same birthday, then the policy with the earlier inception date is primary. If John and Mary both have birthdays on July 12, and the policy for John started August 1, 2004, and the

policy for Mary started December 1, 2003, Mary's policy is primary for their dependent children.

For children of divorced parents who are covered under both parents' policies, the policy of the custodial parent usually is primary unless divorce papers stipulate which parent is responsible.

Explanation of Benefits. The insurance carrier generates an **explanation of benefits (EOB)**, which is mailed to each patient. The EOB is a statement summarizing how the insurance carrier determined the reimbursement for services received by the patient. The backside of the EOB addresses questions frequently asked and defines the terms used within the EOB. The EOB is not to be considered a bill; it simply details information as to how the claim was processed by the insurance carrier. Figure 17-1 shows an example of an EOB.

Remittance Advice. The provider's office receives a **remittance advice** (or **remit**) from the insurance carrier. The provider's remit summarizes all of the benefits paid to the provider within a particular period of time. The remit includes all of the patients covered by a specific insurance for that time period.

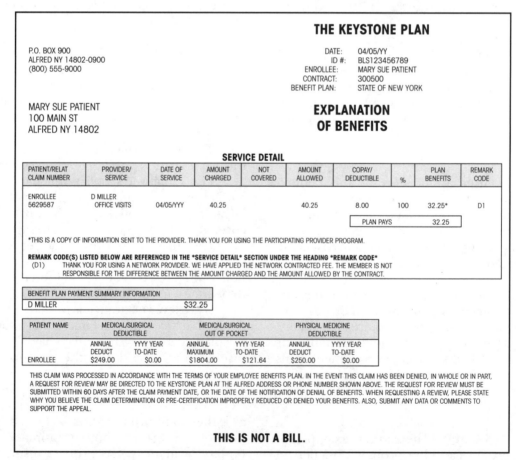

Figure 17-1   Explanation of benefits (EOB) sample.

The difference between the provider's charges and the amount paid by the insurance carrier may be billed to the patient. Figure 17-2 shows an example of a remittance advice.

Terminology Specific to Billing Insurance Carriers

There is specific terminology that one must understand when submitting insurance claims for medical benefits. Most ambulatory care settings bill all appropriate insurance carriers to ascertain that the claim is made and the provider receives payment.

Many policies require **preauthorization** before certain procedures or before a visit can be made to a specialist or a physical therapist. In these cases, the medical assistant must contact the insurance carrier with all of the diagnosis information and the proposed course of treatment. For instance, a patient with a diagnosis of cholecystitis, preauthorization requires notification and approval before referring that patient to a surgeon for possible cholecystectomy. If this is not done, the surgery may not be covered.

A claim occurs when patients, having received treatment, wish to receive reimbursement under their insurance policies for charges for treatment. The patient (or the center's billing office) sends the claim to the insurance carrier for the amount of the treatment. This is done via a claim form, the most common of which is the CMS-1500 (08-05) (Figure 17-3). The Medicare regional carrier can be found at http://www.cms.hhs.gov/contractinggeneralinformation/. When this page opens, scroll down the page and click on Downloads: Intermediary-Carrier Directory. A PDF file listing all Medicare regional carriers will open.

The completed claim form is sent to the insurance carrier by mail, electronically, or through a holding system that batches and transmits claims at timed daily intervals. The most common and expeditious method for submitting claims is electronically. Depending on the policy language and the **assignment of benefits,** payment is sent either directly to the provider (known as direct payment) or to the patient/insured but payable to both the insured and the provider (known as indirect payment).

TYPES OF MEDICAL INSURANCE COVERAGE

In today's health care environment, medical assistants need to be aware of the different types of medical insurance policies.

Traditional Insurance

Traditional insurance provides coverage on a fee-for-service basis. There is usually a deductible and a co-payment or coinsurance amount. The health care provider submits bills to the insurance carrier, and after any deductible has been met, the health care provider or the patient, if the patient has already satisfied the bill, is paid in agreement with the terms of the insurance policy. The patient may be responsible for fees in excess of the contracted amount if the health care provider is not a preferred or participating provider. In the case of a preferred or participating provider, the health care provider has agreed to a discounted fee for different types of procedures performed on patients insured by the carrier. The provider then writes off the difference, and the patient is not responsible for that amount.

```
ABC INSURANCE COMPANY
100 MAIN STREET
ALFRED NY 14802
1-800-555-1234                          REMITTANCE ADVICE

DAVID MILLER, M.D.                                      PROVIDER #: 123456
101 NORTH STREET                                        PAGE #: 1 OF 1
                                                        DATE: 04/05/YY
ALFRED, NY 14802                                        CHECK/EFT #: 000235698

PERF PROV  SERV DATE  POS NOS  PROC  MODS BILLED  ALLOWED DEDUCT    COINS GRP/RC AMT PROV PD
_____
NAME BAKER, JENNY   HIC 235962541         ACNT BAKE1234567-01      ICN 1235626589651   ASG Y MOA MA01
236592ABC  0405 0405YY 11  1 99213     75.00     50.00  0.25      0.00   CO-42 15.00   50.00
PT RESP 10.31      CLAIM TOTALS         75.00     50.00  0.25      0.00         15.00

                                                                             NET    50.00
_____
  TOTALS: # OF    BILLED    ALLOWED    DEDUCT    COINS     TOTAL    PROV PD    PROV     CHECK
    CLAIMS         AMT        AMT        AMT     RC AMT      AMT    ADJ AMT     AMT       AMT
      1           75.00      50.00      0.25     15.00     65.25    50.00     0.00      50.00
```

Figure 17-2   Remittance advice (single claim) sample.

1500

HEALTH INSURANCE CLAIM FORM

APPROVED BY NATIONAL UNIFORM CLAIM COMMITTEE 08/05

PICA · PICA

1. MEDICARE MEDICAID TRICARE CHAMPUS CHAMPVA GROUP HEALTH PLAN FECA BLK LUNG OTHER	1a. INSURED'S I.D. NUMBER (For Program in Item 1)

(Medicare #) (Medicaid #) (Sponsor's SSN) (Member ID#) (SSN or ID) (SSN) (ID)

2. PATIENT'S NAME (Last Name, First Name, Middle Initial)

3. PATIENT'S BIRTH DATE   MM DD YY   SEX   M   F

4. INSURED'S NAME (Last Name, First Name, Middle Initial)

5. PATIENT'S ADDRESS (No., Street)

6. PATIENT RELATIONSHIP TO INSURED   Self   Spouse   Child   Other

7. INSURED'S ADDRESS (No., Street)

CITY   STATE

8. PATIENT STATUS   Single   Married   Other

CITY   STATE

ZIP CODE   TELEPHONE (Include Area Code) (   )

Employed   Full-Time Student   Part-Time Student

ZIP CODE   TELEPHONE (Include Area Code) (   )

9. OTHER INSURED'S NAME (Last Name, First Name, Middle Initial)

10. IS PATIENT'S CONDITION RELATED TO:

11. INSURED'S POLICY GROUP OR FECA NUMBER

a. OTHER INSURED'S POLICY OR GROUP NUMBER

a. EMPLOYMENT? (Current or Previous)   YES   NO

a. INSURED'S DATE OF BIRTH   MM DD YY   SEX   M   F

b. OTHER INSURED'S DATE OF BIRTH   MM DD YY   SEX   M   F

b. AUTO ACCIDENT?   YES   NO   PLACE (State)

b. EMPLOYER'S NAME OR SCHOOL NAME

c. EMPLOYER'S NAME OR SCHOOL NAME

c. OTHER ACCIDENT?   YES   NO

c. INSURANCE PLAN NAME OR PROGRAM NAME

d. INSURANCE PLAN NAME OR PROGRAM NAME

10d. RESERVED FOR LOCAL USE

d. IS THERE ANOTHER HEALTH BENEFIT PLAN?   YES   NO   If yes, return to and complete item 9 a-d.

READ BACK OF FORM BEFORE COMPLETING & SIGNING THIS FORM.

12. PATIENT'S OR AUTHORIZED PERSON'S SIGNATURE I authorize the release of any medical or other information necessary to process this claim. I also request payment of government benefits either to myself or to the party who accepts assignment below.

SIGNED   DATE

13. INSURED'S OR AUTHORIZED PERSON'S SIGNATURE I authorize payment of medical benefits to the undersigned physician or supplier for services described below.

SIGNED

14. DATE OF CURRENT: MM DD YY   ILLNESS (First symptom) OR INJURY (Accident) OR PREGNANCY(LMP)

15. IF PATIENT HAS HAD SAME OR SIMILAR ILLNESS. GIVE FIRST DATE   MM DD YY

16. DATES PATIENT UNABLE TO WORK IN CURRENT OCCUPATION   MM DD YY   FROM   TO   MM DD YY

17. NAME OF REFERRING PROVIDER OR OTHER SOURCE

17a.

17b. NPI

18. HOSPITALIZATION DATES RELATED TO CURRENT SERVICES   MM DD YY   FROM   TO   MM DD YY

19. RESERVED FOR LOCAL USE

20. OUTSIDE LAB?   YES   NO $ CHARGES

21. DIAGNOSIS OR NATURE OF ILLNESS OR INJURY (Relate Items 1, 2, 3 or 4 to Item 24E by Line)

1.   3.

2.   4.

22. MEDICAID RESUBMISSION CODE   ORIGINAL REF. NO.

23. PRIOR AUTHORIZATION NUMBER

24. A. DATE(S) OF SERVICE						B. PLACE OF SERVICE	C. EMG	D. PROCEDURES, SERVICES, OR SUPPLIES (Explain Unusual Circumstances) CPT/HCPCS MODIFIER	E. DIAGNOSIS POINTER	F. $ CHARGES	G. DAYS OR UNITS	H. EPSDT Family Plan	I. ID. QUAL.	J. RENDERING PROVIDER ID. #
From MM	DD	YY	To MM	DD	YY									
1													NPI	
2													NPI	
3													NPI	
4													NPI	
5													NPI	
6													NPI	

25. FEDERAL TAX I.D. NUMBER   SSN EIN

26. PATIENT'S ACCOUNT NO.

27. ACCEPT ASSIGNMENT? (For govt. claims, see back)   YES   NO

28. TOTAL CHARGE $

29. AMOUNT PAID $

30. BALANCE DUE $

31. SIGNATURE OF PHYSICIAN OR SUPPLIER INCLUDING DEGREES OR CREDENTIALS (I certify that the statements on the reverse apply to this bill and are made a part thereof.)

SIGNED   DATE

32. SERVICE FACILITY LOCATION INFORMATION

a. NPI   b.

33. BILLING PROVIDER INFO & PH # (   )

a. NPI   b.

NUCC Instruction Manual available at: www.nucc.org

APPROVED OMB-0938-0999 FORM CMS-1500 (08/05)

CARRIER · PATIENT AND INSURED INFORMATION · PHYSICIAN OR SUPPLIER INFORMATION

Figure 17-3 CMS-1500 (08/05) claim form.

Traditional insurance is sometimes marketed as two types depending on the coverage. Basic insurance covers specific dollar amounts for provider's fees, hospital care, surgery, and anesthesia. Generally, they will not cover examinations to diagnose or treat fertility problems, but more carriers are covering routine physical and preventive care. Major medical insurance covers catastrophic expenses resulting from illness or injury.

Some traditional insurance carriers and most managed care insurance carriers require the patient to select a **primary care provider** or **PCP**. The PCP becomes the first medical practitioner caring for the patient, also known as the gatekeeper, and is responsible for making referrals for further treatment by specialists or for hospital admission. The insurance carrier frequently will refuse payment for treatments not referred by the PCP.

Blue Cross and Blue Shield (BC/BS).

Whereas many traditional policies are offered by commercial carriers, the "Blues" are a well-known type of traditional, or independent, health insurance. Blue Cross was originally established to cover the cost of hospital admission and stay, radiology, and other basic coverage under the health plan. Blue Shield covered the major medical portion, picking up provider's fees, medications, and other charges not covered on the basic portion of the plan. Today, both entities offer a full range of health care coverage. BC/BS plans are locally based in all 50 states, the District of Columbia, Canada, Puerto Rico, and Jamaica. They function independently in their own service area and are flexible enough to meet and satisfy the needs of the local community. They may be organized as not-for-profit corporations or as for-profit companies.

A BC/BS participating provider (PAR) chooses to sign a member contract and receives an incentive. PARs agree to accept the BC/BS reimbursement as payment in full for covered services. BC/BS agrees to reimburse providers directly and in a shorter turnaround time.

Each policyholder is given a card with the subscriber's name and a three-character letter prefix identification number. The letter prefix is important because it indicates under which BC/BS plan the person is insured. This identification number must be included on each claim form submitted to BC/BS; if it is not included, the claim will be denied.

Managed Care Insurance

Managed Care Insurance involves a **Managed Care Organization (MCO)** that assumes the responsibility for the health care needs of a group of enrollees.

The MCO can be a health care plan, hospital, provider group, or health system. The MCO contracts with an insurance carrier, or is itself the carrier, to take care of the medical needs of the enrolled group for a fixed fee per enrollee for a fixed period, usually a calendar year. This payment system is called **capitation.** If the medical costs exceed the fixed fee, the MCO/provider loses income; conversely, if the costs are less than the fixed fee, the MCO/provider makes a profit. An MCO relies on as large an enrollee base as possible to average the cost of medical care.

MCOs were established in an attempt to curb medical costs and provide for more efficient use of medical resources. Almost all MCOs use PCPs as case managers or utilization management services to control what medical resources are used for each patient and to strictly control treatment plans and discharge planning. This policy has led to disputes over quality of care, and many states have enacted laws requiring external quality reviews by independent organizations. The quality-control programs include government oversight, patient satisfaction surveys, review of grievances, measurement of the health status of the enrolled group, and reviews by accreditation agencies. Medicare has established measurable standards for MCOs through its program, Quality Improvement System for Managed Care (QISMC). The federal government requires providers to disclose incentive packages with MCOs to avoid conflicts of interest resulting in reduced level of care solely for the purpose of reducing costs or treatment, thus recognizing a profit at the expense of patient care.

Six models exist for managed cared organizations. They are:

1. **Exclusive Provider Organizations (EPOs).** Enrollees must obtain their medical services from a network of providers or health care facilities that are under exclusive contract to the EPO. The state insurance commissioner regulates EPOs.

2. **Integrated delivery systems (IDSs).** Enrollees obtain medical services from an affiliated group of service providers. The service providers consist of private practices and hospitals that share practice management and services to reduce overhead. An IDS may also be called one of the following: integrated service network, delivery system, horizontally integrated system, vertically integrated system or plan, health delivery network, and accountable health plan.

3. HMO. Enrollees obtain medical services from a network of providers who agree to fixed fees for services but are not under exclusive contract to the insurance carrier.

4. **Point-of-Service (POS) Plan.** The enrollee has the freedom of obtaining medical services from an HMO provider or by self-referral to non-HMO providers. In the case of self-referral, the enrollee will have to pay greater deductibles and coinsurance charges.

5. **Preferred Provider Organization (PPO).** Enrollees obtain services from a network of providers and hospitals that have contracted their services at a discounted fee to an insurance company on a nonexclusive basis.

6. **Triple Option Plan.** Enrollees have the option of traditional, HMO, or PPO health plans.

Table 17-1 lists differences between traditional and managed care policies.

Health maintenance organizations, or HMOs, are probably the most familiar managed care organizations. Originally, HMOs were designed to provide a full range of health care services under one roof. More recently, the HMO without walls has become established, which is typically a network of participating providers within a defined geographic area.

Originally, the HMO with walls was conceived to provide patients with comprehensive health care services at one facility. Today, as managed care and managed competition sweep the health care industry, other arrangements include the preferred provider organization (PPO), where providers network to offer discounts to employers and other purchasers of health insurance, and the Independent Physician Association (IPA), of which the members agree to treat patients for an agreed-upon fee.

The Impact of Managed Care

The emergence of managed care in today's society provides new administrative and clinical challenges to members of the health care team as they struggle to provide the best health care while working within limitations often imposed by insurance carriers. Virtually all health care settings, whether they are individual practices or urgent care centers, are experiencing the impact of managed care, where providers network and compete to serve patients better and more cost-efficiently.

Under managed care, critics charge, health care dollars have grown scarce, providers must strive to provide the same quality for reduced reimbursement, preapprovals must be obtained for many services, and some services may be denied because they are not considered cost-effective.

Clinically, managed care may set limits on services or length of services. Second opinions are encouraged and sometimes required. In some systems, the patient selects a primary care provider, who is considered the gatekeeper and who must provide a referral for specialist care. Critics of managed care point out that restricting or denying services may lead to an increase in professional liability.

Administratively, paperwork and documentation have become increasingly important to ensure proper reimbursement. Although it is the patient's responsibility to understand the conditions of the insurance policy, these are often difficult to understand or interpret. The medical staff must be fully aware of when a preapproval or treatment plan is required, when a second opinion is necessary for reimbursement, and of other clauses and restrictions that affect care and reimbursement for care.

At the same time, although managed care is challenging even the most resilient of providers, the very real need to keep costs down has also generated considerable creativity and energy among the health care profession as providers seek to use technology more efficiently; as they collaborate on new, cost-effective delivery methods; and as everyone involved in health care—insurers, providers, and patients—works together to contain costs by emphasizing prevention and lifestyle changes. Procedure 17-1 provides the steps involved in applying managed care policies and procedures.

Table 17-1 Differences between Traditional and Managed Care Policies

Traditional	Managed Care
Usually can go outside provider network	Usually must stay inside provider network
Coinsurance	Co-pay each visit
Annual deductible	No annual deductible
Illness or injury only	Preventive treatment, as well as illness and injury
Premium paid monthly to company by employer or subscriber	Premium paid monthly to company by employer or subscriber
Provider paid by fee for service	Provider paid by capitation

Critical Thinking

Do you agree with the policy that managed care may set limits on services or length of services? Why or why not? Give your rationale.

Medicare Insurance

Medicare Insurance is the largest medical insurance program in the United States. Most individuals 65 years and older, individuals with a disability that keeps them from working, and individuals with chronic kidney disease are eligible for Medicare. Medicare coverage consists of Parts A, B, C, and D. Part A is the original Medicare program for hospitalization and requires no monthly premiums. Parts B, C, and D require monthly premiums to be paid by the patient, with the amount depending upon income and specific plans selected. Medicare and Medicaid are administered by *Centers for Medicare and Medicaid Services (CMS)* which is an agency within the U.S. Department of Health and Human Services.

Medicare Part A. **Medicare Part A** covers hospital admission and stay, home health care, and hospice care. It has a substantial deductible and a limit to the number of hospital days per stay and the total number of hospitalizations per year. Medicare Part A pays only a portion of a patient's hospital expenses, which are calculated on a **benefit period** basis. A benefit period begins with the first day of hospital stay and ends when the patient has been out of the hospital for 60 consecutive days. Many individuals subscribe to supplemental insurance (called Medigap policies) to cover the substantial deductible.

Individuals not yet 65 years old who already receive retirement benefits from Social Security, the Railroad Retirement Board, or disability are automatically enrolled in Part A and Part B. For all other qualified individuals, Medicare becomes effective the month of their 65th birthday. Three months before their 65th birthday, or the 24th month of disability, individuals are sent an initial enrollment package containing information about Medicare and a Medicare card. If both Medicare Parts A and B are desired, they simply sign the Medicare card and keep it in a safe place for use when needed. Figure 17-4 shows a sample Medicare card.

Medicare Part B. **Medicare Part B** covers outpatient expenses that include providers' fees, physical therapy, laboratory tests, radiologic studies, ambulance services, and charges for durable medical equipment. Durable medical equipment includes items such as canes, crutches, walkers, commode chairs, blood glucose monitors, and so on. Part B does not cover medications *except* certain diabetic testing supplies. Medicare Part B requires a monthly premium, which is adjusted annually and can be dependent on income level.

Currently, the patient must pay an annual deductible of $131 before Medicare Part B will begin to pay its share of the bills. Medicare then reimburses 80% of the Medicare fee schedule

Critical Thinking

A Medicare patient has an office visit and is seen by a PAR provider. The allowed charge for the visit is $150. An insurance claim form is submitted to the local Medicare **fiscal intermediary** to apply against the deductible. At the next visit, the allowed charge is $75. This bill also is submitted to Medicare. How much of the bill will insurance pay after the deductible has been subtracted? How much does the patient owe?

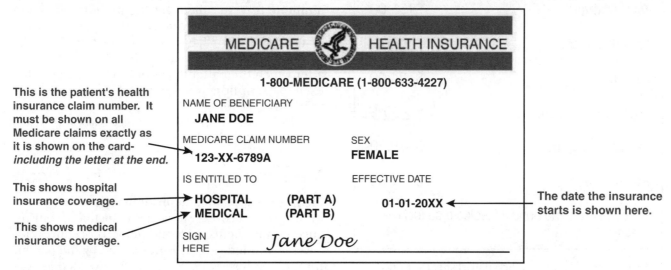

This is the patient's health insurance claim number. It must be shown on all Medicare claims exactly as it is shown on the card—*including the letter at the end.*

This shows hospital insurance coverage.

This shows medical insurance coverage.

The date the insurance starts is shown here.

Figure 17-4   Medicare health insurance card.

for medical care and 100% for laboratory fees. Medicare's fee schedule was adopted in 1992 and is based on the **resource-based relative value scale (RBRVS).** The RBRVS was developed using values for each medical and surgical procedure based on work, practice, and malpractice expenses and is factored for regional differences.

Figure 17-5 shows how the Medicare worksheet would look if there were no exclusions or deductions.

Medical service providers can elect to accept Medicare fee schedules and become a PAR, or they may accept assignment on a case-by-case basis as a nonparticipating provider (non-PAR). Billing of Medicare is done through the regional carrier that is selected by a competitive bidding process. Medical providers are required to bill Medicare as a service to the patient. The regional carrier will file claims with supplemental insurers for PARs, but non-PARs must file claims with the supplemental insurer. The patient cannot be billed for the difference between the participating provider's charges and the Medicare allowed fee. Providers can drop out of Medicare and enter into a contract with their Medicare patients that allows them to charge what they wish for services, but they must not bill Medicare for any services for the next 2 years, except in cases of emergency or urgent care.

Allowed Charges	
Office visit	$105.00
Return visit	+ 50.00
Total Charges	$155.00
Less deductible	−131.00
Subtotal	$ 24.00
Apply 80% coinsurance	x 80%
Insurance Payment	$ 19.20
Patient Owes	$ 4.80*
*In addition to the annual Medicare deductible	

Figure 17-5 Sample Medicare worksheet with no exclusions or deductions.

In the example shown in Figure 17-6, the RBRVS allowed charge is applicable to both the participating and nonparticipating provider in computing the benefits Medicare pays to the provider. However, the non-PAR provider is limited to 95% of the RBRVS allowed charge in computing the amount of coinsurance. The difference between the provider charge in the case of non-PAR, and the RBRVS allowed charge in the case of PAR provider, less the coinsurance is the amount the patient must pay. The PAR provider must write off the difference between what the provider charges for the procedure and the Medicare allowed charge as a courtesy adjustment. In the case of the non-PAR provider, the patient must pay the amount of the courtesy adjustment out of pocket in addition to the amount owed after Medicare has paid its share. This example assumes the yearly Medicare deductible has been met. The yearly deductible is the patient's responsibility to pay out of pocket.

Medicare Part C. Medicare Part C is commonly referred to as Medicare advantage plans. The plans are approved by Medicare and are run by private companies. Advantage plans provide Part A and Part B coverage and may also include Part D coverage. They require a monthly premium and may have restrictions on approved providers and hospital facilities. The medical office should always check the patient's Medicare card to verify the type of plan and effectiveness as this can affect billing procedures.

Medicare Part D. Medicare Part D offers prescription drug coverage for everyone covered by Medicare. Part D requires a monthly premium that varies depending on the plan selected. In the case of advantage plans, the cost of Part D may be administered by private companies.

Part D prescription drug coverage plans have a unique feature called the "**donut hole**" or coverage gap. All plans provide coverage until the total drug costs reach $2,400, then the patient is totally responsible for the next $3,051.25 of drug costs, after which the patient pays only a small co-pay for each prescription until the end of the calendar year. Drug coverage plans vary greatly. Selection should be based on convenience, cost, and drugs covered by the plan.

Medicare Supplemental Insurance

Medicare supplemental insurance is a secondary insurance that covers Medicare deductibles, coinsurance requirements, and additional procedures not covered by Medicare. It is purchased by the patient through an insurance carrier or is provided as part of an employee retirement package. Supplemental

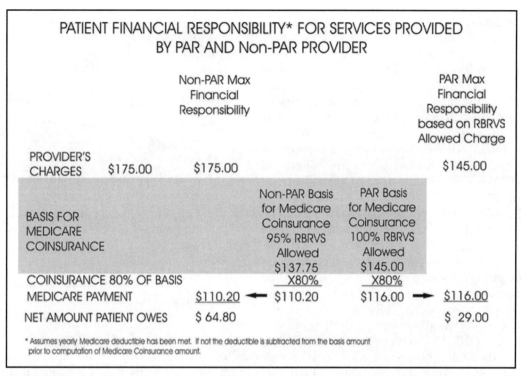

PATIENT FINANCIAL RESPONSIBILITY* FOR SERVICES PROVIDED BY PAR AND Non-PAR PROVIDER

		Non-PAR Max Financial Responsibility			PAR Max Financial Responsibility based on RBRVS Allowed Charge
PROVIDER'S CHARGES	$175.00	$175.00			$145.00
BASIS FOR MEDICARE COINSURANCE			Non-PAR Basis for Medicare Coinsurance 95% RBRVS Allowed $137.75	PAR Basis for Medicare Coinsurance 100% RBRVS Allowed $145.00	
COINSURANCE 80% OF BASIS			X80%	X80%	
MEDICARE PAYMENT		$110.20 ←	$110.20	$116.00	→ $116.00
NET AMOUNT PATIENT OWES		$ 64.80			$ 29.00

* Assumes yearly Medicare deductible has been met. If not the deductible is subtracted from the basis amount prior to computation of Medicare Coinsurance amount.

Figure 17-6 RBRVS allowed charge applicable to both the participating and the nonparticipating provider in computing the benefits Medicare pays to the provider.

Medigap policies are filed with the carrier by the Medicare regional carrier. The regional carrier is not required to file claims for employee retirement plan supplemental packages on behalf of the patient. Supplemental insurance frequently requires the patient to seek treatment with specific providers and hospitals. Different programs have different coverage, which is dependent on the carrier and state requirements and should be determined when scheduling an appointment.

Medicaid Insurance

Medicaid insurance covers medical care for certain qualifying low-income individuals. It is funded by the federal government and is administered by each state's department of Supplemental Security Income (SSI). Pregnant single women with income below the poverty level; those who cannot work because of emotional, mental, or physical difficulties; and people who are on Aid to Families with Dependent Children qualify for this program. Recipients have an identification card for the program. Not all providers accept Medicaid patients. When referring a patient to a specialist or another provider, it is wise to ascertain whether that provider accepts Medicaid patients. A referral form prepared by the PCP or referring provider usually is required.

Because Medicaid is always secondary to any supplemental insurance, billings to Medicaid are considered only after all other insurance payments have been made. When a person has both Medicare and Medicaid, charges are submitted first to Medicare and last to Medicaid.

 Both Medicare and Medicaid are federal programs, and errors in billing could be construed as fraud, for which there are criminal penalties. It is therefore imperative that all billing practices conform to the legal requirements of these programs.

TRICARE

TRICARE, formerly the Civilian Health and Medical Program for Uniformed Services (CHAMPUS), is medical insurance for active duty, activated

Critical Thinking

A patient has an office visit and is seen by a provider whose office does not accept the Medicare assignment. The charges are $150; however, the Medicare allowable amount is $100. A return office visit is charged at $90, with a Medicare allowable amount of $70. The $131 deductible has not yet been satisfied for the year. How much does the patient owe?

guard, reserves, retired members of the military, and their families and survivors. Active duty, guard, and reserve service members are automatically enrolled in TRICARE Prime. Retirees and dependents must enroll in one of the three TRICARE options: Prime, Extra, or Standard (original CHAMPUS). TRICARE Prime provides treatment mainly through military hospital facilities. TRICARE Extra provides care primarily through contracted civilian providers called *preferred providers*. TRICARE Standard provides care through traditional fee-for-service providers. Preferred providers receive a fee based on TRICARE Allowable Charges (TAC). Fee-for-service providers can charge up to 15% more than the TAC values, for which the patient is responsible. Primary care managers direct the care of TRICARE Prime and Extra patients, and referrals are required for treatment by a specialist. TRICARE Extra and Standard options usually require a deductible and co-payments. TRICARE patients are issued identification cards providing information on the type of plan in which they are enrolled. Qualifying subscribers must be listed in the Defense Department's **Defense Enrollment Eligible Reporting System (DEERS)**. The TRICARE insurance program is managed by three regional centers in the United States and by a TRICARE overseas center.

Civilian Health and Medical Program of the Veterans Administration

Civilian Health and Medical Program of the Veterans Administration (CHAMPVA) is medical insurance for spouses and unmarried dependent children of a veteran with permanent total disability resulting from a service-related injury and for the surviving spouse and children of a veteran who died of a service-related disability. The patient has an identification card for the program. The program is administered by the Health Administration Center in Denver, Colorado.

Workers' Compensation Insurance

Workers' Compensation Insurance is medical and paycheck insurance for workers who sustain injuries associated with their employment. In some instances, the insurance covers family members in the case of death of the worker. The employer usually pays the premium to the state or an insurance carrier designated by the state. Some large employers assume the insurance risk and are self-insured. Federal and state laws define minimum standards for Workers' Compensation programs. Workers' Compensation

covers 100% of associated medical expenses. Claims are filed with the insurance carrier. Although most workers are insured under state programs, federal programs exist for the following specific groups:

- Office Workers' Compensation Programs (OWCP)
- Energy Workers' Occupational Illness Compensation Program
- Federal Black Lung Program
- Federal Employees' Compensation Act Program (FECA)
- Longshore and Harbor Workers' Compensation Program
- Mine Safety and Health Administration (MSHA)

Self-Insurance

Large companies, nonprofit organizations, and governments frequently use **self-insurance** to reduce costs and gain more control of their finances. Each self-insured plan differs in coverage and claim filing requirements. The plan administrator should be contacted before scheduling a patient appointment.

Medical Tourism Insurance

Medical tourism is an unusual option being added to conventional insurance plans in an effort to control rising health care costs. It consists of health-provider networks paying the insured client to go abroad for treatment at internationally accredited hospitals. This insurance option has several potential disadvantages that may outweigh the reduced costs. Safety of blood supplies for transfusions and tissue for bone grafts are questionable in some countries, long distance travel may be dangerous to some patients, and returning patients may find it difficult to obtain follow-up care due to concerns of providers about exposure to possible malpractice lawsuits. Medical tourism options are quite new to the industry. At this time, whether it will become the new wave in insurance or will disappear from the future of insurance is uncertain.

SCREENING FOR INSURANCE

It is the responsibility of the medical assistant to screen all new patients for their insurance. New patients should be asked to arrive 15 to 20 minutes earlier than their appointment time to complete a patient registration form. The form requests vital information that enables the medical office to contact the patient, process their billing and insurance claims, know who to contact in case of emergency, authorize payment of insurance benefits, and record method of payment. Commercial forms are available for purchase or can be designed by office management personnel for this purpose.

The medical assistant should review each section of the patient registration form to verify that all information is complete and legible. Many offices make a photocopy of the patient's driver's license and attach it to the registration form. This procedure helps in identifying the correct person through photo identification should it be necessary. It is important to verify the spelling of all patient names: first, middle, and last.

Ask the patient to show his or her health insurance card and verify the effective date and pertinent information. Most offices make a photocopy of both sides of the card to maintain in the patient's chart. In most cases, the back of the card contains information about any deductible, copayment, and preapproval requirements, as well as the insurance company's name, address, and telephone number. It also shows any special claim submission instructions.

Each time a patient checks in, the medical assistant should ask questions to verify the following insurance information:

- Request DOB to establish correct patient.
- Confirm the patient's current address.
- Confirm the patient's insurance carrier and plan.
- Ask for the patient's insurance card and verify information and effective dates.
- Determine whether the insurance carrier covers the procedure.
- Determine that the patient's PCP is performing the procedure.
- Confirm whether a referral is required and whether an authorization number or authorization code is required. Confirm evidence of qualifying has been secured.
- Establish proof of eligibility.

When screening patients for insurance, it is important to understand the philosophy of the medical office. Some see patients regardless of ability to pay; responsible medical assistants will investigate all avenues for reimbursement first. Some situations include the patient who is eligible for Medicaid but has not yet applied, or the patient who has applied for Medicaid but has not yet received notification of qualification. Procedure 17-2 provides the steps for screening for insurance.

The medical assistant should investigate and verify that all avenues have been taken to achieve the proof of eligibility that the office needs to receive reimbursement from Medicaid. This may include calling the Medicaid office to verify eligibility or going online and printing a proof of eligibility directly from the Medicaid system. This electronic data exchange system is called an *envoy*. Proof of eligibility cards are distributed to recipients and are in effect for at least 1 year. However, the most common avenue to ensure that services will be reimbursed is not to see any patient who does not have proof of Medicaid coverage. Medicaid sends their eligibility Medical Assistance Identification (MAID) (medical coupons) to the patient the first day of the month. This coupon guarantees the ambulatory care center payment for the services provided. Unless it is an emergency, some offices will not schedule Medicaid patients before the fifth of each month. This allows ample time for the beneficiary to receive the medical coupon. If the patient presents for an appointment without a medical coupon, and proof of eligibility cannot be determined elsewhere, it is common practice to have that patient reschedule the appointment. The exception is an emergency.

Medical assistants with responsibility for billing are key to the success of a thriving ambulatory care center. Billing the insurance carriers promptly, completing claim forms properly, billing patients as needed, and keeping track of aging accounts will do much to ensure a flow of adequate income. In all insurance matters, be available to patients with questions regarding their insurance or accounts because a friendly attitude helps patients feel positive about the care they receive and establishes a long-term relationship.

REFERRALS AND AUTHORIZATIONS

When a PCP refers a patient to a specialist, the term **referral** is used by managed care facilities. Referrals may be denied because of incomplete information contained on the referral form or because a medical necessity was not established. Referrals are generally categorized as one of three types:

- *Regular:* Usually takes 3 to 10 working days to review procedures and approve
- *Urgent:* Usually takes about 24 hours for approval
- *STAT:* May be approved via telephone after faxing the information to the utilization review department

The most common referral used by managed care plans is the regular referral. The Member Services department must be contacted to check the status of a referral. It is important to never tell the patient that the referral has been approved until you have obtained a hard copy of the *authorization* (a managed care term for approved referrals).

Preauthorizations or *precertification* are terms used to determine whether a service or procedure is covered and if the insurance plan approves it as medically necessary. Preauthorization is required for some services, hospital admissions, inpatient and outpatient surgeries, and most elective procedures (Procedure 17-3). Once approved, an authorization number will be provided. The patient also receives a letter containing the authorization number and the approved services. The patient must present this letter to the specialist's office on the day the service is provided.

When questions arise regarding preauthorization, precertification, or referral procedures, the medical assistant should call the plan's contact number for specific information. Many offices find it helpful to maintain a reference log regarding these requirements. Information to maintain includes:

- Name of the insurance plan
- Address and telephone number
- Name and telephone number of contact person or the person with whom you spoke
- Co-payment amount and deductible information
- Inpatient and outpatient surgery benefits
- Preauthorization requirements, second-opinion options
- Participating hospitals, radiology service providers, laboratories, and physicians

The authorization number and referral numbers are entered in Box 23 of the CMS-1500 form when billing for services.

DETERMINING FEE SCHEDULES

A provider charges for services using a variety of means for computing a fee schedule. Although all of the fee computation plans vary and give somewhat different results, they all have common elements. For example,

- *The overhead or practice expenses for the clinic or office.* This category includes rental of the physical building or office space and equipment; utilities; cost of medical supplies inventory; and salaries of nurses, medical assistants, bookkeepers, and other personnel who are paid on a salary or contract basis. It also includes cost of employee benefits such as retirement plans, sick leave, and vacation time.

- *The cost of medical malpractice insurance.* This is separated from general insurance, which is included in the preceding category, because of the significant portion of the fee attributed to this item and because it varies greatly for different types of services. OB/GYN procedures are probably the greatest for the entire medical community, including surgical procedures.

- *Hourly rate for the services provided by the provider.* This rate varies depending on the skill and training required for the procedure, the cost of living in the area, and the rate charged by other providers in the area. (The law of supply and demand applies here as in any other economic arena.) Surgeons charge a greater rate than providers in general practice, rates are greater in a metropolitan area than in a rural area, and experience level commands greater rates.

All of these cost elements are derived on an hourly basis. The sum of the above elements combined with the time required is used to arrive at the fee schedule for a procedure or service.

The advent of insurance plans, Medicare, and managed care plans has resulted in specific formulas being developed and accepted by the different plans to establish a fee schedule acceptable to the carrier. Several of the fee schedule systems in common usage are discussed in the following sections. All of them, however, incorporate the preceding three elements (practice expenses, malpractice expenses, and provider's experience).

Usual, Customary, and Reasonable Fees

Usual, Customary, and Reasonable (UCR) fee schedule is a fee system that defines allowable charges that will be accepted by insurance carriers. The actual rate may vary from one carrier to another, but the process is the same.

- Usual fee is the provider's average fee for a service or procedure. This fee is based on the economic analysis of the practice described earlier in this section.
- Customary fee is the average or range of fees within the geographic area that an insurance carrier will accept. It is frequently tied to a national average for a similar metropolitan or rural setting.

- Reasonable fee is the generally accepted fee for services or procedures that are extraordinarily difficult or complicated and require more time and effort by the provider.

An example of the operation of the UCR system is as follows. An insurance carrier operating on the UCR fee schedule may have determined a customary fee range for a new patient office visit with history and physical examination to be $140 to $225 for that region. If the amount billed by the provider were $160, the provider would be reimbursed for the service in full. Had the provider billed $250, the reimbursement would be $225, and the provider would have to write off the $25 nonallowed charge. The amount the provider would have to write off is often referred to as an **adjustment**. Providers who participate in UCR systems cannot bill the patient for the nonallowable charge.

Resource-Based Relative Value Scale (RBRVS)

Medicare has used the RBRVS since 1992. Under this system, provider's services are reimbursed based on relative value units (RVUs). Each service, procedure, or medication is assigned a code compiled from the *Current Procedural Terminology* (CPT) manual issued by the American Medical Association for procedures and the *International Classification of Diseases, 9th Revision, Clinical Modification* (ICD-9-CM) manual for diagnoses issued by the World Health Organization. Medicare then issues three RVUs for each code in the *Medicare Fee Schedule* (MFS) manual issued each year. The RVUs are for provider's work, practice expenses, and malpractice expenses. The practice expense is further differentiated based on location, that is, whether the work was done in a hospital (facility)

or in a clinic or office (nonfacility). The nonfacility practice expense further differentiates between whether the nonfacility is transitioned or fully implemented. A geographic practice cost index (GPCI) related to the geographic area where the provider is located is issued for each RVU category. The GPCI is based on zip code for the address of the practice or wherever the service is performed. The payment for service is then established from the sum of the geographically adjusted RVUs multiplied by a nationally uniform conversion factor for services. The complex formula calculation is given in Table 17-2. RBRVS units and formula for payment are subject to frequent changes. The prudent medical assistant will verify that they have current information.

Hospital Inpatient Prospective Payment System (IPPS)

The IPPS is a reimbursement system for hospitals based on similar diagnostically related groups (DRGs) of inpatients discharged. Rather than the traditional method of payment based on actual costs incurred in providing care, DRGs are based on an average cost for treatment of a patient's condition. The hospital is reimbursed for each discharge according to a predetermined rate for each DRG.

Hospital Outpatient Prospective Payment System (OPPS)

OPPS is a reimbursement system for hospital outpatients, certain Part B services furnished to hospital inpatients who have no Part A coverage, and partial hospitalization services furnished by community mental health centers. All services are classified into groups called Ambulatory Payment Classifications (APCs). Payments are established

Table 17-2 Medicare Formula for Payment of Services

Code	Description of Procedure	Factor	Work	Practice Expense (PE)	Malpractice (MP)
38206	Stem cell collection @ transitioned nonfacility	RVU	1.5	0.61	0.07
		GPCI 2007 (King County, Seattle, WA)	1.014	1.109	.755

Budget Neutrality Adjuster (BNA) = 0.8806
RVU Conversion Factor (CF) for 2008 = $38.0870
Medicare Allowable = MA
MA = [(RVU$_{work}$ × BNA)* × GPCI$_{work}$ + RVU$_{PE}$ × GPCI$_{PE}$ + RVU$_{MP}$ × GPCI$_{MP}$] × RVU CF
MA = [(1.5 × 0.8806)* × 1.014 + 0.61 × 1.109 + 0.07 × 0.755] × $38.0870 = $78.76
*Rounded to two decimal places. 1.32

Critical Thinking

The purpose of this exercise is to understand how to determine the provider's fee by two different methods: (1) RVU calculations, and (2) looking it up in tables provided by the regional Medicare carrier. Determination of procedure codes used in this exercise is explained in this chapter. Use the following factors to calculate the provider's fee billed to Medicare.

METHOD 1

Factor Procedure Code 11401	Work	Practice or Facility Overhead	Malpractice	Conversion Factor
RVU*	1.25	2.12	0.10	38.0870
GCPI†	1.014	1.109	0.755	0.8806

*Procedure performed in a transitioned nonfacility.
†Values of GCPI for King County, Seattle, Washington, 2008.

METHOD 2

Using the Internet:

- Go to the home page of the regional carrier: http://www.noridianmedicare.com.
- Select: Washington Part B.
- Accept End User Agreement for Providers.
- Go to: News/Publications and Select: Fee Schedules.
- Select year: 2008.
- Select: 2008 Medicare Physician Fee Schedule (MPFS).
- Select: Washington – Locality 02 and desired file format PDF.
- Find procedure code 11401 in the table. (Do not use the code with the # sign as it is designated for a procedure performed in a facility).

Alternate Internet site using HCPC codes (interchangeable with CPT codes).

- Go to www.cms.hhs.gov/PFSlookup/.
- Select: Physicians Fee Schedule.
- Accept license agreement.
- Select year: 2008, Single HCPC Code, and Pricing Information.
- Select: Specific Locality and Default Fields
- Enter HCPC Code 11401.
- Select: All Modifiers and Locality (Seattle, King County).
- Click: Submit.
- Scroll down for answer.

The fee generated using either Web site (Method 2) should be the same as the fee calculated using Method 1.

for each APC, and the hospital is reimbursed for each patient. Depending on the services provided, hospitals may be paid for more than one APC for an encounter.

Capitation

Capitation is a payment system used primarily by managed care organizations. A fixed dollar amount is reimbursed to the provider for patients enrolled during a specific period. The payment per patient is independent of services or procedures provided to a patient. To be financially responsible, this system requires enrollment of a large number of patients so that a few patients do not unduly skew an average cost. This type of system requires extensive practice of preventative medicine to be cost effective. Procedure 17-4 provides steps for computing the Medicare allowable few schedule.

LEGAL AND ETHICAL ISSUES

Most Medicare claims are now required to be submitted electronically, and private payers in growing numbers are also using electronic claims submission. In a computerized system, everything related to billing and reimbursement is computerized and transmitted electronically. If the office is participating in CMS's Electronic Data Interchange (EDI), it will be assigned a unique identifier number that constitutes its legal electronic signature. Be cautious with this electronic signature, because the office is responsible for any and all claims made with it. The Health Insurance Portability and Accountability Act (HIPAA) of 1996 (specifically title II, subtitle F) regulates the security and privacy of transmitted health care information. Review HIPAA's regulations in Chapters 11 and 15.

Many legal and ethical issues related to insurance issues face the medical assistant on a daily basis; therefore, it is important that each patient be treated equally and fairly. As mentioned in Chapter 4, it is critical that patients not be stereotyped, regardless of whether they have multiple insurance plans or are not covered by any insurance plan at all. Every patient must be cared for objectively, with respect, and in a professional manner.

Medical personnel are bound by law to maintain the confidentiality of all medical information and must be able to recognize information that is protected by privacy rules and understand how it is to be handled. Protected health information (PHI) may be considered "individually identifiable health information." This includes information that describes the health status of an individual, including basic demographics and the use of medical services, as well as information that either identifies or can be used to identify an individual. Medical personnel must remember that informed consent is not consent to use and disclose personal information.

HIPAA Implications

HIPAA privacy requirements specifically address issues of confidentiality. These requirements include:

- Providing the patient with a notice of privacy protocols form that outlines a provider's privacy practices, and obtaining the patient's acknowledgment of receipt of the notice

- Obtaining a patient's specific authorization to use or disclose personal information for purposes that are not covered by the consent

- Providing the patient, on request, with an accounting of disclosures of PHI

- Giving the patient access to his or her PHI and providing an opportunity to amend the information

HIPAA regulations apply to PHI that is created, transmitted, received, or stored in an electronic form. The federal regulation uses the phrase "electronic PHI." Four legal obligations defined by the security rule under federal law for medical practices that are covered entities include:

- Ensure the confidentiality, integrity, and availability of electronic PHI.

- Protect against any reasonably anticipated threats or hazards to the security or integrity of such information.

- Protect against any reasonably anticipated uses or disclosures of such information that are not permitted or required by law.

- Ensure compliance with this subpart by its workforce.

One technical exception is verbal information that is transmitted in a telephone call or printed information that is faxed over a telephone line. In both cases, the information is being transmitted electronically, but it was not in electronic form before being transmitted. If the information transmitted by voice or fax was produced from information that was stored electronically, it is subject to the security rule. The security rule establishes obligations for medical practices that include:

- Complying with the security standards, including all "required" implementation specifications and all "addressable" implementation specifications to the extent that they apply to the medical practice.

- Reviewing and modifying security measures as needed to ensure the continued "reasonable and appropriate" protection of electronic PHI.

- Including provisions in business associate contracts that ensure the security of electronic PHI the business associate creates, receives, maintains, or transmits on behalf of the provider.

- Implementing reasonable and appropriate policies and procedures to comply with the standards, implementation specifications, and other requirements of the security rule.

- Documenting the policies and procedures implemented to comply with the security requirements—including any action, activity, or assessment the standards require to be documented.

Insurance Fraud and Abuse

 Insurance **fraud** and **abuse** may be involved in more than 10% of submitted medical claims according to the Insurance Information Institute. These estimates include both intentional as well as accidental coding and billing irregularities and, if detected and proven, can result in legal action against the practice or clinic and personnel responsible for or having knowledge of the irregularities. Personnel involved in coding and billing should be alert for both accidental and intentional coding and billing irregularities and bring them to the attention of responsible managers. If no corrective action is taken, they are legally responsible to report the irregularities to the insurance carrier. Examples of fraudulent insurance activities include but are not limited to:

- Coding to a higher level of service to increase revenue
- Misrepresenting the diagnosis to justify payment
- Billing for services, equipment, or procedures that were never provided
- Charging uninsured patients less than insured patients
- Receiving rebates or any type of compensation for referrals

Insurance abuse involves activities that are inconsistent with accepted business practices. Some examples of abuse include but are not limited to:

- Charging for services that are not medically necessary
- Overcharging for services, equipment, or procedures
- Improper billing practices
- Violating participating provider agreements with insurance companies

Heavy penalties, including a $10,000 fine per claim form plus three times the fraudulent claim amount, may be sanctioned on individuals who knowingly and willfully misrepresent information submitted on insurance claim forms to gain greater payments or benefits.

To protect yourself and the medical practice from committing insurance fraud and abuse, you should begin by identifying risk areas based on

errors in the past history of billing and insurance claims processing. Practice internal audits to monitor compliance with written protocols. Participate in seminars and in-service programs to keep current with coding and billing practices. Be sure to use only the current year's coding manuals to ensure accuracy. Code only what is documented in the medical record, and ask for clarification when needed.

PROFESSIONAL CAREERS IN INSURANCE

 To be successful in the field of health insurance specialists, training and entry-level requirements are essential. An opportunity for employment in these specialties is greater for those with a college degree that includes coursework in medical terminology, anatomy and physiology, pharmacology, insurance and coding procedures, and communication skills.

Personal attributes that enhance employment possibilities as health insurance specialists include, but are not limited to, the following: self-motivated, works well independently, detail oriented, a critical thinker, ethical, maintains confidentiality, cooperative, reliable, and adaptable.

The following Internet links will help you explore a variety of health insurance specialist career opportunities.

- American Academy of Professional Coders (AAPC) at http://www.aapc.com
- American Health Information Management Association (AHIMA) at http://www.ahima.org
- American Medical Billing Association (AMBA) at http://www.ambanet.net
- National Association of Claims Assistance Professionals (NACAP) at http://www.medicalcodingandbilling.com
- National Electronic Billers Alliance (NEBA) at http://www.nebazone.com

Procedure 17-1

Applying Managed Care Policies and Procedures

PURPOSE:

To apply managed care policies and procedures that the provider and/or medical facility has partnership agreements with.

EQUIPMENT/SUPPLIES:

Managed care contracts
Managed care policies and procedures manuals
Patient record
Authorized forms from managed care organizations
Clerical supplies

PROCEDURE STEPS:

1. Determine which managed care organization the patient has contracted with. RATIONALE: To ensure that the correct policies and procedures are applied to the correct organization.

2. Contact the insurance carrier(s) via telephone to:

   a. verify the patient has insurance in effect and is eligible for benefits

   b. confirm any exclusions or noncovered services

   c. determine deductibles, co-payments, or any other out-of-pocket expenses that the patient is responsible for paying

   d. ask if preauthorization is required for referrals to specialists or for any procedures and/or services. RATIONALE: Ascertains that insurance is viable and what benefits and patient expenses are established within the contract.

3. Record the name, title, and telephone number and extension of the insurance person contacted. RATIONALE: Documents the name of the individual providing the information. If questions arise at a later date, a contact is readily available.

4. Collect any forms necessary to process the patient claims. RATIONALE: Submitting correct forms to managed care organization expedites the process.

5. Document the information collected in the patient's medical record and on the Verification of Eligibility and Benefits form. RATIONALE: Provides a record of what has taken place.

6. Attend seminars and workshops offered by managed care organization or in-service training sessions. RATIONALE: Promotes obtaining up-to-date information regarding managed care policies and procedures.

Procedure 17-2

Screening for Insurance

PURPOSE:

To verify insurance coverage and obtain vital information required for processing and billing insurance claim forms.

EQUIPMENT/SUPPLIES:

Patient registration forms
Clipboard and black ink pen
Patient's chart

PROCEDURE STEPS:

1. When scheduling the first appointment, ask the patient to bring his or her insurance card and to arrive 15 to 20 minutes before the appointment time to complete the patient registration form. RATIONALE: The insurance card is required to verify effective dates and pertinent information relative to insurance coverage. The registration

continues

form also requests vital information necessary for patient care and insurance billing.

2. When the patient turns in the completed registration form, review it immediately to be sure that all information has been collected and that it is legible. RATIONALE: It is important that all information has been included on the registration form and that the medical assistant can read it clearly when processing the insurance claim forms. If information is omitted from the claim form or is incorrect, the insurance carrier may deny the claim.

3. Ask the patient for his or her insurance card and make a photocopy of both sides of the card to be maintained in the patient's chart. RATIONALE: The insurance card provides vital information, including correct spelling of patient's name, insurance plan numbers, effective dates, telephone numbers to call regarding referrals and preauthorizations, and information about any deductible and co-payment.

4. Verify proof of eligibility for Medicaid patients. The patient should have his or her proof of eligibility card with him or her, or you may need to make a telephone call directly to Medicaid or use the online electronic data exchange system to determine proof of eligibility. RATIONALE: This information is required for Medicaid reimbursement.

5. Each time a patient checks in, whether established or new, the following information should be verified:

- Address. Confirm the patient's current address and telephone number. RATIONALE: Patients may have moved and may not realize they had not reported their new address and telephone number to the office.

- Verify insurance coverage. RATIONALE: This information is required for correct claims processing and billing procedures.

- Ask for the patient's insurance card and verify information and effective dates. Also be sure that a photocopy of the card is maintained in the patient's chart. RATIONALE: This is a means of keeping insurance records current for billing purposes.

- Determine whether the insurance carrier covers the procedure. RATIONALE: If the carrier does not cover the procedure, reimbursement will need to come from a third party or the patient.

- Determine that the patient's PCP is performing the procedure. RATIONALE: This information is needed for reimbursement purposes.

- Determine whether a referral is required and whether an authorization number or code is needed. RATIONALE: Reimbursement by the carrier cannot take place without the proper documentation and authorization number.

- Confirm that evidence of qualifying has been secured. RATIONALE: Proof of eligibility must be verified for reimbursement from Medicaid.

Procedure 17-3

Obtaining Referrals and Authorizations

PURPOSE:
To ascertain coverage by the insurance carrier for specific medical services, hospital admissions, inpatient or outpatient surgeries, elective procedures, or when the PCP elects to refer the patient to another provider.

EQUIPMENT/SUPPLIES:
Patient's medical chart and copy of his or her insurance card
Name and telephone number of the contact person for the carrier
Completed referral form
Telephone/fax machine
Pen/pencil

continues

PROCEDURE STEPS:

1. Collect all necessary documents and equipment (patient's chart/record, insurance carrier's information and telephone number). RATIONALE: Allows for efficient use of time in acquiring the referral or authorization.

2. Determine the service or procedure requiring preauthorization. You will also need to know the name and telephone number of the specialist involved and the reason the request is being sought. RATIONALE: This information is required to complete the referral form to obtain authorization from the patient's insurance carrier.

3. Complete the referral form, being sure to include all pertinent information. RATIONALE:

The request may be denied if all information has not been included.

4. Proofread the completed form. RATIONALE: Because of the importance of this step, accuracy is critical.

5. Fax the completed form to the insurance carrier. RATIONALE: It appraises the carrier of the patient's medical condition, requests preauthorization for treatment, requests a verification or authorization number, and confirms the treatment plan.

6. Maintain a completed copy of the referral form in the patient's chart. RATIONALE: The form can be accessed in the future should questions arise.

Procedure 17-4

Computing the Medicare Fee Schedule

PURPOSE:
To compute the Medicare allowable (MA) payment for services.

EQUIPMENT/SUPPLIES:
CPT book
Computer
Calculator

PROCEDURE STEPS:

1. Using the *Current Procedural Terminology* (CPT) book, obtain the CPT code for the exact procedure or service for which a fee schedule is being computed. RATIONALE: Accurate code must be obtained to ensure correct billing.

2. Using the Medicare Fee Schedule, which is issued each year, determine the relative value units for (a) provider's time (work), (b) practice expense (PE), and (c) costs of malpractice insurance (MP) listed for the CPT code in Step 1. These factors represent the relative amount of a fee allocated to each item.

3. Using the Medicare Fee Schedule, determine the geographic practice cost index (GPCI). This factor accounts for different cost of living values for urban versus rural and geographic locations in the United States.

4. Using the Medicare Fee Schedule, determine the Budget Neutrality Adjuster (BNA). This number is a factor that attempts to reduce Medicare fees to match the amount budgeted by Congress.

5. Using the Medicare Fee Schedule, determine the relative value unit (RVU) conversion factor (CF). This factor converts RVU units to dollars based on an average for the entire United States.

6. Compute the Medicare allowable fee for the procedure or service using the following equation:

$$MA = [(RVU_{work} \times BNA)* \times GPCI_{work} + RVU_{PE} \times GPCI_{PE} + RVU_{MP} \times GPCI_{MP}] \times CF$$

*Round product of numbers to two decimal places.

Case Study 17-1

Review the scenario at the beginning of the chapter.

CASE STUDY REVIEW

1. Identify ways that Jane O'Hara, CMA (AAMA), can stay abreast of policy changes regarding reimbursement.
2. List options for Jane to take in order to be up to date with insurance coverage in order to help patients understand their responsibility, if any, for payment.
3. Recall steps for screening patients for insurance. Why is this so important?

Case Study 17-2

Jane O'Hara, CMA (AAMA), is responsible for all patient insurance billing procedures. Jane has the following information:

	Total Charges	Allowed Charges
Office visit	$100.00	$90.00
Return visit	$70.00	$65.00

Deductible has not been satisfied.

CASE STUDY REVIEW

1. Calculate the patient's correct billing if the provider accepts assignment.
2. Calculate the patient's correct billing if the provider does not accept assignment.

DOCUMENTATION

Documentation must support all claims submitted. Failure to document a service translates into nonperformance of that service from the perspectives of quality patient care, legal safeguards, and reimbursement issues. In other words, a deed not documented is a deed not done ————————

SUMMARY

An understanding of medical insurance terminology and various types of coverage is vital to a thriving ambulatory care setting. The astute medical assistant will perceive the challenges involved in understanding his or her role in the management of medical office insurance. The medical assistant must be able to explain insurance procedures to the patient and know how to make contact with appropriate representatives to determine eligibility and coverage questions.

STUDY FOR SUCCESS

To reinforce your knowledge and skills of information presented in this chapter:

- Review the Key Terms
- Practice the Procedures
- Consider the Case Studies and discuss your conclusions
- Answer the Review Questions
  ○ Multiple Choice
  ○ Critical Thinking
- Navigate the Internet by completing the Web Activities
- Practice the StudyWARE activities on the textbook CD
- Apply your knowledge in the Student Workbook activities
- Complete the Web Tutor sections
- View and discuss the DVD situations

REVIEW QUESTIONS

Multiple Choice

1. The most common avenue to ensure that services will be reimbursed is:
   a. not see any patient who does not have proof of Medicaid coverage
   b. complete an envoy
   c. go online and print a proof of eligibility directly from the system
   d. ask patients if they are covered
2. The most common insurance claim form is the:
   a. UB92 form
   b. ICD-9-CM
   c. CMS-1500 (08-05) form
   d. CPT
3. Medicare:
   a. was created by Title 19 of the Social Security Act
   b. covers most persons 65 years and older
   c. is designed to cover prescriptions
   d. is handled separately by each state
4. If the RBRVS allowable is $150 and the deductible has not been met, Medicare will pay:
   a. $20
   b. $40
   c. $120
   d. 80% of RBRVS allowable after $131 deductible
5. There are _____ primary MCO models operating across the country.
   a. four
   b. three
   c. six
   d. eight

6. Medicaid insurance:
   a. is funded by the federal government and administered by each state's department of SSI
   b. requires a Medigap policy
   c. consists of Part A, Part B, Part C, and Part D
   d. requires PARs to accept assignment
7. BC/BS:
   a. are locally based in all 50 states in the United States
   b. operate like MCOs
   c. recognize Medicare Part B
   d. are part of CHAMPVA
8. TRICARE:
   a. is part of CHAMPVA
   b. is part of OWCP, MSHA, and FECA programs
   c. is a self-insurance program
   d. was formerly the Civilian Health and Medical Program for Uniformed Services

Critical Thinking

1. When children of married parents are covered under both parents' policies, how is the birthday rule used to determine which policy is primary?
2. Your Medicare patient has an office visit with a $200 provider's charge ($150 RBRVS allowable) and a follow-up visit with a $100 provider's charge ($75 RBRVS allowable). Your provider–employer does not accept assignment. This is the first visit of the calendar year and the Medicare deductible has not been satisfied. How will you determine the amount owed by the patient?

3. You are the medical assistant working the front desk and one of your responsibilities is to screen patients for insurance. What questions will you ask when collecting these data, and how will you word each question so that accurate information is received from the patient?

4. An established patient is seen by the provider today, who determines that a liver scan is necessary to determine a diagnosis. You must ascertain if this procedure is a covered benefit, determine what the payment rate will be by the carrier, and secure preapproval if necessary. How will you go about collecting this information?

5. You must establish proof of eligibility for a patient. How will you go about doing this?

WEB ACTIVITIES

Mr. Jones is in reasonably good health and incurs drug expenses less than $1,000 per year. Review the Medicare drug plans for your area and select the optimum plan for Mr. Jones. If his prescription drug costs increased to $1,800 per year, how would this change the plan selection? (Visit http://www.medicare.gov on the Internet and select "Compare" under "Prescription Drug Plans.")

REFERENCES/BIBLIOGRAPHY

Green, M. A. (2007). *3-2-1 Code It!* Clifton Park, NY: Delmar Cengage Learning.

Green, M. A., & Rowell, J. C. (2006). *Understanding health insurance: A guide to billing and reimbursement* (8th ed.). Clifton Park, NY: Delmar Cengage Learning.

ingenix. (2003). *HIPAA tool kit.* Salt Lake City, UT: St. Anthony Publishing/Medicode.

Moisio, M. A. (2006). *A guide to health insurance billing* (2nd ed.). Clifton Park, NY: Delmar Cengage Learning.

Medical Insurance Coding

KEY TERMS

Bundled Codes

Claim Register

CMS-1500 (08-05)

**Current Procedural
Terminology (CPT)**

Down-coding

E Codes

Encounter Form

**Explanation of Benefits
(EOB)**

**Healthcare Common
Procedure Coding
System (HCPCS)**

**International Classification
of Diseases, 9th Revision,
Clinical Modification
(ICD-9-CM)**

M Codes

Modifier

**Point-of-Service
(POS) Device**

Unbundling Codes

Uniform Bill 04 (UB-04)

Up-coding

V Codes

OUTLINE

OBJECTIVES

*The student should strive to meet the following performance objectives and
demonstrate an understanding of the facts and principles presented in this
chapter through written and oral communication.*

1. Define the key terms as presented in the glossary.

2. Define terminology necessary to understand and code medical
   insurance claim forms.

3. Understand the process of procedure and diagnosis coding.

4. Code a sample claim form.

5. Discuss third-party guidelines.

6. Recognize common errors in completing insurance claim
   forms.

7. Explain the difference between the CMS-1500 (08-05) and the
   UB-04 forms.

OBJECTIVES (continued)

8. Describe the way computers have altered the claims process.

9. Discuss why claims follow-up is important to the ambulatory care setting.

10. Discuss legal and ethical issues related to coding and insurance claims processing.

Scenario

At Inner City Health Care, a multiprovider urgent care center in a large city, medical assistant Jane O'Hara, CMA (AAMA), is responsible for all patient billing procedures, including insurance claim forms. Jane stresses with her assistants the fact that coding is the basis for information exchanged between the health care providers and various agencies that compile health care statistics as well as third-party payers for health care services rendered to patients. Understanding medical terminology, anatomy, physiology, and how to code medical procedures and diagnoses accurately is a must. Using the computer to complete insurance forms, while considering common errors that may lead to denial of a claim, and transmitting the claims electronically are reviewed during in-service meetings. Jane emphasizes that accurate coding must always reflect services actually performed and documented within the patient's chart.

INTRODUCTION

Coding is the basis for the information on the claim form. Medical coding is mandatory for the accurate transmission of procedures and diagnosis information between health care providers and various agencies that compile health care statistics and the insurance companies that act as third-party payers for health care services rendered to patients. To code accurately, the medical assistant must have a good understanding of medical terminology, especially of those medical specialties found in the ambulatory care setting.

The use of computers to generate the insurance claim form and to transmit the form to the third-party payer is commonplace today. Computers are able to compute and compare numbers only. Letters that are in a sequence, such as the alphabet, are able to be compared as to their relativity to each other. For instance, A comes before B in the alphabet, thus a computer can compare those two values. For that reason, all charges, patient accounts, insurances, diagnoses and procedures, and even various categories are assigned letters or numbers (alphanumeric). The letters/numbers assigned to diagnoses and procedures (services) are called insurance codes. People whose jobs are to check accuracy of insurance codes and assign billing parameters (such as code modifiers) are called medical coders. (See Professional Careers in Insurance section at the end of Chapter 17 for more information).

INSURANCE CODING SYSTEMS OVERVIEW

The process of translating written or spoken description of diseases, injuries, medical procedures, services, and supplies into numeric or alphanumeric format is called *coding*. The following coding systems are used within the United States and throughout most of the world:

- **Current Procedural Terminology (CPT)** system was developed by the American Medical Association (AMA) to convert commonly accepted descriptions of medical procedures into a five-digit numeric code with two-digit numeric **modifiers** when required. This system is used to code medical procedures.

- **Healthcare Common Procedure Coding Sysytem (HCPCS)** was developed by Medicare as a supplement to the CPT system for procedures not defined with sufficient specificity. This system uses a five-digit alphanumeric code with an additional two-digit modifier if required.

- **International Classification of Diseases, 9th Revision, Clinical Modification (ICD-9-CM)** system was developed by the World Health Organization (WHO) to classify all known diseases to assist in maintaining statistical records of morbidity (sickness) and mortality (death). Although not originally designed as a reimbursement system, it has been adopted in the United States for this purpose. This system is used for both diagnostic and procedure coding. The current ICD-9-CM code consists of a three-digit code with one or two numeric modifiers. The modifiers are separated from the three-digit code by a decimal point. The document is revised periodically and is updated yearly. The book is in its ninth revision. As of January 2009 the 10th revision is in final draft. Implementation will be based on the process for adoption of standards under HIPAA 1996. A 2-year implementation window will be provided once the final notice to implement has been published in the Federal Register. The 10th revision will use alphanumeric codes consisting of up to seven characters. This format results in much more detailed description of medical conditions and increases the number of codes by nearly a factor of five.

CODING OF MEDICAL PROCEDURES

When billing, medical assistants are expected to adhere to ethical standards and legal practices. All codes reported must be supported by documentation in the patient chart. Understanding medical terminology, anatomy, physiology, and procedures is critical to coding accuracy. It is also important to maintain coding skills by attending Continuing Education activities that discuss changes in codes and present guidelines and regulation requirements necessary for accurate coding. Networking with other medical coders is another valuable method of staying current with what is happening in this profession.

CPT Manual Organization and Use

The CPT manual, issued every October, is used to code medical procedures and services of all kinds—office, hospital, nursing facility, and home services. The current volume, which is the fourth edition, is divided into seven sections that are discussed in the following paragraphs.

To determine the CPT code, turn to the Category I section of the CPT codebook and select one of the sections that constitutes the general classification of the procedure being coded (e.g., Surgery, Radiology, etc). Then select the name of the procedure or service that accurately identifies what you are looking for. Do not select a CPT code that only approximately defines the service performed. If you cannot find a name that exactly defines the service provided, report the service using the appropriate unlisted code. Unlisted codes are found at the end of each subsection in the CPT codebook. The five-digit code for unlisted services end in 99. When using an unlisted code, a special report must be submitted with an insurance claim form to avoid denial or rejection. Unlisted codes should not be used if a Category III code is available. This section is found in the back of the codebook and gives temporary codes for emerging technologies, services, and procedures. The 2007 edition of the CPT codebook provides codes for the treatment of patients with the tools of the virtual office (communication with the patient via the Internet).

HIPAA

Under HIPAA, a code set is any set of codes used for encoding data elements that may include but is not limited to the following medical categories: tables of terms, medical concepts, medical diagnoses, and medical procedures. Nonmedical code sets may be used to define state abbreviations, provider specialty, and remittance remarks to explain adjustments on a remittance.

Evaluation and Management. The Evaluation and Management section takes every possible combination of visits into consideration and assigns each its own number. For instance, Mary O'Keefe, a new patient, is seen for a period of 45 minutes during which the provider takes a detailed history, examines the patient, and makes a medical decision of moderate complexity. The CPT code for this visit (99204) is found by looking under office services, new patient, time and service provided. In another instance, Abigail Johnson, an established patient, is seen in the hospital for several days. These visits (99231, 99232, or 99233) would be found under hospital services, subsequent hospital care, and the time and service provided. Codes for any type of evaluation or management are found in this section. In many offices, the provider determines the level or charge for visits; however, the medical assistant must be familiar with all of the codes to make certain that billings are correct and that codes match the provider's documentation.

Anesthesia. The Anesthesia section includes all codes for anesthesia required for any procedure. The codes begin with the head and continue down the body to the legs and feet, concluding with anesthesia for radiologic procedures. If you want to find the correct code for anesthesia during a total hip replacement, you will find "Anesthesia" in the index, look for "hip" and refer to the codes listed: 01200–01215. When you refer back to the Anesthesia section, you find:

01200	Anesthesia for all closed procedures involving hip joint
01202	Anesthesia for arthroscopic procedures of hip joint
01210	Anesthesia for open procedures involving hip joint; not otherwise specified
01212	hip disarticulation
01214	total hip arthroplasty
01215	revision of total hip arthroplasty

As you read through the codes, you see that the correct code is 01214.

Surgery. The section on Surgery divides codes according to system. It begins with the skin, subcutaneous and areolar tissues, and continues through subsequent systems ending with ocular and auditory systems. The codes are very specific. For instance, a simple laceration repair is found as:

12001	Simple repair of superficial wounds of scalp, neck, axillae, external genitalia, trunk and/or extremities (including hands and feet): 2.5 cm or less
12002	2.6 cm to 7.5 cm
12004	7.6 cm to 12.5 cm
12005	12.6 cm to 20.0 cm
12006	20.1 cm to 30.0 cm
12007	over 30.0 cm

Thus, the exact length of the laceration and complexity of repair can be found and coded correctly on the claim form.

Radiology, Nuclear Medicine, and Diagnostic Ultrasound. Coding in the Radiology section covers each procedure done and each specific alteration to the procedure. For instance,

75889	Hepatic venography, wedged or free, with hemodynamic evaluation, radiological supervision, and interpretation
75891	Hepatic venography, wedged or free, without hemodynamic evaluation, radiological supervision, and interpretation

Radiologic procedures are not often done in the provider's office, although they may be in larger urgent care centers. Occasionally, chest X-rays are done or, in an orthopedic specialty, many skeletal X-rays may be done. More often, though, radiologic studies are ordered by the provider through a local facility that bills the insurance company directly, using the diagnosis the provider has provided.

Pathology and Laboratory. The Pathology and Laboratory section includes every test and combination of laboratory tests that can be ordered, as well as a section on surgical pathology. This latter section includes specimens sent for examination, such as Pap smears, analysis of biopsy tissue from surgical sites, and tissue typing. Following is an example of a laboratory procedure code for hepatitis B that illustrates the complete selection of tests that may be ordered:

87340	Hepatitis B surface antigen (HBsAg)

86704 Hepatitis B core antibody
(HBcAb); total

86705   IgM antibody

86706 Hepatitis B surface antibody
(HBsAb)

87350 Hepatitis Be antigen (HBeAg)

86707 Hepatitis Be antibody (HBeAb)

The medical assistant should be aware of laboratory codes because when a laboratory test is ordered, the laboratory may call to clarify the order. If the coding is correct, the laboratory should have no questions.

For surgical pathology, the codes are different. The level of examination for the item determines the code. The provider usually determines these levels or the charge for these services.

Medicine. The section of the CPT entitled Medicine includes codings for immunizations, injections, dialysis, allergen immunotherapy, and chemotherapy, as well as ophthalmologic, cardiovascular, pulmonary, and neurological procedures, to name a few. As in the earlier sections, there is a comprehensive breakdown of each procedure. Under Cardiography, for example:

93000 Electrocardiogram, routine ECG
with at least 12 leads; with interpretation and report

93005 tracing only, without interpretation and report

93010 interpretation and report only

Under Chemotherapy Administration:

96409 Chemotherapy administration, intravenous, push technique

96413 infusion technique, up to one hour

+96415 infusion technique, one to eight hours, each additional hour

96416 infusion technique, initiation of prolonged infusion (more than eight hours), requiring the use of a portable or implantable pump

The plus symbol before the CPT code indicates that the procedure is an add-on to a previously described procedure. For example, 96413 would be used to describe the service and the time administered up to 1 hour. Anything longer than 1 hour would be listed as +96415 for each additional 1 hour administration took place.

Index. The final portion of the CPT codebook is a comprehensive index listing every procedure alphabetically. The proper use of the CPT involves looking for the procedure in the index and then checking the number given to determine the precise code.

Each code found in the CPT has five numeric digits. Note that there are no letter codes and no decimal points in these codes. Each five-digit code stands for a specific procedure not duplicated elsewhere.

Modifiers

Occasionally, a service or procedure needs to be modified. In that case, there are two-digit alphanumeric modifiers that can be applied to the five-digit code. These modifiers can indicate unusual procedural services (-22), bilateral procedure (-50), multiple procedures (-51), two surgeons (-62), surgical team (-66), or repeat procedure by same provider (-76). When any of these or other modifiers are used and a full five-digit code for the modifier is desired, use 099 before the modifier code. Thus, they become 09922, 09950, 09962, and so on. The modifiers are delineated in the front of each section of the CPT to alert the coder to modifiers available for that section.

If more than two modifiers are needed for a procedure, use (-99) before any other modifier. Thus, if a procedure required a modifier of -22 and -51, code -99 before the other modifiers. For instance, "33411 Replacement, aortic valve; with aortic annulus enlargement, noncoronary cusp," becomes 33411-99. This can also be written 33411 and 09999, indicating multiple modifiers.

See Procedure 18-1 for instructions on CPT coding.

Critical Thinking

In which code book would you look to find the code for upper gastrointestinal endoscopy, simple primary examination (e.g., with small-diameter flexible endoscope) (separate procedure)? Which code did you select?

HEALTHCARE COMMON PROCEDURE CODING SYSTEM (HCPCS)

In 1983, Medicare created HCPCS (pronounced "hick picks"), the Healthcare Common Procedure Coding System. These codes are used as supplements to the basic CPT system and are required when reporting services and procedures provided to Medicare and Medicaid beneficiaries (patients). HCPCS uses the basic system (Level I) with two additional levels (II and III) as required. Level II provides codes to enable the provider to report nonprovider services such as durable medical equipment, supplies and medications (particularly injectable drugs), and ambulance services. Two-digit alphanumeric or letter modifiers are used in Level II codes to provide greater detail on procedures and medical supplies. (*NOTE:* The use of CPT code 99070 defining supplies and materials provided by the provider over and above those normally included in the office visit should be avoided, and Level II codes, which are more detailed, should be used.) Level III codes are defined by the Medicare regional Part B carriers. Local codes are five-digit alphanumeric codes and use letters *S* and *W* through *Z*.

CODING OF MEDICAL DIAGNOSES

The ICD-9-CM is published annually, available October 1, by the National Center for Health Statistics (NCHS) and Centers for Medicare and Medicaid (CMS).

ICD-9-CM Resource Manual Organization and Use

The ICD-9-CM was created by the WHO to provide a diagnostic coding system for the compilation and reporting of morbidity and mortality statistics for ICD-9-CM reimbursement purposes in the United States. A quarterly publication, *Coding Clinic for ICD-9-CM,* is available as the official guideline for ICD-9-CM. A similar publication should be available when the 10th revision is adopted. The guidelines given are applicable to all settings; provider's office and hospital inpatient, outpatient, and clinical settings.

ICD-9-CM is broken into three volumes:

- *Volume I,* also known as the Tabular List, lists all diagnostic codes in numeric order.

- *Volume II* is an alphabetic listing of all known diagnoses (Index to Diseases). It includes symptoms, accidents and their causes, and concurrent diagnosis. Volume II also contains a table of drugs and chemicals, a neoplasm table, and a list of external causes for injuries. Volume II is the recommended starting point to identify diagnostic codes.

- *Volume III* lists procedures in tabular form. It is not extensively used in the United States, where the procedure codes of the CPT are more commonly used. Information in Volume III can, however, be helpful in identifying a procedure in the CPT.

Step 1 in coding a diagnosis is to enter Volume II using the main reason or condition (main term) that brought the patient into the medical facility. This could be a "soreness in the throat" or a "broken leg," among other symptoms. The lookup entry (main term) in Volume II would never include the anatomical term of "throat" or "leg," but would list "sore" or "fracture." The main term is shown in boldface type in the upper left of the page in the margin. Information in parentheses following the main term is called a nonessential modifier. The presence or absence of nonessential modifiers does not affect the code assignment.

Step 2 is to identify subterms that further identify the condition. Subterms are indented two spaces from the main term identified in step 1. Sometimes there is too much information to fit on the subterm line and it will be included on a carryover line that is indented two spaces from the subterm line.

Step 3 consists of selecting the main or subterm that matches the diagnosis and obtaining the code. The code is then entered into the tabular list of Volume I (Classification of Diseases and Injuries) to verify that it identifies the proper diagnosis. The tabular listing is broken into 17 chapters that are grouped according to cause or body system. Sometimes the code identified from Volume II will not be found in the tabular list of Volume I because of space constraints. When this occurs, the code identified from Volume II should be checked; if found to be correct, that code should be used. Alternatively, sometimes more specific identification is provided in the tabular index in the form of fourth or fifth digits. When a more specific code is found, it should be used.

External Cause Codes (E Codes)

When the cause of a patient's visit is not due to a disease but rather to an injury or poisoning, an additional code is required to identify the reason

Critical Thinking

In which code book would you look to determine the code for hypoparathyroidism that is induced surgically? Which code did you select?

for the visit or the cause of the injury. These codes are called **E Codes** and are found in Volume II. In the case of the broken leg, listed earlier, if the patient had fallen from a ladder, the code would be E881.0; if the patient had fallen from a scaffold, the code would be E881.1. Diagnosis codes are quite precise.

Supplementary Health Factor Codes (V Codes)

When the patient comes to the medical facility for a reason other than sickness or injury, a supplementary health factor code is used. These are called **V Codes.** Had the patient simply come in for a test, such as a TB skin test, a supplementary health factor code would be required. In this case the V Code from Volume II would be V74.1, Screening for Pulmonary Tuberculosis.

Morphology Codes (M Codes)

M Codes (morphology codes) are used primarily with cancer registries. They are used to further identify behavior and the cell type of a neoplasm. This code is used in conjunction with neoplasm codes for the main classification.

Code References

Sometimes a diagnostic code has the notation NEC or NOS attached to it. NEC means "not elsewhere classified" and is used if there is not enough information to find a more specific code. NOS means "not otherwise specified."

See Procedure 18-2 for instructions on ICD-9-CM coding.

CODING ACCURACY

Accuracy in coding is important. Imprecise coding can affect how quickly the provider is reimbursed and also the amount of the reimbursement. Codes must be appropriate to the documentation.

Insurance carriers always **down-code** if documentation or codes are ambiguous and reimburse the provider for the lowest possible fee. Following are the three primary reasons why down-coding happens:

- The coding system used on the claim form does not match the coding system used by the insurance carrier. The carrier's computer will convert the submitted claim code to the closest recognized code. In most cases, the reimbursement amount will be less.
- If a Workers' Compensation claims examiner has to convert a CPT code to a relative value scale (RVS) code, the examiner will select the lowest-paying code. When billing Workers' Compensation, always use the RVS system used by that carrier and match the code to the best description of the CPT code.
- When attached documentation does not match the written description of the procedure, the reimbursement will always be the lowest paying code that fits the written description.

Up-coding, also known as code creep, over-coding, or overbilling, occurs when the insurance carrier is deliberately billed a higher rate service than what was performed to obtain greater reimbursements. Computer software programs have been developed to detect this practice easily. Often, complete audits are performed to assess the extent of up-coding practices. Sanctions and penalties are imposed on offenders.

The Medicare program, in particular, often uses CPT codes, which are **bundled codes.** A bundled code is a grouping of several services that are directly related to a specific procedure and are paid as one. For example, surgical dressings and reading test results may be bundled into evaluation and management codes. **Unbundling** refers to separating the components of a procedure and reporting them as billable codes with charges to increase reimbursement rates. This procedure may also be termed *fragmentation, exploding,* or *à la carte medicine.* This practice is considered fraud and may lead to audit, sanctions, and penalties.

The more accurate the coding on the claim form, the less chance there is for error, the more quickly the provider is reimbursed, and the better the chance that the provider's reimbursement will reflect the actual charge. Many insurance carriers keep a fee profile of each provider's charges. This profile reflects the amount of each charge for each service and can affect the provider's reimbursement for those services.

Critical Thinking

The provider operates as part of a clinic in an integrated medical facility with radiology, laboratory, and surgical facilities in the same building. The clinic is located in Philadelphia, Pennsylvania, with the provider operating as a participating provider in the Medicare System.

A healthy, 65-year-old man presents at the clinic with a chief complaint of a badly bruised left hand and an apparent dislocation of the metacarpophalangeal joint. He had been putting up Christmas lights at his home using a 20-foot aluminum ladder. The ladder had fallen, striking his left thumb as he tried to catch the ladder. He is an established patient.

The provider orders anteroposterior, lateral, and oblique radiographs of the hand to rule out fractures. The radiographs show no evidence of fractures. The diagnosis is dislocation of the metacarpophalangeal joint. The joint is bruised and extremely painful. The procedure performed is a closed treatment of the metacarpophalangeal dislocation with manipulation and requires anesthesia.

Determine the diagnostic and procedures codes. Should you consider E codes? Why or why not? Determine the provider's fee to be billed to Medicare.

Do not guess when coding. The coding that is used becomes a permanent part of the patient's medical record with the insurance carrier. If an incorrect code is used, that coded diagnosis will stay with that patient. This can be a difficult problem for insured persons if they change insurance carriers or if other health problems occur.

Consider a patient with hip pain. She has a history of ovarian cancer for which she has had radiology treatments. The hip pain is thought to be possible metastases from the original cancer site. When ruling out this possibility, the provider indicates the following code for the claim form:

> 198.89 Secondary malignant neoplasm of other specified sites: hip.

When the pain is finally discovered to be arthritis and it is determined that the patient needs a hip replacement, the insurance carrier denies coverage for this operation for the following reason: The patient's condition is terminal, and the company does not want her to spend her last months having surgery and recovering from surgery when she is already in poor health. And, of course, there is the cost factor to consider in the eyes of the insurance carrier.

Incorrect coding can be a problem with ruling out a diagnosis. For instance, a patient presents many symptoms of peptic ulcer disease. Do not immediately code that patient as having that disease until the diagnosis is confirmed. Instead, code the symptoms. When the tests come back and a specific diagnosis of peptic ulcer can be made, then code the disease as:

> 533.70 chronic without mention of hemorrhage or perforation without mention of obstruction.

When coding:

- Be as precise as possible.
- Do not guess.
- Do not code what is not there.

CODING THE CLAIM FORM

For the insurance company to understand what is being billed, the claim form is completed by the medical assistant or billing clerk in the ambulatory care setting. The provider completes an **encounter form** at the time of the visit. This encounter form (Figure 18-1) includes the date of service, the visit or consultation code, diagnoses for this visit, procedures done and laboratory tests ordered, and, if necessary, the date the patient is to return. This information is then translated onto the claim form.

The **CMS-1500 (08-05)** is the claim form accepted by most insurance carriers (Figure 18-2). This form is prepared using words and CPT codes for procedures performed and ICD-9-CM codes for diagnoses. Keep in mind that the codes must correlate; for instance, if a person had an ICD-9-CM diagnosis code of earache, otitis media, or 382.9, and the CPT procedure code indicated was 69090, ear piercing, the insurance company would question the claim and reject it for payment. The person completing the claim form must be *as precise as possible*. If the coding is wrong, the claim will be denied and the provider will not receive payment. Coding must correlate with the provider's note in the chart; otherwise, fraud is committed.

Coding the claim form is a precise way to communicate with the insurance carrier. Coding

PATIENT INFORMATION

| PATIENT'S LAST NAME | FIRST | INITIAL | BIRTHDATE | SEX ☐ MALE ☐ FEMALE | TODAY'S DATE |

| ADDRESS | CITY | STATE | ZIP | RELATIONSHIP TO SUBSCRIBER | INJURY DATE |

| SUBSCRIBER OR POLICYHOLDER | INSURANCE PAYER |

| ADDRESS | CITY | STATE | ZIP | INS. I.D.   COVERAGE CODE   GROUP |

ASSIGNMENT AND RELEASE: I HEREBY AUTHORIZE MY INSURANCE BENEFITS TO BE PAID DIRECTLY TO THE UNDERSIGNED PHYSICIAN. I AM FINANCIALLY RESPONSIBLE FOR NON-COVERED SERVICES. I ALSO AUTHORIZE THE PHYSICIAN TO RELEASE ANY INFORMATION REQUIRED.

OTHER HEALTH COVERAGE   YES ☐   NO ☐   IDENTIFY

DISABILITY RELATED TO:
☐ ACCIDENT ☐ INDUSTRIAL ☐ ILLNESS ☐ OTHER

SIGNED _____ Date _____
(PATIENT, OR PARENT, IF MINOR)

DATE SYMPTOMS APPEARED, INCEPTION OF PREGNANCY, OR ACCIDENT OCCURRED:

✓ DESCRIPTION	CPT/MD	FEE	✓ DESCRIPTION	CPT/MD	FEE	✓ DESCRIPTION	CPT/MD	FEE
OFFICE VISITS	NEW PT		LABORATORY (Cont'd.)			PROCEDURES		
Level III	99203		Wet Mount	87210		EKG	93000	93005
Level IV	99204		Pap Smear	88141		Resp. Function Test	94010	
Level V	99205		Handling	99000		Ear Lavage	69210	
OFFICE VISITS	EST. PT		Hemoccult Stool	82270		Injection Inter. Jt.	20605	
Level I	99211		Glucose	82948		Injection Major Jt.	20610	
Level II	99212		INJECTIONS			Anoscopy	46600	
Level III	99213		Vitamin B12/B Complex	J3420		Sigmoidoscopy	45355	
Level IV	99214		ACTH	J0800		I & D	10060	
Level V	99215		Depo-Estradiol	J1000		Electrocautery	17000	
CONSULTATIONS	OFFICE		Depo Testosterone	J1070		Thromb Hemor.	46320	
Level III	99243		Imferon	J1750		Inj. Tendon	20550	
Level IV	99244							
HOME	EST. PT		Influenza Vaccine - Flu	90658		MISCELLANEOUS		
Level II	99348		Pneumococcal Vaccine	90732		Drugs, Supplies, Materials	99070	
ER			TB Tine Test	86585		Special Reports	99080	
Level III	99283		Aminophyllin	J0280		Services After Hrs.	99050	
Level IV	99284		Terbutaline Sulf.	J3105		Services 10pm - 8am	99052	
LABORATORY			Demerol HCL	J2175		Services Sun. & Holidays	99054	
Urinalysis - Complete	81000		Compazine	J0780		Counseling	99403	
Hemoglobin	85018		Injection Therapeutic	90782				
Culture, Strep/Monilia	87081		Estrone Susp.	J1410				

DIAGNOSIS:

☐ Allergic Rhinitis	477.9	☐ CHF	428.0	☐ Gout	274.9	☐ Parkinsonism	332.0
☐ Anemia	280.9	☐ Cholecystitis	575.10	☐ HCVD	429.2	☐ Peripheral Vascular Dis	443.9
☐ Angina Pectoris	413.9	☐ Chronic Fatigue Synd.	300.5	☐ Headache, Vascular	784.0	☐ Pharyngitis	462
☐ Anxiety	300.00	☐ COPD	496	☐ Headache, Migraine	346.90	☐ Pneumonia, Bacterial	482.9
☐ Aortic Stenosis	424.1	☐ Costochondritis	733.99	☐ Hemorrhoids	455.6	☐ Pneumonia, Viral	480.9
☐ ASCVD	429.2	☐ CVA	431	☐ Hiatal Hernia	553.3	☐ Rectal Bleeding	569.3
☐ ASHD	414.9	☐ Cystitis	595.9	☐ Hiatal Hernia & Reflux	530.10	☐ Renal Failure, Chronic	585
☐ Asthma	493.90	☐ Deg. Disc. Disease, CX	722.4	☐ HVD	402.10	☐ Rheumatoid Arthritis	714.0
☐ Atrial Fibrillation	427.31	☐ Deg. Disc. Dis., Lumbar	722.52	☐ Hyperlipidemia	272.4	☐ Sinusitis	461.9
☐ Bigeminy	427.89	☐ Depression, Endogenous	296.20	☐ Hypothyroidism	244.9	☐ Supraventr. Tachycardia	427.0
☐ BPH	600.__	☐ Dermatitis	692.9	☐ Impacted Cerumen	380.4	☐ T.I.A.	435.9
☐ Bronchitis, Acute	466.11	☐ Diabetes Mellitus, Adult	250.00	☐ Influenza, Viral	487.1	☐ Tachycardia	426.89
☐ Bronchitis, Chronic	491.9	☐ Diarrhea	558.9	☐ Irritable Bowel Syndrome	564.1	☐ Tendinitis	726.90
☐ Bursitis	726.__	☐ Diverticulitis	562.11	☐ Laryngitis	464.00	☐ Tonsillitis	463
☐ Cardiomyopathy	425.4	☐ Esophagitis	530.10	☐ Menopausal Syndrome	627.2	☐ URI	465.9
☐ Carotid Artery Disease	433.10	☐ Fibrocystic Breast Disease	610.1	☐ Mitral Insufficiency	396.2	☐ UTI	599.0
☐ Cerebral Vascular Disease	437.9	☐ Fissure in Ano	565.0	☐ Neuritis	729.2	☐ Vaginitis	616.10
		☐ Gastroenteritis	558.9	☐ Otitis Media	382.9	☐ Vertigo	780.4

| DIAGNOSIS: (IF NOT CHECKED ABOVE) | | REF. DR. & # |

| DOCTOR'S SIGNATURE / DATE | **NO SERVICES PURCHASED** | SERVICE PERFORMED | ACCEPT ASSIGNMENT | TODAY'S FEE |

INSTRUCTIONS TO PATIENT FOR FILING INSURANCE CLAIMS

MAIL THIS FORM DIRECTLY TO YOUR INSURANCE COMPANY.
ATTACH YOUR OWN INSURANCE COMPANY'S FORM.

PLEASE REMEMBER THAT PAYMENT IS YOUR OBLIGATION, REGARDLESS OF INSURANCE OR OTHER THIRD PARTY INVOLVEMENT.

OFFICE ☐   YES ☐   AMT. REC'D TODAY

E.R. ☐   NO ☐

HOME ☐   TOTAL DUE

Figure 18-1   Encounter form. (Courtesy of Bibbero Systems, Inc., Petaluma, CA, 800-242-2376, http://www.bibbero.com)

1500

HEALTH INSURANCE CLAIM FORM

APPROVED BY NATIONAL UNIFORM CLAIM COMMITTEE 08/05

PICA   PICA

1. MEDICARE (Medicare #)   MEDICAID (Medicaid #)   TRICARE CHAMPUS (Sponsor's SSN)   CHAMPVA (Member ID#)   GROUP HEALTH PLAN (SSN or ID)   FECA BLK LUNG (SSN)   OTHER (ID)   1a. INSURED'S I.D. NUMBER (For Program in Item 1)

2. PATIENT'S NAME (Last Name, First Name, Middle Initial)

3. PATIENT'S BIRTH DATE MM DD YY   SEX M F

4. INSURED'S NAME (Last Name, First Name, Middle Initial)

5. PATIENT'S ADDRESS (No., Street)

6. PATIENT RELATIONSHIP TO INSURED   Self   Spouse   Child   Other

7. INSURED'S ADDRESS (No., Street)

CITY   STATE

8. PATIENT STATUS   Single   Married   Other   Employed   Full-Time Student   Part-Time Student

CITY   STATE

ZIP CODE   TELEPHONE (Include Area Code) ( )

ZIP CODE   TELEPHONE (Include Area Code) ( )

9. OTHER INSURED'S NAME (Last Name, First Name, Middle Initial)

10. IS PATIENT'S CONDITION RELATED TO:

11. INSURED'S POLICY GROUP OR FECA NUMBER

a. OTHER INSURED'S POLICY OR GROUP NUMBER

a. EMPLOYMENT? (Current or Previous) YES NO

a. INSURED'S DATE OF BIRTH MM DD YY   SEX M F

b. OTHER INSURED'S DATE OF BIRTH MM DD YY   SEX M F

b. AUTO ACCIDENT? YES NO   PLACE (State)

b. EMPLOYER'S NAME OR SCHOOL NAME

c. EMPLOYER'S NAME OR SCHOOL NAME

c. OTHER ACCIDENT? YES NO

c. INSURANCE PLAN NAME OR PROGRAM NAME

d. INSURANCE PLAN NAME OR PROGRAM NAME

10d. RESERVED FOR LOCAL USE

d. IS THERE ANOTHER HEALTH BENEFIT PLAN? YES NO *If yes,* return to and complete item 9 a-d.

READ BACK OF FORM BEFORE COMPLETING & SIGNING THIS FORM.

12. PATIENT'S OR AUTHORIZED PERSON'S SIGNATURE I authorize the release of any medical or other information necessary to process this claim. I also request payment of government benefits either to myself or to the party who accepts assignment below.

SIGNED _____ DATE _____

13. INSURED'S OR AUTHORIZED PERSON'S SIGNATURE I authorize payment of medical benefits to the undersigned physician or supplier for services described below.

SIGNED _____

14. DATE OF CURRENT: MM DD YY   ILLNESS (First symptom) OR INJURY (Accident) OR PREGNANCY(LMP)

15. IF PATIENT HAS HAD SAME OR SIMILAR ILLNESS. GIVE FIRST DATE MM DD YY

16. DATES PATIENT UNABLE TO WORK IN CURRENT OCCUPATION FROM MM DD YY TO MM DD YY

17. NAME OF REFERRING PROVIDER OR OTHER SOURCE   17a.   17b. NPI

18. HOSPITALIZATION DATES RELATED TO CURRENT SERVICES FROM MM DD YY TO MM DD YY

19. RESERVED FOR LOCAL USE

20. OUTSIDE LAB? YES NO $ CHARGES

21. DIAGNOSIS OR NATURE OF ILLNESS OR INJURY (Relate Items 1, 2, 3 or 4 to item 24E by Line)
1.   3.
2.   4.

22. MEDICAID RESUBMISSION CODE   ORIGINAL REF. NO.

23. PRIOR AUTHORIZATION NUMBER

24. A. DATE(S) OF SERVICE From MM DD YY To MM DD YY   B. PLACE OF SERVICE   C. EMG   D. PROCEDURES, SERVICES, OR SUPPLIES (Explain Unusual Circumstances) CPT/HCPCS MODIFIER   E. DIAGNOSIS POINTER   F. $ CHARGES   G. DAYS OR UNITS   H. EPSDT Family Plan   I. ID. QUAL.   J. RENDERING PROVIDER ID. #

1 NPI
2 NPI
3 NPI
4 NPI
5 NPI
6 NPI

25. FEDERAL TAX I.D. NUMBER SSN EIN

26. PATIENT'S ACCOUNT NO.

27. ACCEPT ASSIGNMENT? (For govt. claims, see back) YES NO

28. TOTAL CHARGE $

29. AMOUNT PAID $

30. BALANCE DUE $

31. SIGNATURE OF PHYSICIAN OR SUPPLIER INCLUDING DEGREES OR CREDENTIALS (I certify that the statements on the reverse apply to this bill and are made a part thereof.)

SIGNED _____ DATE _____

32. SERVICE FACILITY LOCATION INFORMATION   a. NPI   b.

33. BILLING PROVIDER INFO & PH # ( )   a. NPI   b.

NUCC Instruction Manual available at: www.nucc.org

APPROVED OMB-0938-0999 FORM CMS-1500 (08/05)

Figure 18-2   CMS-1500 (08-05) health insurance claim form.

indicates the complexity of the visit, the diagnosis for the visit, and the specific procedures performed during the visit. This results in little confusion, and a minimum of communication is needed between the carrier and the provider's office because all information is contained in the codes.

For instance, Leo McKay, a regular patient, is seen for an extended visit to determine the cause of his abdominal pain. Symptoms include diarrhea, fever, nausea, and anorexia. An abdominal ultrasound is ordered, as well as laboratory tests, and the results are unknown at the time of the insurance billing. The visit lasts 30 minutes and includes a full physical examination and a history of the present illness.

The CPT procedure coding for this visit is 99214, which reflects the examination and time spent with the patient, the history taken of this illness, and a medical decision of moderate complexity.

The ICD-9-CM diagnosis coding for abdominal pain is 789.0, for diarrhea 787.91, for nausea 787.02, and for anorexia 783.0. The claim form is submitted to the insurance carrier with these codes, and even though they are all symptoms, the claim will be paid because the visit and the tests ordered interrelate.

When the test results are known, they show a positive diagnosis of Giardia lamblia. The diagnosis code is changed to 007.1. Any further charges sent to the insurance carrier while Leo McKay is being treated for this problem are coded 007.1. The symptom codes from the first submission are dropped.

 Many electronic health records (EHRs) use encoder programs that are available on CD-ROM or as Internet downloads. Encoder programs are coding software programs that allow the user to locate CPT, ICD-9-CM, and HCPCS codes quickly. Many of the encoder programs permit the placement of bookmarks or notes for quick reference.

THIRD-PARTY GUIDELINES

Because patient information is easily accessed through medical charts, EHRs, and the human factor, security and confidentiality measures must be in place in medical offices. When patients schedule an appointment and are seen by the provider, they enter into a contract for specific services. The first party is the person receiving the contracted service. The second party is the person or organization providing the service. A third party is one that is not involved in the patient–provider relationship but rather with reimbursement procedures.

 The patient has a right to expect that his or her health information will not be disseminated to others without written permission to do so. Confidentiality issues involve restricting the health information to only those individuals who need to know. Compliance with Health Insurance Portability and Accountability Act (HIPAA) of 1996 regulations is one way to safeguard protected health information (PHI). Chapters 11, 12, 13, 14, 15, and 17 all place emphasis on HIPAA as it relates to PHI. You may want to review those chapter sections again.

Authorization to release necessary medical information to payers, such as insurance carriers, must be obtained from the patient, the parent, or the guardian *before* any information is released. A breach of confidentiality is the release of unauthorized PHI to a third party. One way to prevent this when processing insurance claims forms is to ask the patient, parent, or guardian to sign an "Authorization to Release Medical Information" statement *before* the claim form is completed. The CMS-1500 (08-05) form provides space for this signature in Block 12.

Some medical offices, especially those that send claim forms electronically, develop their own specialized "Authorization for Release of Medical Information" form. The customized form must contain the specific name of the insurance company and must be signed by the patient, parent, or guardian. This form is generally valid for 1 year. The insurance company may request a copy of the signed form. When completing the CMS-1500 (08-05), Block 12 may contain the words "SIGNATURE ON FILE" or the abbreviation "SOF."

Three authorization exceptions are allowed by the federal government. The first two exceptions apply to Medicaid and Workers' Compensation. In these instances, the patient becomes a third-party beneficiary in the contract between the health care provider and the government agency sponsoring the insurance program. Providers agree to accept the program's payment as payment in full, and the patient may only be billed if the payer does not cover services rendered or if the patient is ineligible for benefits. The third exception is related to hospital admission. The patient must sign a release of medical information *before* being seen by the provider or receiving treatment in a hospital.

Most states have specific laws related to release of medical information regarding mental health services and federally assisted alcohol and drug abuse programs. Patients being screened for HIV infection or AIDS must sign an additional authorization statement *before* information may be released regarding their status. See Procedure 18-3 for specific steps involved in authorization to release PHI to third-party payers.

COMPLETING THE CMS-1500 (08-05)

The CMS-1500 (08-05) form is completed using data from the patient's EHR in most offices today (Figure 18-3). In the few cases where the office does not use EHR, the paper encounter form is used by the billing specialist to complete the form. Each insurance carrier has its own thoughts on how the form is completed and no two companies agree entirely on the information required, the boxes checked, and the rationale about what information goes in which boxes.

With the transition to an increase in electronic claims submission and the HIPAA regulations, the National Uniform Claim Committee (NUCC) established a standardized dataset for

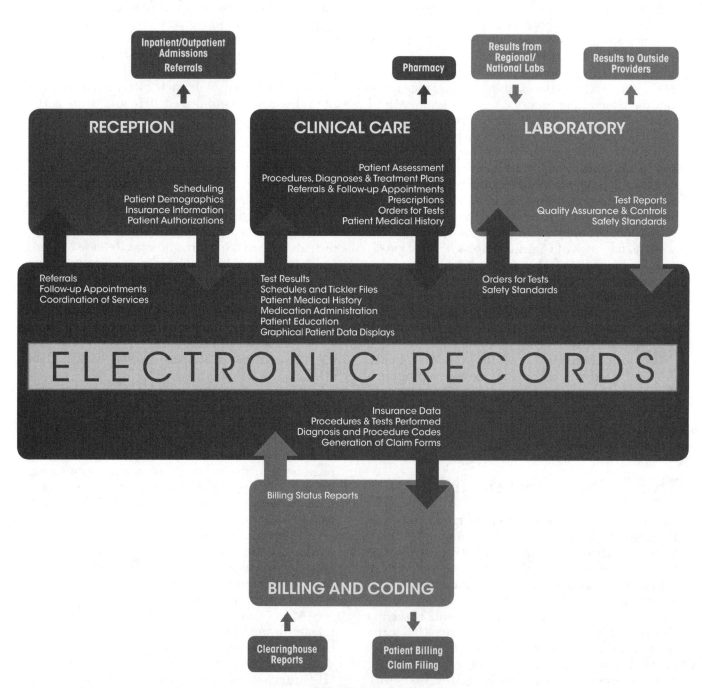

Figure 18-3 How the EHR can be used in processing insurance procedures.

use in an electronic environment as well as with paper claim form standards. The NUCC continues to monitor how insurance carriers use the various claim form fields. Additional changes to the CMS-1500 (08-05) form may be required in the future as the NUCC works to create standardized national instructions for completing the form.

To illustrate the completion of a claim form, a fictitious insurance carrier will be used. Insurance carriers often change their rules and regulations for submitting claims constantly. To avoid out-of-date material, we sent this claim for payment to How Much Insurance Company. Using the example given of Leo McKay in the coding section, the CMS-1500 (08-05) in Figure 18-4 shows the properly completed claim form.

Remember, many insurance carriers require some of the boxes to be filled in and others left blank. The billing person for the medical office needs to comply with the current requirements of the insurance carrier that is being billed. There is no right or wrong answer for every insurance carrier. If there is a question about billing, check with that carrier about its requirements.

The CMS-1500 (08-05) claim form contains all of the identification information that the carrier needs to process or analyze the claim for payment. The new form is distinguishable from the old form in that the 1500 symbol and the date approved by the NUCC appear in the top left margin. When completing the PATIENT AND INSURED INFORMATION section, use commas to separate the last name, first name, and middle initial. A hyphen can be used for hyphenated names. Do not use periods within the name. Do not use commas, periods, or other punctuation in the address. When entering the 9-digit zip code, include the hyphen. Do not use a hyphen or space as a separator within the telephone number. The top right-hand space, identified as CARRIER, provides space for the carrier's name and address to be keyed in. Procedure 18-4 gives instructions for completing a Medicare claim form. Before completing claims for carriers other than Medicare, the medical assistant should verify with a carrier's representative exactly which blocks are required for that particular carrier. In the next chapter, Procedure 19-4 simulates sending an electronic claim to an insurance carrier after procedure and diagnostic codes have been posted to a patient's account.

Uniform Bill 04 Form

 The NUCC has also updated the CMS-1450 claim form, also known as **Uniform Bill 04 (UB-04),** to accommodate reporting the National Provider Identifier (NPI) number. The NPI, a requirement of HIPAA legislation, must be used by all HIPAA-covered entities. Figure 18-5 shows a sample of the UB-04 form.

The UB-04 form is the standard form used for inpatient admissions, outpatient and emergency department services and procedures, psychiatric facilities, drug and alcohol facilities, clinical and laboratory services, walk-in centers, nursing facilities, home health care agencies, hospice centers, and long-term care benefits under a health plan.

Using the Computer to Complete Forms

 The CMS-1500 (08-05) claim form is designed to accommodate optical scanning of paper claims. A scanner is used to convert printed or handwritten characters into text that can be viewed by the optical character reader (OCR). This technology greatly increases claims processing productivity, with some claims being paid within 7 to 10 days.

Practice management software may require data be entered using uppercase and lowercase letters and other data be entered without regard to OCR guidelines. The computer program converts the data to the OCR format when the claim is printed or electronically transmitted to the carrier. Always use the software program's test pattern program to verify alignment of forms. Be sure the *X*s are completely within the designated boxes. You may need to check this alignment each time a new batch of claims is inserted into the printer.

While completing the claim form on the computer, remember not to interchange a zero (0) with the alpha character (o). A substitute space should be used in place of the following keystrokes:

- Dollar sign or decimal in all charges or totals
- Decimal point in a diagnosis code number
- Dash in front of a procedure code modifier
- Parentheses surrounding the area code in a telephone number
- Hyphens in Social Security numbers

When a fee is expressed in whole dollars, always enter two zeros in the cent column. Birth dates should be entered using eight digits (MM/DD/YYYY). Two-digit code numbers are used for months (i.e., January 01, February 02, and so on). If the day of the month number is less than 10, add a zero before the day (i.e., 03 for the third day of the month, and so forth).

1500

HEALTH INSURANCE CLAIM FORM

APPROVED BY NATIONAL UNIFORM CLAIM COMMITTEE 08/05

PICA | | | | | | PICA

1. MEDICARE (Medicare #) MEDICAID (Medicaid #) TRICARE CHAMPUS (Sponsor's SSN) CHAMPVA (Member ID#) GROUP HEALTH PLAN (SSN or ID) FECA BLK LUNG (SSN) OTHER ☒ (ID)

1a. INSURED'S I.D. NUMBER (For Program in Item 1)
555-55-555

2. PATIENT'S NAME (Last Name, First Name, Middle Initial)
MCKAY, LEO M

3. PATIENT'S BIRTH DATE MM 04 DD 01 YY 1963 SEX M ☒ F ☐

4. INSURED'S NAME (Last Name, First Name, Middle Initial)
MCKAY, LEO M.

5. PATIENT'S ADDRESS (No., Street)
123 W FIRST STREET

6. PATIENT RELATIONSHIP TO INSURED
Self ☒ Spouse ☐ Child ☐ Other ☐

7. INSURED'S ADDRESS (No., Street)
123 W FIRST STREET

CITY: ANYWHERE   STATE: PA

8. PATIENT STATUS
Single ☒ Married ☐ Other ☐
Employed ☐ Full-Time Student ☐ Part-Time Student ☐

CITY: ANYWHERE   STATE: PA

ZIP CODE: 11666   TELEPHONE (Include Area Code) (824) 556-6189

ZIP CODE: 11666   TELEPHONE (Include Area Code) (824) 556-6789

9. OTHER INSURED'S NAME (Last Name, First Name, Middle Initial)

10. IS PATIENT'S CONDITION RELATED TO:

11. INSURED'S POLICY GROUP OR FECA NUMBER
1122334

a. OTHER INSURED'S POLICY OR GROUP NUMBER

a. EMPLOYMENT? (Current or Previous) ☐ YES ☒ NO

a. INSURED'S DATE OF BIRTH MM 04 DD 01 YY 1963 SEX M ☒ F ☐

b. OTHER INSURED'S DATE OF BIRTH MM DD YY SEX M ☐ F ☐

b. AUTO ACCIDENT? ☐ YES ☒ NO   PLACE (State)

b. EMPLOYER'S NAME OR SCHOOL NAME
ABC MANUFACTURING COMPANY

c. EMPLOYER'S NAME OR SCHOOL NAME

c. OTHER ACCIDENT? ☐ YES ☒ NO

c. INSURANCE PLAN NAME OR PROGRAM NAME
HOW MUCH INSURANCE COMPANY

d. INSURANCE PLAN NAME OR PROGRAM NAME

10d. RESERVED FOR LOCAL USE

d. IS THERE ANOTHER HEALTH BENEFIT PLAN? ☐ YES ☒ NO If yes, return to and complete item 9 a-d.

READ BACK OF FORM BEFORE COMPLETING & SIGNING THIS FORM.

12. PATIENT'S OR AUTHORIZED PERSON'S SIGNATURE I authorize the release of any medical or other information necessary to process this claim. I also request payment of government benefits either to myself or to the party who accepts assignment below.
SIGNED Signature on File   DATE 01/14/XXXX

13. INSURED'S OR AUTHORIZED PERSON'S SIGNATURE I authorize payment of medical benefits to the undersigned physician or supplier for services described below.
SIGNED Signature on File

14. DATE OF CURRENT: MM 01 DD 10 YY XXXX ILLNESS (First symptom) OR INJURY (Accident) OR PREGNANCY(LMP)

15. IF PATIENT HAS HAD SAME OR SIMILAR ILLNESS. GIVE FIRST DATE MM DD YY

16. DATES PATIENT UNABLE TO WORK IN CURRENT OCCUPATION FROM MM DD YY TO MM DD YY

17. NAME OF REFERRING PROVIDER OR OTHER SOURCE
17a.
17b. NPI

18. HOSPITALIZATION DATES RELATED TO CURRENT SERVICES FROM MM DD YY TO MM DD YY

19. RESERVED FOR LOCAL USE

20. OUTSIDE LAB? ☐ YES ☐ NO $ CHARGES

21. DIAGNOSIS OR NATURE OF ILLNESS OR INJURY (Relate Items 1, 2, 3 or 4 to Item 24E by Line)
1. 789.0
2. 558.9
3. 783.0
4.

22. MEDICAID RESUBMISSION CODE   ORIGINAL REF. NO.

23. PRIOR AUTHORIZATION NUMBER

24. A. DATE(S) OF SERVICE From MM DD YY	To MM DD YY	B. PLACE OF SERVICE	C. EMG	D. PROCEDURES, SERVICES, OR SUPPLIES CPT/HCPCS	MODIFIER	E. DIAGNOSIS POINTER	F. $ CHARGES	G. DAYS OR UNITS	H. EPSDT Family Plan	I. ID. QUAL.	J. RENDERING PROVIDER ID. #
1 01 10 XXXX		3		99214		1,2,3	85 00	1		NPI	1543298760
2 01 10 XXXX		3		82270		1,2	13 00	1		NPI	1543298760
3										NPI	
4										NPI	
5										NPI	
6										NPI	

25. FEDERAL TAX I.D. NUMBER 91-1234432 SSN ☐ EIN ☒

26. PATIENT'S ACCOUNT NO. MCK111

27. ACCEPT ASSIGNMENT? ☐ YES ☒ NO

28. TOTAL CHARGE $ 98 00

29. AMOUNT PAID $

30. BALANCE DUE $ 98 00

31. SIGNATURE OF PHYSICIAN OR SUPPLIER INCLUDING DEGREES OR CREDENTIALS (I certify that the statements on the reverse apply to this bill and are made a part thereof.)
SIGNED Mark Wos MD   DATE 01/14/XXX

32. SERVICE FACILITY LOCATION INFORMATION
a. NPI b.

33. BILLING PROVIDER INFO & PH # (814) 555-1155
INNER CITY HEALTH CARE
222 S FIRST AVE
CANTON PA 11666
a. R09876543 b.

NUCC Instruction Manual available at: www.nucc.org

APPROVED OMB-0938-0999 FORM CMS-1500 (08/05)

Figure 18-4   Completed CMS-1500 (08-05) claim form.

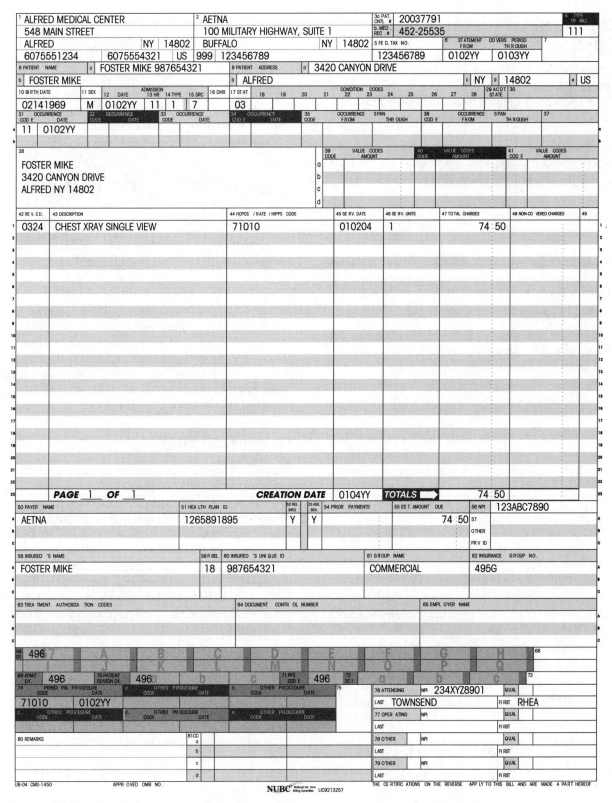

Figure 18-5 UB-04 claim containing sample patient data (with highlighted form locators that contain ICD-9-CM and CPT codes).

EHR The Administrative Simplification Compliance Act (ASCA), which went into effect July 5, 2005, specifies that no payment may be made under Part A or Part B of the Medicare program for any expenses incurred for items or services for which a claim is submitted in a nonelectronic form. Simply stated, paper claims submitted to Medicare will not be paid. Some exceptions to this rule can be found in the *Medlearn Matters* article MM3440 available at the CMS Web site (http://cms.hhs.gov/medlearn/matters).

Common Errors in Completing Claim Forms

Once the claim form has been completed, it should be proofread for accuracy and to make certain that all information has been filled in correctly. The following list provides common errors:

- Eliminate typographic errors. Check all numbers carefully to be sure they have not been transposed or entered incorrectly.
- Eliminate incorrect information. The name of the patient and the name of the policyholder must be the same.
- Verify that all blanks have been completed accurately. Specifically check that units of service are entered, hospital admission and discharge date are included, and procedure service date is provided.
- Verify that each procedure links correctly with the correct diagnosis (Block 24E).
- Verify that the procedure was medically necessary.
- Include the patient's name and policy identification information on each page of all attachments.
- Do not use staples when submitting paper claims, because the form cannot feed through the OCR if it is defaced or creased.
- Verify that the printer alignment was properly set and that all claim information is contained within its proper field.
- Be sure the claim form is signed appropriately.

BENEFITS OF SUBMITTING CLAIMS ELECTRONICALLY

Submitting claims electronically has many benefits, which may include, but are not limited to, the following:

- Standardized electronic claim format ensures consistency, reducing errors.
- Submitters can exchange electronic data with multiple payers using the same data format.
- Supplies required (e.g., paper, postage) and administrative costs are reduced.
- Cash flow can be significantly improved because Medicare pays 14 days after receipt of electronically submitted claims (paper claims may take a minimum of 29 days to process).

MANAGING THE CLAIMS PROCESS

Once the claim form has been coded, a series of events take place. The medical assistant, who may have used a referral number generated by a point-of-service device, enters the claim into the office register of submitted claims; the insurance carrier processes the claim; an explanation of benefits is sent to the insured person; and, if necessary, follow-up procedures are instituted if payment is not received from the carrier within a specified time period. Each of these events is discussed in detail in the following sections.

Documentation of Referrals

Many insurance plans require that a referral be preapproved by the plan before scheduling an appointment with other than the primary care provider. This is particularly true for managed care plans. The medical assistant working in both the primary care facility and specialist facility must make sure that when an approval is required, the necessary authorization has been obtained and referral number recorded in the patient's file. The referral number must be submitted as part of the claim submitted to the carrier by the specialist.

Point-of-Service Device

An electronic device available to some health care providers is a **point-of-service (POS) device.** This device provides immediate and direct access to patient eligibility information and managed care functions through an electronic network connecting the medical office and the health plan's computer.

The POS is a small card-swipe box similar in design and function to a credit card terminal (Figure 18-6). It allows medical office personnel to:

- Record a patient visit
- Check eligibility for patients in the health plan

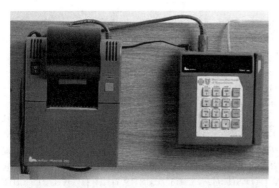

Figure 18-6   Point-of-service device. (Right) To enter information, the patient's insurance card is swiped through the machine, or the patient's identification number is entered on the keypad together with specific transaction code numbers. (Left) Responses from the plan's computer are printed directly in the medical office.

- Enter referrals for patients in managed care plans
- Verify referral information
- Check authorization status
- Enter inpatient authorization requests
- Enter outpatient authorization requests

After the information is input by the medical assistant, the POS communicates with the health plan's computer system. The computer then returns an acknowledgment to the medical office confirming the transaction or giving an error message code. For example, when visits are recorded accurately, a reference number is generated that is used as the medical office's confirmation that the transaction is complete. On successful entry of a referral, a referral number is generated. Specialists may use this number on claims they submit for services they render under the referral.

Maintaining a Claims Registry

When claim forms are sent to the appropriate insurance carrier, it is wise and necessary for the medical office personnel to keep a diary or register of submitted claims (Figure 18-7). This **claim register** should include the patient's name, the insured's name if it is different from the patient's name, the dates of service for which the claim is being made, the amount of the claim, and the date the claim is submitted. When payment is received, the date of payment should be entered. When aging and reconciling accounts, the bookkeeper then can check the diary to note where the claim is in the process.

Following Up on Claims

Occasionally, claims are denied because the claim form was not properly coded. However, if there is no payment from the carrier and no other notification after a period of 4 to 6 weeks, it is necessary to follow up on the claim. The claim register will enable the office to keep track of the progress of claims (Figure 18-7).

To follow up, a toll-free number is provided by most carriers. The necessary information to have on hand before making the call includes a copy of the claim form and the patient's name and insurance identification number. The carrier should be able to give the status of the claim. If payment is delayed, the carrier should be able to give the date when it can be expected. It is possible that payment was sent to the insured person, in which case a statement should be sent to the patient. If there is a problem with the claim, the medical assistant may need to investigate the cause of the error and submit a revised claim.

See Chapter 20 for information on billing and collection procedures.

INSURANCE CLAIMS STATUS

ACTION DATE	LAST NAME	FIRST NAME	INSURANCE COMPANY	ORIGINAL BILLING DATE	TOTAL CHARGES $	AMOUNT RECEIVED	STATUS / ACTION TAKEN
1/30/2008	McKay	Leo	Nationwide	1/30/2008	$ 88.00	$ -	Submitted
2/14/2008	Lovelace	Terry	World Health	9/24/2007	$ 128.00	$ -	Add'l data submitted
4/15/2008	Taxman	William	US Health	12/15/2007	$ 640.00	$ 640.00	Paid in full
5/1/2008	Fooler	April	Surprise Health	4/1/2007	$ 375.98	$ -	Collection
5/16/2008	Zonker	James	Gotcha Covered	4/3/2008	$ 236.00	$ 136.00	Patient billed $100.00
7/5/2008	Stripes	Stanley	Bangor Insurance				

Figure 18-7   Sample claim register.

THE INSURANCE CARRIER'S ROLE

On receipt of the claim form, the claims processor at the insurance carrier checks the codes to confirm that the procedures and accompanying diagnoses agree. The processor then analyzes the information to confirm that:

1. The coverage was in force at the time of treatment
2. The provider has contracted with the insurance carrier
3. There are no exclusions or restrictions on the policy for payment of that diagnosis
4. There are no preexisting condition restrictions
5. The diagnosis and procedures done are medically necessary and reasonable

The processor also checks to make sure that the billed amount falls within the usual, customary, and reasonable fee that the insurance carrier has developed for that specific procedure.

Explanation of Benefits

On completion of the processing of the claim, the insurance company sends an **Explanation of Benefits (EOB)** to the insured person. Figure 17-1 shows a sample EOB. This form includes the dates; charges; amounts applied toward the deductible; amounts not covered either because of an exclusion or excess over the usual, customary, and reasonable charge; and the amount the company is paying for this claim. Some Explanation of Benefits forms even serve as a "bill" or "notice" in that they indicate the amount the insured must forward to the provider for payment of the account in full.

LEGAL AND ETHICAL ISSUES

 Issues of insurance fraud and abuse must be understood before accurate codes can be assigned to medical procedures and diagnosis of disease. See Chapter 17 for a complete discussion regarding insurance fraud and abuse.

Coding errors pose another type of legal and ethical issue. The Omnibus Budget Reconciliation Acts of 1986 and 1987 state that providers can be assessed civil penalties if they "know of or should know that claims filed with Medicare or Medicaid on their behalf are not true and accurate representations of the items or services actually provided." This means that providers can be held responsible not only for negligent mistakes they make but also for mistakes made on their behalf by their medical assistants who complete insurance claim forms. The penalties assessed are usually in the form of a monetary fine and may also involve exclusion from Medicare and Medicaid programs for a period.

Compliance Programs

Compliance programs based on guidelines issued by the Office of the U.S. Inspector General are not mandatory; however, they help prevent violations that can be financially costly and that may carry criminal penalties for the provider and office personnel. Participation in a compliance program demonstrates that the practice is making a good faith effort to submit claims appropriately and is considered equivalent to practicing preventative medicine. The following are basic elements of a compliance program:

1. Have a designated compliance officer.
2. Develop and use written standards and procedures for coding.
3. Develop a plan for communicating coding standards and procedures.
4. Train personnel in standards and procedures.
5. Conduct periodic audits.
6. Respond to detected violations and notify appropriate government agencies.
7. Make personnel aware that they have an ethical duty to report suspected or observed fraudulent or erroneous coding practices so that they can be corrected. Publicize and enforce disciplinary standards on coding violations.

Procedure 18-1

Current Procedural Terminology Coding

PURPOSE:
To convert commonly accepted descriptions of medical procedures (services) and visits of all types—office, hospital, nursing facility, home services—into a five-digit numeric code with two-digit numeric modifiers when required.

EQUIPMENT/SUPPLIES:
CPT code book for the current year
Copy of the encounter form and access to the patient's chart
Pencil and paper

CASE SCENARIO
Mary O'Keefe, a new patient, is seen for 10 minutes, during which the provider takes a focused history and completes a problem-focused examination. A routine urinalysis, nonautomated and without microscopy, is performed and a straightforward medical decision is made. Mary's preliminary diagnosis is painful urination. The urinalysis confirms a urinary tract infection. The provider writes her a prescription for an antibiotic and asks her to make an appointment in 10 days for another urinalysis to confirm the infection has cleared.

PROCEDURE STEPS:
1. Using the CPT code book, look in the Evaluation and Management section, Office or Other Outpatient Services, New Patient. Carefully read through the options until the code matching the described scenario has been found. RATIONALE: This section of the CPT code book provides codes used to report evaluation and management services provided in the provider's office or in an outpatient or other ambulatory care facility. You should have selected 99201.

2. Continue with the CPT code book, turn to the Index again, and look up Urinalysis, Routine. The code given is 81002. RATIONALE: This provides you with a code to investigate and determine its appropriateness.

3. Continue in the CPT code book and turn to the Pathology and Laboratory section. Follow the codes until you locate code 81002. Be sure the description provided there matches what the provider has documented in the patient's chart. RATIONALE: To verify that the code is correct and matches documentation.

Procedure 18-2

International Classification of Diseases, 9th Revision, Clinical Modification Coding

PURPOSE:
The ICD-9-CM code books provide a diagnostic coding system for the compilation and reporting of morbidity and mortality statistics for reimbursement purposes.

EQUIPMENT/SUPPLIES:
Volumes 1 and 2 of the ICD-9-CM code books for the current year
Copy of the encounter form and access to the patient's chart
Pencil and paper

CASE SCENARIO
Mary O'Keefe, a new patient, presents at the office today reporting painful, frequent urination. She is seen for 10 minutes, during which the provider takes a focused history and completes a problem-focused examination. A routine urinalysis, nonautomated and without microscopy, is performed and a straightforward medical decision is made. Mary's preliminary diagnosis is painful urination. The urinalysis confirms a urinary tract infection. The provider writes her a prescription for an antibiotic and asks her to make an appointment in 10 days for another urinalysis to confirm the infection has cleared.

continues

Procedure 18-2 (continued)

PROCEDURE STEPS:

1. Using Volume II of the ICD-9-CM code book, the alphanumeric Index to Diseases, look up the main symptom or condition that brought the patient to the facility or the specific diagnosis confirmed by test results. In this case, the laboratory results confirmed a urinary tract infection. Code 599.0 RATIONALE: Use alphanumeric Volume II first to close in on the section of Vol-

ume I for specificity. *NOTE:* Enter the Tabular List, Volume I, with the first three digits of the code determined (599).

2. Using Volume I, look up code 599. Read through all of the 599 listings to determine the appropriate code having the highest level of specificity. RATIONALE: To establish the most accurate code: urinary tract infection, site not specified. 599.0 .

Procedure 18-3

Applying Third-Party Guidelines

PURPOSE:
To obtain written authorization to release necessary medical information to third-party payers.

EQUIPMENT/SUPPLIES:
Patient chart
CMS-1500 (08-05) claim form

PROCEDURE STEPS:

1. When the patient signs in at the reception desk, check his or her chart to ascertain whether an "Authorization to Release Medical Information"

form has been signed and is currently valid. RATIONALE: PHI cannot be released without written authorization from the patient.

2. If there is no record of SIGNATURE ON FILE, have the patient sign Block 12 of the CMS-1500 (08-05) claim form or the offices' customized "AUTHORIZATION TO RELEASE MEDICAL INFORMATION" form. RATIONALE: PHI cannot be released without written authorization from the patient.

Procedure 18-4

Completing a Medicare CMS-1500 (08-05) Claim Form

PURPOSE:
To complete the CMS-1500 (08-05) insurance claim form for Medicare for reimbursement.

EQUIPMENT/SUPPLIES:
Patient information
Patient account or ledger card
Copy of patient's insurance card
Insurance claim form
Computer and printer

PROCEDURE STEPS:
1. The CARRIER section of the CMS-1500 (08-05) is in the upper portion of the form. The bar code that contained the carrier's name and address has been eliminated. Use the blank space at the top right of the section marked CARRIER to enter the name and address of the payer to whom this claim is being sent. The payer is the carrier, health plan, third-party administrator, or other payer who will handle the claim. The format for this information should be as follows:

Key on line 4: first line — Name

Key on line 5: second line — First line of address

Key on line 6: third line — Second line of address

Key on line 7: fourth line — City, state (2 letters) and zip code

Do not use commas, periods, or other punctuation in the address. When entering a 9-digit zip code, include the hyphen. When printing page numbers on multiple-page claims (generally done by clearinghouses when converting the electronic claim form to the CMS 1500 claim form), print the page numbers in the Carrier Block on Line 8 beginning at column 32. Page numbers are to be printed as Page XX of YY.

RATIONALE: The claims processor must know who the claim is from.

2. The PATIENT AND INSURED INFORMATION section asks for specific information related to the patient and his or her health insurance plan. The following information is required for this section. Complete each block as directed. RATIONALE: These blocks must be accurately completed or the claim may be denied.

Block 1   Indicate the type of health insurance coverage applicable to this claim by placing an X in the Medicare box. Only one box can be marked.

Block 1a   Enter insured's ID number as shown on insured's ID card for the payer to whom the claim is being submitted. RATIONALE: The insured's ID number is the identification number of the person who holds the policy. This information identifies the patient to the payer.

Block 2   Enter the patient's full last name, first name, and middle initial in this block.

Block 3   Enter the patient's 8-digit birth date (MM/DD/CCYY). Enter an X in the correct box to indicate sex of the patient. Only one box can be marked. If gender is unknown, leave blank.

Block 4   Enter the insured's full last name, first name, and middle initial.

Block 5   Enter the patient's mailing address and telephone number.

Block 6   Enter an X in the correct box to indicate the patient's relationship to insured when Block 4 has been completed. Only one box can be marked.

1500
HEALTH INSURANCE CLAIM FORM
APPROVED BY NATIONAL UNIFORM CLAIM COMMITTEE 08/05
PICA   PICA
CARRIER

continues

Procedure 18-4 (continued)

1. MEDICARE ☐ (Medicare #)	MEDICAID ☐ (Medicaid #)	TRICARE CHAMPUS ☐ (Sponsor's SSN)	CHAMPVA ☐ (Member ID#)	GROUP HEALTH PLAN ☐ (SSN or ID)	FECA BLK LUNG ☐ (SSN)	OTHER ☐ (ID)	1a. INSURED'S I.D. NUMBER (For Program in Item 1)

2. PATIENT'S NAME (Last Name, First Name, Middle Initial)

3. PATIENT'S BIRTH DATE MM DD YY   SEX   M ☐ F ☐

4. INSURED'S NAME (Last Name, First Name, Middle Initial)

5. PATIENT'S ADDRESS (No., Street)

6. PATIENT RELATIONSHIP TO INSURED   Self ☐ Spouse ☐ Child ☐ Other ☐

7. INSURED'S ADDRESS (No., Street)

CITY   STATE

8. PATIENT STATUS   Single ☐ Married ☐ Other ☐

Employed ☐ Full-Time Student ☐ Part-Time Student ☐

CITY   STATE

ZIP CODE   TELEPHONE (Include Area Code) ( )

ZIP CODE   TELEPHONE (Include Area Code) ( )

9. OTHER INSURED'S NAME (Last Name, First Name, Middle Initial)

10. IS PATIENT'S CONDITION RELATED TO:

11. INSURED'S POLICY GROUP OR FECA NUMBER

a. OTHER INSURED'S POLICY OR GROUP NUMBER

a. EMPLOYMENT? (Current or Previous)   YES ☐ NO ☐

a. INSURED'S DATE OF BIRTH MM DD YY   SEX   M ☐ F ☐

b. OTHER INSURED'S DATE OF BIRTH MM DD YY   SEX   M ☐ F ☐

b. AUTO ACCIDENT?   YES ☐ NO ☐   PLACE (State)

b. EMPLOYER'S NAME OR SCHOOL NAME

c. EMPLOYER'S NAME OR SCHOOL NAME

c. OTHER ACCIDENT?   YES ☐ NO ☐

c. INSURANCE PLAN NAME OR PROGRAM NAME

d. INSURANCE PLAN NAME OR PROGRAM NAME

10d. RESERVED FOR LOCAL USE

d. IS THERE ANOTHER HEALTH BENEFIT PLAN?   YES ☐ NO ☐   *If yes*, return to and complete item 9 a-d.

READ BACK OF FORM BEFORE COMPLETING & SIGNING THIS FORM.
12. PATIENT'S OR AUTHORIZED PERSON'S SIGNATURE I authorize the release of any medical or other information necessary to process this claim. I also request payment of government benefits either to myself or to the party who accepts assignment below.

SIGNED _____   DATE _____

13. INSURED'S OR AUTHORIZED PERSON'S SIGNATURE I authorize payment of medical benefits to the undersigned physician or supplier for services described below.

SIGNED _____

PATIENT AND INSURED INFORMATION

Block 7 Enter the insured's address and telephone number. If Block 4 has been completed, then this field should also be completed.

Block 8 Enter an X in the box for the patient's marital status and in the box for the patient's employment or student status. Only one box on each line can be marked.

Block 9 If Block 11d is marked yes, complete fields 9 and 9a–d, otherwise leave blank. When additional group health coverage exists, enter other insured's full last name, first name, and middle initial of the enrollee in another health plan if it is different from that shown in Block 2.

Block 9a Enter the policy or group number of the other insured. Do not use a hyphen or space as a separator within the policy or group number.

Block 9b Enter the 8-digit date of birth (MM/DD/CCYY) of the other insured and an X to indicate the sex of the other insured. Only one box can be marked. If gender is unknown, leave blank.

Block 9c Enter the name of the other insured's employer or school.

Block 9d Enter the other insured's insurance plan or program name.

Blocks 10a–10c When appropriate, enter an X in the correct box to indicate whether one or more of the services described in Block 24 are for a condition or injury that occurred on the job or as a result of an automobile or other accident. Only one box on each line can be marked. The two-letter state abbreviation must be shown if YES is marked in 10b. RATIONALE: Any item marked YES indicates there may be other applicable insurance coverage that would be primary.

Block 10d Refer to the most current instructions from the applicable public or private payer regarding the use of this field.

Block 11 Enter the insured's policy or group number as it appears on the insured's health care ID card. If Block 4 has been completed, then this field should also be completed.

Block 11a Enter the 8-digit date of birth (MM/DD/CCYY) of the insured and an X to indicate the sex of the insured. Only one box can be marked. If gender is unknown, leave blank.

continues

Block 11b   Enter the name of the insured's employer or school.

Block 11c   Enter the insurance plan or program name of the insured. (Some payers require an ID number of the primary insurer rather than the name in this field.)

Block 11d   When appropriate, enter an X in the correct box. If marked YES, complete Blocks 9 and 9a–d. Only one box can be marked.

Block 12   Enter "Signature on File," "SOF," or legal signature. When legal signature, enter date signed in 6- or 8-digit format. If there is no signature on file, leave blank or enter "No Signature on File." RATIONALE: The patient's or authorized person's signature indicates there is an authorization on file for the release of any medical or other information necessary to process and/or adjudicate the claim.

Block 13   Enter "Signature on File," "SOF," or legal signature. If there is no signature on file, leave blank or enter "No Signature on File." RATIONALE: The insured's or authorized person's signature indicates that there is a signature on file authorizing payment of medical benefits.

3.   The PHYSICIAN OR SUPPLIER INFORMATION section must be accurately completed or the claim may be denied.

Block 14   Enter the 6- or 8-digit date of the first date of the present illness, injury, or pregnancy. For pregnancy, use the date of the last menstrual period (LMP) as the first date.

NUCC Instruction Manual available at: www.nucc.org   APPROVED OMB-0938-0999 FORM CMS-1500 (08/05)

Block 15   Enter the first date the patient had the same or a similar illness. Enter the date in the 6- or 8-digit format. Previous pregnancies are not a similar illness. Leave blank if unknown.

Block 16   If the patient is employed and is unable to work in current occupation, a 6- or 8-digit date must be shown for the "from–to" dates that the patient is unable to work. RATIONALE: An entry in this field may indicate employment-related insurance coverage.

Block 17   Enter the name (first name, middle initial, last name) and credentials of the professional who referred, ordered, or supervised the service(s) or supply(s) on the claim. Do not use periods or commas within the name. A hyphen can be used for hyphenated names.

Block 17a   The two-digit qualifier code is entered in the small box. Qualifiers are as follows:

0B   State License Number

1B   Blue Shield Provider Number

1C   Medicare Provider Number

1D   Medicaid Provider Number

1G   Provider UPIN Number

1H   CHAMPUS Identification Number

E1   Employer's Identification Number

G2   Provider Commercial Number

LU   Location Number

N5   Provider Plan Network Identification Number

SY   Social Security Number (the Social Security number may not be used for Medicare)

X5   State Industrial Accident Provider Number

ZZ   Provider Taxonomy

The other ID number of the referring, ordering, or supervising provider is reported in the larger space.

Block 17b   Enter the NPI number of the referring, ordering, or supervising provider. RATIONALE: The NPI number refers to the HIPAA National Provider Identifier number.

Block 18   Enter the inpatient 6- or 8-digit hospital admission date followed by the discharge date (if discharge has occurred). If not discharged, leave discharge date blank.

Block 19   Refer to the most current instruction from the applicable public or private payer regarding the use of this field.

Block 20   Complete this field when billing for purchased services. Enter an X in "YES" if the reported service(s) was performed by an entity other than the billing provider. If "YES," enter the purchased price under charges. RATIONALE: A "YES" indicates that an entity other than the entity billing for the service performed the purchased services. A "NO" indicates that no purchased services are included on the claim. When "YES" is indicated, Block 32 must be completed. Only one box can be marked.

Block 21   Enter the patient's diagnosis/condition. List up to four ICD-9-CM diagnosis codes. Relate lines 1, 2, 3, and 4 to the lines of service in Block 24E by line number. Use the highest level of specificity. Do not provide a narrative description in this field. When entering the number, include a space between the two sets of numbers.

Block 22   Enter the original reference number for resubmitted claims. Refer to the most current instruction from the applicable public or private payer regarding the use of this field.

Block 23   Enter any of the following: prior authorization number, referral number, mammography precertification number, or CLIA number, as assigned by the payer for the current service. Do not enter hyphens or spaces within the number.

Block 24A   Enter date(s) of service, from and to. If one date of service only, enter that date under "From." Leave "To" blank or reenter "From" date.

Block 24B   Enter appropriate two-digit code from the Place of Service Code list for each item

Block 24C This block was originally titled "Type of Service" and is no longer used. Check with trading partner to determine if emergency indicator is necessary. If required, enter Y for "YES" or leave blank if "NO". RATIONALE: The definition of emergency would be defined by either federal or state regulations or programs or payer contracts, or as defined in the electronic 837 Professional 4010A1 implementation guide.

Block 24D Enter the CPT or HCPCS code(s) and modifier(s), if applicable, from the appropriate code set in effect on the date of service.

Block 24E Enter the diagnosis code reference number as shown in Block 21 to relate the date of service and the procedures performed to the primary diagnosis. When multiple services are performed, the primary reference number for each service should be listed first; other applicable services should follow. Enter the numbers left justified in the field. Do not use commas between the numbers.

Block 24F Enter number right justified in the dollar area of the field. Do not use commas when reporting dollar amounts. Negative dollar amounts are not allowed. Dollar signs should not be entered. Enter 00 in the cents area if the amount is a whole number.

Block 24G Enter the number of days or units. This field is most commonly used for multiple visits, units of supplies, anesthesia units or minutes, or oxygen volume. If only one service is performed, the numeral 1 must be entered. Enter numbers right justified in the field. No leading zeros are required. If reporting a fraction of a unit, use the decimal point.

Block 24H For Early & Periodic Screening, Diagnosis and Treatment-related services, enter the response as follows: If there is no require-

The text at the top of column two begins: used or service performed. Place of Service Codes are available at www.cms.hhs.gov/PlaceofServiceCodes/Downloads/POSDataBase.pdf.

ment to report a reason code for EPDST, enter Y for "YES" or N for "NO" only.

Block 24I Enter the qualifier identifying if the number is a non-NPI. The Other ID# of the rendering provider is reported in block 24J. The NUCC defines the same qualifiers as listed for Block 17a.

Block 24J Enter the non-NPI ID number in the top portion of the field. Enter the NPI number in the lower area of the field.

Block 25 Enter the provider of service or supplier federal tax ID or Social Security number. Enter an X in the appropriate box to indicate which number is being reported. Only one box can be marked. Do not enter hyphens with numbers. Enter numbers left justified in the field.

Block 26 Enter the patient's account number assigned by the provider of service's or supplier's accounting system. Do not enter hyphens with numbers. Enter numbers left justified in the field.

Block 27 Enter an X in the correct box. Only one box can be marked.

Block 28 Enter total charges for the services (total of all charges in Block 24F). Enter number right justified in the dollar area of the field. Do not use commas when reporting dollar amounts. Negative dollar amounts are not allowed. Dollar signs should not be entered. Enter 00 in the cents area if the amount is a whole number.

Block 29 Enter total amount the patient or other payers paid on the covered services only. Enter number right justified in the dollar area of the field. Follow instructions given for Block 28 for format.

Block 30 Enter total amount due. Enter number right justified in the dollar area of the field. Do not use commas when reporting dollar amounts. Negative dollar amounts are not allowed. Dollar signs should not be entered. Enter 00 in the cents area if the amount is a whole number.

continues

Procedure 18-4 (continued)

Block 31	Enter the legal signature of the practitioner or supplier, signature of the practitioner or supplier representative, "Signature on File," or "SOF." Enter either the 6- or 8-digit date or alphanumeric date the form was signed. RATIONALE: The signature refers to the authorized or accountable person and the degree, credentials, or title.
Block 32	Enter the name, address, city, state, and zip code of the location where the services were rendered. Providers of service must identify the supplier's name, address, zip code, and NPI number when billing for purchased diagnostic tests. When more than one supplier is used, a separate claim form should be used to bill for each supplier. Follow previously outlined format for entering address information.

Block 32a	Enter the NPI number of the service facility location.
Block 32b	Enter the two-digit qualifier identifying the non-NPI number followed by the ID number. Use the same qualifiers as listed in Block 17a.
Block 33	Enter the provider's or supplier's billing name, address, zip code, and phone number. The phone number is to be entered in the area to the right of the field title. Follow previously outlined format for entering address information.
Block 33a	Enter the NPI number of the billing provider.
Block 33b	Enter the two-digit qualifier identifying the non-NPI number followed by the ID number as listed in Block 17a.

Case Study 18-1

Review the scenario at the beginning of the chapter.

CASE STUDY REVIEW

1. Explain why coding accurately is important to health care providers and insurance companies that act as third-party payers for health care services rendered to patients.

2. List ways to ensure accurate coding.
3. Recall common errors in completing insurance claim forms.

Case Study 18-2

Leo McKay, an established patient at Inner City Health Care, schedules a visit, reporting nausea and severe abdominal pain. Dr. Mark Woo spends 30 minutes taking a history and doing an examination. He suspects an ulcer and orders laboratory tests (CBC complete, guaiac, lipid panel, and UA) to be done in the office and sends Mr. McKay for an upper GI series. Mr. McKay returns in 10 days to learn that the test results show a duodenal ulcer.

CASE STUDY REVIEW

1. What are the proper diagnosis codes for Mr. McKay?
2. What are the proper procedure codes for Mr. McKay?
3. In coding the claim form for Mr. McKay's visit, what ethical principle and legal principle should guide the medical assistant?

SUMMARY

Much material has been covered in this chapter. Remember, you can be the person to make a difference in insurance billing. By checking and double-checking your work, you make certain that the provider's time is being billed at the appropriate rate, that all procedures are billed with the proper diagnoses and CPT codes, and that the billing is sent to the correct insurance carrier. It takes much less time to double-check work once and have it correct *before* it is sent out than to send it out with errors that cause difficulty in the future.

An understanding of medical insurance coverages and coding procedures is vital to a thriving ambulatory care setting. The astute medical assistant will perceive the challenges involved in proper coding techniques and will understand his or her role in the management of the provider's office.

STUDY FOR SUCCESS

To reinforce your knowledge and skills of information presented in this chapter:

- Review the Key Terms
- Practice the Procedures
- Consider the Case Studies and discuss your conclusions
- Answer the Review Questions
  - ○ Multiple Choice
  - ○ Critical Thinking
- Navigate the Internet by completing the Web Activities
- Practice the StudyWARE activities on the textbook CD
- Apply your knowledge in the Student Workbook activities
- Complete the Web Tutor sections
- View and discuss the DVD situations

REVIEW QUESTIONS

Multiple Choice

1. CPT codes:
   a. are for diagnosis coding
   b. have five digits and may have two-digit modifiers
   c. have three-digit codes with a decimal point and one to two additional digits
   d. are updated semiannually
2. When coding a diagnosis, go first to:
   a. CPT
   b. Volume I of ICD-9-CM
   c. Volume II of ICD-9-CM
   d. E codes in ICD-9-CM
3. Level II of HCPCS:
   a. provides codes to enable the provider to report nonprovider services
   b. is the same as the regular CPT system

   c. is assigned by the fiscal intermediary
   d. uses the letter codes W, X, Y, and Z
4. The ICD-9-CM codes:
   a. were developed by the AMA as uniform descriptions of medical, surgical, and diagnostic services
   b. are divided into seven sections
   c. use modifiers
   d. code every disease, illness, condition, injury, and cause of injury known
5. Most insurance carriers accept which claim form?
   a. UB-04
   b. CMS-1500 (08-05)
   c. CPT
   d. HCFA-1450

6. Claim registers are used to:
   a. anticipate claims to be sent to insurance companies for processing
   b. check how many claims are sent to Medicare
   c. monitor claims that have been sent to insurance companies for processing
   d. help in aging accounts
7. Information to be included in the CARRIER section of the CMS-1500 (08-05) insurance claim form includes all of the following *except:*
   a. the payer's name
   b. the patient's name
   c. the payer's address
   d. the payer's city, state, and zip code
8. Information to be included in the PATIENT AND INSURED section of the CMS-1500 (08-05) insurance claim form includes all of the following *except:*
   a. health insurance plan
   b. patient's name and address
   c. insured's name and address
   d. NPI number of the billing provider
9. Differentiate the following as either CPT or IC-9-CM codes and the code you assign to each:
   a. irregular menstrual cycle

   _____   _____

   b. biopsy, soft tissue of neck

   _____   _____

   c. dissection of the renal artery

   _____   _____

   d. adenitis, lymph gland, except mesenteric

   _____   _____

   e. thyroid hormone (T3 or T4) uptake

   _____   _____

   f. hearing aid examination and selection; monaural

   _____   _____

Critical Thinking

1. Electronic claims filing is mandatory for Medicare. Karen recently graduated from an accredited medical assisting program and is employed in the insurance department of a busy medical practice. She has asked her supervisor how she can gain more knowledge in coding and electronic billing procedures and how she might decrease the number of rejected claims. How would you respond to her if you were the supervisor?
2. The supervisor has given Karen a number of rejected claim forms and asks her to determine why the claims were denied and to maintain a log of these reasons to be discussed at the next staff meeting. How should Karen proceed with this assignment?
3. Karen finds that many claim forms were rejected because important information was omitted. How might Karen suggest corrections for these omissions?
4. The policy at Inner City Health Care is to request that the patient assign benefits by signing Block 13 of the CMS-1500 (08-05) claim form if he or she does not pay for services on the day rendered. One of the patients is hesitant to comply with this policy. How should Karen explain this policy to the patient?
5. How might a compliance program benefit Inner City Health Care and what basic elements should it address?

WEB ACTIVITIES

 Mr. Jones is in reasonably good health and incurs drug expenses less than $1,000 per year. Review the Medicare drug plans for your area and select the optimum plan for Mr. Jones. If his prescription drug costs increased to $1,800 per year, how would this change the selection? Visit http:// www.Medicare.gov on the Internet and select "Compare" under "Prescription Drug Plans.")

REFERENCES/BIBLIOGRAPHY

American Medical Association. (2007). *Current procedural terminology.* Chicago: American Medical Association.

American Medical Association. (Oct. 2007). *International classification of diseases, clinical modifications* (2nd ed., 9th rev.). Chicago: American Medical Association.

Greene, M. A. (2007). *3-2-1 code IT !* Clifton Park, NY: Delmar Cengage Learning.

ingenix. (2003). *HIPAA tool kit.* Salt Lake City, UT: St. Anthony Publishing/Medicode.

ingenix. (2007). *HCPCS level II.* Salt Lake City, UT: St. Anthony Publishing/Medicode.

Moisio, M. A. (2006). *A guide to health insurance billing* (2nd ed.). Clifton Park, NY: Delmar Cengage Learning.

Office of Inspector General, U.S. Department of Health and Human Services. (2000). *Compliance program guide for individual and small group physician practices.* Retrieved March 1, 2003 from http://oig.hhs.gov/authorities/docs/physcian.pdf.

Chapter 19

Daily Financial Practices

OUTLINE

KEY TERMS

Accounts Payable
Accounts Receivable
Adjustments
Balance
Cashier's Check
Certified Check
Credit
Day Sheet
Debit
Encounter Form
Guarantor
Ledger
Money Market Account
Notary
Payee
Pegboard System
Petty Cash
Posting
Traveler's Check
Voucher Check

OBJECTIVES

The student should strive to meet the following performance objectives and demonstrate an understanding of the facts and principles presented in this chapter through written and oral communication.

1. Define the key terms as presented in the glossary.
2. Understand the importance of communication in regard to establishing patient fees.
3. Identify circumstances that require adjustment of fees and post accordingly.
4. Develop a knowledge of various credit arrangements for patient fees.
5. Differentiate between manual and computerized bookkeeping systems.
6. Describe the pegboard system.
7. State the advantages of computerized systems for financial practices.
8. List six good working habits for financial records.

OBJECTIVES (continued)

9. Describe the encounter form.

10. Identify the parts of the patient account or ledger.

11. Discuss preparation of patient receipts.

12. Describe month-end activities.

13. Demonstrate a knowledge of banking procedures, including types of accounts and services.

14. Show proficiency in preparing deposits and checks and reconciling accounts.

15. Explain the process of purchasing equipment and supplies for the ambulatory care setting.

16. Demonstrate proficiency in establishing and maintaining a petty cash system.

Scenario

At the offices of Drs. Lewis and King, many different types of patients are seen. Most have some kind of insurance, either a traditional plan or an HMO plan, some are on Medicare, a few on Medicaid, and occasionally a patient does not have any insurance or any financial resources to pay for treatment. Whoever schedules the first patient appointment also opens a courteous discussion with the patient about provider fees and the patient's anticipated method of payment. Initiating this discussion of fees at the beginning of the provider–patient relationship keeps patients informed of their responsibility for payment and helps the medical assistants at Drs. Lewis and King's practice make any necessary credit arrangements with the patient before treatment begins.

INTRODUCTION

Ambulatory care settings are primarily designed to serve the patient. However, without sound financial practices, patient care will suffer and the practice will not thrive and grow. The health care industry is complex and complicated. The impact of managed care and the many detailed insurance plans affect not only the way patients receive treatment, but the manner in which the ambulatory care center is administered from a financial point of view.

The discussion of fees is only a small part of the ambulatory care setting's daily financial practices. Selecting an appropriate system for tracking patient accounts, overseeing banking procedures, managing the purchase of supplies, controlling patient accounts, and establishing a petty cash system all are important to the smooth functioning of today's ambulatory care setting.

PATIENT FEES

All providers receive education, training, and experience in diagnosing and treating the concerns of their patients. That is their major concern; therefore, the management of the business details usually becomes the responsibility of the medical assisting staff. Informing the patient about charges, collecting payments, making credit arrangements if necessary, and making certain patients and their providers receive the full benefit of medical insurance becomes the responsibility of the medical assistant staff. An attitude that anticipates that the majority of patients pay their medical bills in a timely and responsible manner is helpful in completing this task.

Helping Patients Who Cannot Pay

There are times when patients may have difficulty paying their bills. The economy changes, and with its fluctuations, individuals lose their jobs and often their medical insurance. The majority of today's employment force does not recall a time without medical insurance when patients expected to pay the total fee for medical services. These same patients may not fully comprehend what medical

Spotlight on Certification

RMA Content Outline
- Financial and bookkeeping

CMA (AAMA) Content Outline
- Equipment and supply inventory
- Bookkeeping systems
- Accounting and banking procedures

CMAS Content Outline
- Managing practice finances
- Bookkeeping systems
- Banking procedures

services cost. They likely do not understand the explanation of benefits (EOB) from their insurance reports. There is also a growing number of "working poor" in society, who may work two or more part-time jobs but never qualify for company insurance benefits and struggle daily to pay necessary bills. Some patients must decide whether to put food on the table or pay the provider. Emergencies can deplete an individual's financial resources as well. These are the times when the administrative medical assistant might make financial arrangements with patients allowing full payment for the services provided. Patients will appreciate the assistance, and the administrative medical assistant can expect the patient to abide by the agreed plan. Such an agreement fosters a climate where patients are less likely to withdraw from any necessary medical treatment when their finances are low.

Determining Patient Fees

Providers place a value on their services. In today's managed care climate, ambulatory care settings have many different arrangements with patients, insurance carriers, and health maintenance organization (HMO) insurance contracts. Managed care contracts pay predetermined fees for specific procedures and services. Providers who practice in a concierge-type medical group collect an additional fee. This usually is a flat fee at the beginning of each year for the specialized service; many do not accept the insurance carrier's required co-payment. Patients who choose concierge medical services are willing to pay the additional fee and generally have the resources to do so. Provider fees for procedures, however, are billed and reimbursed according to standard insurance guidelines. Chapter 17 provides further details on fees.

Discussion of Fees

The manner in which billing is done and fees established varies depending on the type of medical facility, the needs of the practice, and the professional services rendered. Today, the fee for the visit is simply stated, and if a person does not have cash or a check, the option of credit or debit card payment is often provided. If a patient is a member of an HMO, the patient is expected to pay any established co-payment amount at the time of service.

Inherent to the total billing process is the necessity of informing patients of charges and exactly what portion of the bill they are expected to pay. Ideally, the patient should be told the approximate cost of the procedures at the start of treatment. For Medicare and Medicaid patients, a form officially known by Medicare as an Advanced Beneficiary Notification (ABN) or by Medicaid as a waiver is the only legal means a clinic has to collect payment on charges not allowed by Medicare or Medicaid. These forms are to be in writing, should indicate the type of procedure(s), the total responsibility of the patient, and the reason why this is the patient's responsibility.

 Charges for some daily routine visits may be submitted to an insurance carrier, and the office may not always know what portion is covered until information is received from the carrier. The facility may contract with numerous insurance plans, including private carriers, and participation in these plans determines the amount the patient owes. Many misunderstandings can be prevented and subsequent collection of delinquent accounts expedited when the clinic staff is well informed about insurance reimbursement and carefully explains fees to the patients.

Adjustment of Fees

 Providers who accept assignment with Medicare and Medicaid are mandated to charge every patient the same amount for similar services rendered. If a professional courtesy is extended then it is considered insurance

Patient Education

One way to easily provide information to patients regarding fees is to include in the office brochure policies regarding fees, insurance, co-payments, and how third-party payments are handled. If credit and debit cards are allowed, include that information as well.

fraud, because the office would be billing insurance an increased rate than what they charge others. Deductibles are to be collected from patients as part of their premium expectation. Unless you follow government guidelines for establishing when patients are financially unable to pay their portion of the bill, you cannot give discounts to patients for cash payments.

Adjustments may be made for patients with limited income. For example, for patients who recently lost a job or ran into unfortunate financial circumstances, the provider may write off a portion of the bill. This sum will be written off against the provider's income, and the patients do not pay that portion.

Adjustments also may occur with Medicare, Medicaid, Blue Shield, and private health insurance patients. Providers who accept assignment in these programs agree to accept as payment in full what the insurer allows. For instance, a fee of $150 may be charged, but $95 is accepted as payment in full by the provider after deductibles and co-payments are satisfied. The remainder of the bill, $55, is written off so that the patient is not responsible for the nonallowed amount.

Medical assistants must be aware, however, of the pitfalls of adjusting or reducing fees. It is difficult to accept all hardship cases and still remain a viable practice. It is always a helpful resource to patients who cannot pay to be given the names and telephone numbers of local health care clinics that may be able to accept them as patients on a sliding scale or no-fee basis.

Refunds. On rare occasion, a refund will be necessary. It usually occurs when the insurance carrier pays more than anticipated. Notably, there are a few members of the older adult population who may still be a little uncomfortable with Medicare and are accustomed to paying for all their medical expenses out of pocket; therefore, they will pay their entire bill when the statement is received. When Medicare payments arrive, an overpayment is created. The financial transaction required is to prepare a check for the amount due to the patient and enter the transaction on the **day sheet** and patient account. In most cases, such a refund will bring the patient balance to zero.

CREDIT ARRANGEMENTS

If the patient will need to pay a substantial out-of-pocket amount, it is beneficial to make the patient aware of this and discuss different credit arrangements that can be made. Many ambulatory care settings will accept prearranged installment payments, usually without finance charges, to spread the cost of services over a pre-agreed period. This eases the financial burden on the patient and also makes it more likely that the balance due will be collected.

Payment Planning

Medical assistants can help patients plan for anticipated medical expenses (having a baby, surgery, extensive therapy). When patient and provider know in advance that there will be costly medical expenses, the medical assistant should review the patient's insurance coverage. It is helpful to prepare an estimate sheet, which will give the patient an idea of the cost of the medical services for the planned treatment. The estimate may also include the anticipated cost of anesthetist, consultants, and hospital charges.

Many ambulatory care settings accept credit and debit cards as a means of payment. Remember, this service is strictly for the convenience of the patient, and providers cannot increase their charges for patients who wish to use these cards even though the provider is charged a fee for this service. Credit and debit cards are convenient and ensure payment; therefore, the practice may wish to encourage their use.

The one advantage to the ambulatory care setting that accepts credit/debit cards is that monies for fees charged usually are available within 24 hours. Also, the provider is relieved of the responsibility of collection. However, credit card companies do assess a fee for every charge made, which the ambulatory care center must pay.

 When a patient decides to use a credit or debit card, it is extremely important that confidentiality be maintained to the fullest extent possible. When writing a description of the services on the credit card receipt, the medical assistant should be as vague as possible to preserve patient confidentiality. For example, "medical services" is often used.

THE BOOKKEEPING FUNCTION

Daily financial management in the ambulatory care setting is important to the functioning of the clinic, because it directly affects overall accounting and bookkeeping procedures. Accounting generates financial information for the ambulatory care setting and is defined as a system of monitoring the financial status of a facility and the specific results of its activities. Accounting provides financial information for decision making (see Chapter 21). Bookkeeping, the actual daily recording of the accounts or transactions of the business, is a major part of this accounting process. This chapter deals with daily bookkeeping (or recording) functions necessary to manage the income and expenses of an ambulatory care setting.

Managing Patient Accounts

 All businesses must keep careful records of income and expenses for tax and legal purposes. One aspect of this recordkeeping in a medical practice is maintaining patient accounts. Because few patients are able to pay in full each time they are seen by the provider, it is necessary to maintain account records for each individual or family as opposed to simply keeping a record of cash received as is done in many other types of business. The money owed to the clinic by patients is known as **accounts receivable;** this must be carefully monitored to ensure that the provider is paid for services provided in a timely manner and that patients are properly credited for payments made.

There are various ways to track patients' balances. This chapter discusses the two most common methods:

- Computerized financial systems
- The **pegboard system** (also known as the write-it-once method)

 Although the financial records of most practices are fully automated, many practices probably started with some sort of manual system (generally pegboard). Converting from manual to computerized recordkeeping seems cumbersome at the beginning, but it offers great versatility and reduces the need to record and re-record entries.

A knowledgeable medical assistant will understand both the manual and computerized systems.

The Importance of Good Working Habits in Financial Transactions.
In managing the day-to-day finances of the ambulatory care setting, always observe the following guidelines:

1. Always work with care and accuracy; it is extremely easy to transpose numbers (e.g., entering 23 instead of 32) or make other posting errors. A moment of carelessness can result in hours spent trying to find the mistake.

2. The work must be kept current or it may become an overwhelming chore.

3. Double-check all entries made for accuracy.

In a manual bookkeeping system, follow these additional rules:

- Use a consistent ink color; black or blue is preferred.
- Form your numbers and letters carefully, using neat and clear writing.
- Align your columns carefully, preferably using paper with grid lines.
- Write small enough to stay within the columns.
- Be careful when placing or carrying decimal points.
- Double-check all math.
- If a mistake is found, draw one line through the error and write "Corr." or "Correction" above it. Red ink may be used in correcting errors on a paper copy.

Pegboard System.
A complete pegboard or write-it-once system consists of day sheets, ledger cards, **encounter forms** or charge slips, and receipt forms. The forms are designed to work together to simplify the task and to avoid mistakes in patient accounts. All forms have matching columns that align and are held in place on the pegboard when the system is in use (Figure 19-1). The forms are on NCR© (no carbon required) paper, which permits entering of charges, credits, or adjustments, called **posting,** onto the day sheet, encounter form, or receipt and the patient's ledger simultaneously. The day sheet provides complete and up-to-date information about accounts receivable status at a glance. Also, a pegboard system is relatively inexpensive.

Computerized Financial Systems.
The majority of medical facilities use computers for bookkeeping. A number of medical practice software packages

Critical Thinking

Discuss with another student the advantages and disadvantages of adopting a computer system that allows the practice to start with one component and add more components at a later time.

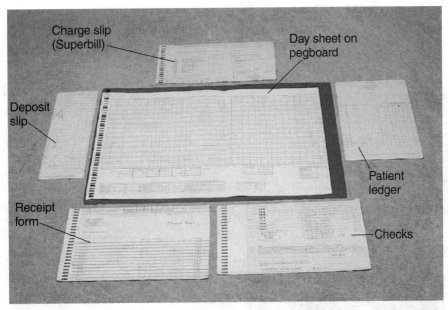

Charge slip
(Superbill)

Day sheet on
pegboard

Deposit
slip

Patient
ledger

Receipt
form

Checks

Figure 19-1   An example of the pegboard system and possible overlays.

are available on the market. These ready-made systems are available for both single- or multiple-provider partnerships and large group practices. Occasionally, a consultant is hired to design a customized program, although this can be more expensive than purchasing mass-produced software. When selecting and using any computer system:

- Be sure the system will meet current needs, and will grow with the practice.
- Consider adopting a system that allows the practice to start with one component, such as scheduling, and to add another component, such as bookkeeping and medical records, at a later date until the entire practice is fully automated (Figure 19-2).

RECORDING PATIENT TRANSACTIONS

The administrative medical assistant is largely responsible for recording patient transactions for the practice. Bookkeeping activities are exact. Either they are right or they are wrong, and in any form of business, they have to be right to be correct and to be "in balance." In the pegboard or manual system, if an error is made during entry, it will carry through to all the other documents, thus compounding the error. In a computerized system, there is the old but true statement, "garbage in, garbage out." *All* entries must be correct; there is no room for just a "slight" mistake.

In one way or another, the forms and procedures discussed in the following sections are common elements to any system of bookkeeping for a medical practice.

Encounter Form

The encounter form, also known as the charge slip, superbill, or multipurpose billing form, is used in both manual and computerized bookkeeping systems. It often is a three-part form that has the following functions:

1. Provides patients one copy with a record of account activity for the day (usually a pink form)
2. Provides a second copy of account activity for possible insurance submission (usually a yellow form)
3. Provides a third copy that serves the office's permanent copy of account activity (usually a white form)

The encounter forms can be custom designed to fit the particular practice, computer system, or pegboard. Information on the form includes the patient's name, address, account number, and necessary insurance information, as well as any previous balance. Often, the encounter form is attached to the patient's chart so that the provider is able to indicate the day's activities and charges; the provider can also indicate a requested return visit. The encounter form also includes procedure and diagnosis codes. The most applicable procedure codes can be preselected and printed on the encounter

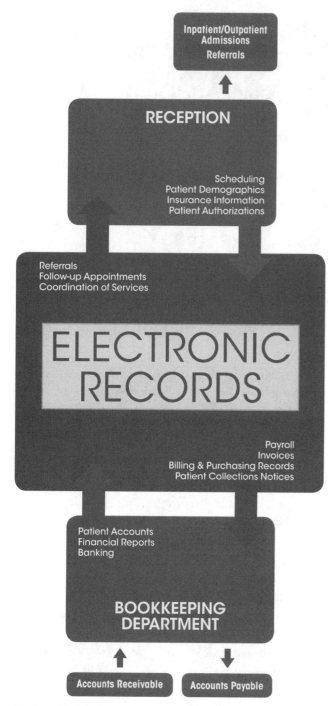

Figure 19-2   Total practice management system diagram illustrating the connection between daily financial practices, patients' electronic medical records, and reception/scheduling activities.

phone number of the practice and the attending provider's National Provider Identifier (NPI).

Encounter forms are designed to fit over the pegs of a pegboard system when a manual system is used. In a computerized system, an encounter form carrying the same information is prepared for the patient, printed, and attached to the patient chart. Some computer systems automatically match the correct charge to the procedure code identified. When a facility is totally automated (including medical records), the provider identifies patient procedures in the medical record on the computer. The computer software assigns appropriate codes and charges to create the encounter form, which can be printed for the patient at the completion of the service.

Patient Account or Ledger

The financial record of the patient is known as that patient's account. All the patient accounts with balances make up the accounts receivable. Patient accounts are recorded in an accounts receivable **ledger.** (Figure 19-3 illustrates a typewritten ledger.) The ledger, or record of services, lists payments and balances due. In family practice, each adult has his or her own ledger or account that carries insurance information, name of subscriber, and patient's relationship to the subscriber. A responsible party is identified for each minor or patient who does not have insurance, and that name also appears on the ledger. Charges for any members of the family seen in the clinic are entered on their own ledger. It is important that charges and credits be applied to the correct family member for insurance purposes and accurate bookkeeping practices.

form to fit the practice, with blank lines added for infrequently used procedures. Often, providers use the form to check the appropriate procedures and diagnoses while with the patient. The encounter form also will carry the name, address, and tele-

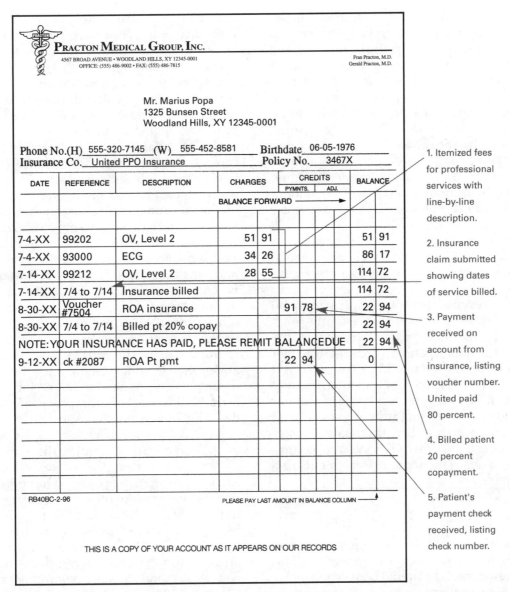

Figure 19-3   Typewritten ledger card illustrating posting of professional services, fees, payments, and balance due.

In cases of divorced parents and blended families, the parent with physical custody of the child is considered to be **guarantor** and the one responsible for payment if the child is not insured with a contracted insurance carrier. This prevents the staff from having to interpret divorce decrees and parenting plan documents. This information should be clearly identified and discussed with the parent when appointments are made.

In the manual system of bookkeeping, ledger cards are used. They have a minimum of three columns for entering figures:

1. **Debit** column is on the left and is used for entering charges and a brief description of services, including a procedure code.

2. **Credit** column is to the right of the debit column and is used for entering payments.

3. **Balance** column is at the far right and is used to record the difference between the debit and credit columns and shows any amount due.

Most ledger cards have space for another column called **adjustments,** which are used to indicate any insurance payments, personal discounts or write-offs, or any other adjustments that need to be recorded.

The adjustment column is a credit column; therefore, entries here normally reduce the balance due. When making an adjustment intended to increase the balance, a negative entry (in parentheses) is made to show that you reverse the function when you balance. (Add instead of subtract the amount.) For example, Edith Leonard had surgery, and because of a hardship, the provider agreed to reduce the fee by half of the balance remaining after insurance has paid. At the time of surgery, a charge of $2,500 is entered on her ledger and the day sheet. Today, payment is received from her insurance company in the amount of $2,000, which would normally leave a balance of $500. However, because the provider agreed to write off half of that amount ($250), you enter $250 in the adjustment column when posting the insurance payment. That amount is subtracted from the previous balance to get the new total of $250.

The ledger is placed under the charge slip or encounter form in a pegboard system and aligned before posting. Never post any patient entry in this manual system without the patient's ledger in place. This prevents recording information on the day sheet while inadvertently omitting it from the patient's ledger. In the computerized system, a patient's account or ledger can be printed with the same information by just entering the patient's name and usually an identification number. The computerized patient account ledger provides more room for helpful detail and is much faster to create than the manual paper ledger. Procedure 19-1 identifies steps in recording/posting patient charges and adjustments in a manual system.

Day Sheet

All financial transactions for professional services are posted daily on a day sheet or daily ledger. This is an important part of the overall bookkeeping process, so absolute accuracy is critical. At the close of each business day, the day sheet is balanced to provide a complete picture of all patient financial activity for that day. Those balances carryover from day to day to provide the accumulated data needed for month-end closing. If more than one day sheet is required to record all the transactions in the pegboard system, pages are numbered and the information is carried forward just as if it were a new day.

There are a number of different styles for the day sheet; some provide a deposit portion to use as a deposit slip and a section used for business analysis. For example, if the provider wants to know the amount of income generated from laboratory services performed in the clinic, the totals can be obtained from the day sheet columns where only laboratory charges were posted. Over time, the laboratory income totals can be compared with the cost for running the laboratory.

The pegboard write-it-once section is where individual transactions are posted, using the ledger card and encounter form on top of the day sheet. The information in this section includes the date, patient name, description of transaction or service, charges, credits, and previous and current balances. At the bottom of the day sheet, transactions are totaled and balanced at the end of the day. This total section includes space to bring forward the previous page balance for a month-to-date total. These totals allow the provider and office manager to monitor totals that assist in predicting the financial status for the practice. The total accounts receivable figure shows how much is owed to the provider by all patients to date, allowing management to see the total outstanding balance at a glance. A major disadvantage to this system, as mentioned earlier, is that an error made in one place is going to carry through to all the other forms. When balancing this financial information, always use a calculator's print function to create a tape of the calculations. These tapes are an invaluable time saver if the initial balance is incorrect and you need to search for mistakes. Procedure 19-2 describes the process for balancing a day sheet in a manual system.

Daily sheets or ledgers in a computerized system require the same data. The patient's name, date, diagnosis, and services provided are posted. The computer system or database matches the correct charge and posts it to the patient account and the accounts receivable ledger. Any error made is quickly changed and corrected throughout. Totals are automatically created for the day-end total, month-end total, and cumulative total from the beginning of the year.

Receipts

Unlike encounter forms, receipt forms used for payments on accounts usually are not customized with other than the name, address, and telephone number of the practice preprinted. The receipt form is used only when someone makes a payment on an account on a day when no services were rendered. In the pegboard system, this transaction is entered on the day sheet and the ledger card at the same time the receipt is filled out. When payments are received by mail, the same system is followed; however, there is no need to create a receipt.

In a computerized system, the receipt is easily printed for the patient as soon as the information has been entered and the patient account updated. If the patient needs a receipt and the payment is not posted right away, a handwritten receipt is acceptable.

The provider may have charges created from emergency department visits, patient hospital visits, surgeries, visits in a convalescent nursing facility, or other out-of-office services. These charges are to be entered on the day sheet and the ledger or patient's account. Some providers produce information manually in a pocket-size notebook, in a calendar, or on a personal handheld computer and give it to the medical assistant on their return to the clinic. The medical assistant then enters the data into the daily sheet and the patient's account. If the provider uses the handheld computer for tracking and recording of office charges, the medical assistant can electronically download the billing information.

Month-End Activities

In the pegboard system, when the last day sheet for the month has been balanced, it is then necessary to verify that the month-end figures on the day sheet agree with patient accounts. Although this may be a time-consuming process in the manual system, it will find mistakes before they grow into major accounting or collection problems.

Reconciling the month-end sheet to the patient ledgers is accomplished by adding all the open balances on the ledgers and verifying that the total agrees with the end-of-month accounts receivable balance on the last day sheet of the month. When these figures agree, the accounts receivable balance is correct.

By following these procedures of "checks and balances," it is likely that all payments have been properly credited to patient accounts and deposited, and that all charges shown as outstanding on the day sheet agree with the outstanding balances of the individual patient accounts. If a payment is somehow misplaced, the deposits will not agree with the credits or with the patient ledgers, and an error will be revealed immediately. Not only does this catch errors, it also eliminates the possibility of loss of a check or undetected theft of funds, because when a mistake is caught immediately, the payer can stop payment on the missing check or credit or debit card slip and a new payment can be made.

Computerized Patient Accounts

A total practice management system offers many advantages in managing patient accounts. The program automatically creates an encounter form the day before the patient is seen or when the administrative medical assistant prints out the schedule. After the patient's examination, the program calculates the charges for the monthly billing statement (Figure 19-4). The management program also creates and updates the patient account, adds new names to the list of patients and to the daily log, and transfers data to produce insurance forms, statements, a list of checks received each day, and deposit slips. In addition, the program automatically ages accounts at each billing cycle and creates billing statements (Figure 19-5). As a result, when patient accounts are computerized, practice collections usually increase.

The computerized patient account contains personal information about each patient, including name, address, and telephone number; email address; the person responsible for payment; and all insurance carriers. The account also lists all previous office visits and the procedures, procedure codes, charges, payments, and adjustments for each visit. Most account management software can be customized to meet the special needs of the individual ambulatory care setting.

As billing information is entered from the encounter forms, the computer automatically updates the account by adding a description of each procedure and procedure code and each diagnosis and diagnosis code. The computer software automatically posts the charges and calculates the balance after credits and adjustments are entered.

Once charges and payments have been entered and the day has been closed, they are not easily removed or changed. This is an important software design because it ensures that monies are not removed from receivables credited to a previous month. This procedure would cause the practice year-end balance to be unresolved. Procedures 19-3, 19-4, 19-5, and 19-6 describe the electronic process for recording patient charges, billing insurance, posting payments and adjustments, credit balances, and refunds.

As useful and efficient as a computerized bookkeeping system can be, it is important to recognize that an inadequate manual system will not get better once computerized. Also, it takes time to move to a computerized system, train personnel, and enter existing patient data. Manual and computer systems may need to run concurrently for a month or two.

BANKING PROCEDURES

Understanding bank accounts and services, making deposits, preparing checks, and reconciling accounts are all a part of daily financial practices. Although many banking services are similar from one bank to another, it is a good idea for the medical assistant in charge of maintaining daily accounts to investigate

Douglasville Medicine Associates
5076 Brand Blvd., Suite 401
Douglasville, NY 01234
Ph: (123) 456-7890
Fax: (123) 456-7891
E-mail: admin@dfma.com
Web site: www.dfma.com

STATEMENT OF ACCOUNT

MANUEL RAMIREZ
1211 Gravel Way
Douglasville, NY 01234

Date: 1/3/20XX
Account No: RAM001

Date	Patient	Description of Service	Total Charges	Patient Payment	Insurance Payment	Adjust-ments	Dedu-ctible	Current Balance
18-Oct-XX	Manuel Ramirez	Established Patient - Level 3 99213	$78.00	$0.00	$47.20	$19.00	$0	$11.80
29-Oct-XX	Manuel Ramirez	Colonscopy 44389	$750.00	$0.00	$0.00	$0.00	$0	$750.00
29-Oct-XX	Manuel Ramirez	Established Patient - Level 5 99215	$176.00	$0.00	$0.00	$0.00	$0	$176.00
		Totals:	$569.00	$0.00	$47.20	$19.00	$0	$937.80

0 to 30 Days Current	31 to 60 Days Past Due	61 to 90 Days Past Due	91+ Days Past Due	BALANCE DUE	$937.80
$0.00	$0.00	$937.80	$0.00		

Important Note:

Figure 19-4 Computerized patient statement

the banking resources of the local community. In an effort to secure new business, many banks compete for customers by offering special services that can be of use to the ambulatory care setting.

Online Banking

Use of the Internet has changed banking and the services it provides. Online banking allows individuals to check account balances, trans-fer funds between accounts, pay bills electronically, check credit card balances, view images of checks and deposits, and download account information 24 hours a day, 7 days a week. Considerable time and expense can be saved with online banking, but remember that any online banking should be completed only through the use of secure and unique passwords granted to only those individuals deemed necessary.

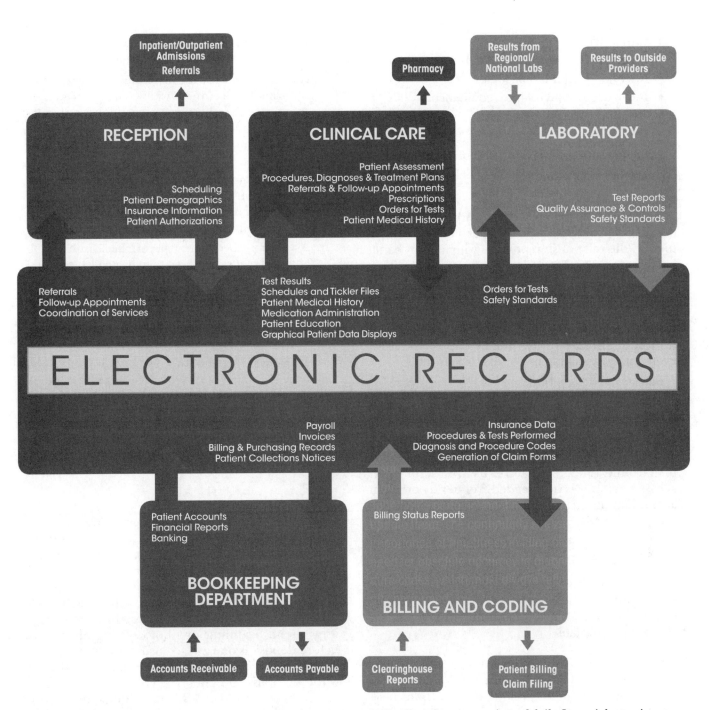

Figure 19-5 Diagram of total practice management system indicating the connection of daily financial practices to insurance billing, clinical care of the patient, reception activities, and laboratory testing.

Types of Accounts

Checking and savings accounts are the two primary types of accounts.

Checking Accounts. The checking account is the primary account type the medical assistant will use in the ambulatory care setting. Today, there are many variations on checking accounts. In the event

that the medical assistant is responsible for establishing a new account, it is worthwhile to investigate features of different checking accounts both within the same bank and at competing banks.

Some features that may differ include:

• Interest paid
• Monthly fees

- Check charges
- Automated teller machine (ATM) access and fees
- After hours deposit capabilities
- Initial deposit and balance requirements
- Overdraft protection
- Fees for checks
- Special services extended free of charge such as **notary,** cashier's checks, traveler's checks, and online banking.

When selecting an account, rather than choosing the account with the lowest fees, consider convenience, the relationship possible with a given bank, bank hours, number of bank locations, and other factors.

Savings Accounts. Savings accounts initially were distinguished from checking accounts because they paid interest on the money deposited. However, many checking accounts pay interest now as well. In either case, the interest is minimal on accounts that give immediate access to the deposit. **Money market accounts** often pay a higher rate of interest, although they may require a higher initial deposit and maintenance of a higher balance. Access to the account may require 24-hour turnaround time. Such accounts are useful when access to money is not needed frequently or when accumulating an amount necessary to invest for long-term goals.

Types of Checks

For the most part, the ambulatory care setting uses a standard business check. However, for special purposes, it is useful to understand the other check types available:

- A **cashier's check** is often used when a check must be guaranteed for the amount in which it is written. Because a cashier's check is the bank's own check drawn against the bank's accounts, the recipient has the assurance that the check will clear. Cashier's checks are obtained at the bank by paying the bank

Critical Thinking

What factors make money market funds a good investment during one period, but provide little return for the investment at another time?

representative cash or sometimes a personal check for the amount of the cashier's check.

- A **certified check** is the depositor's own check that the bank has "certified" with a date and signature to indicate that the check is good for the amount in which it is written.
- Money orders are available from a number of places, even online. The U.S. Postal Service and Western Union are common sites for the purchase of money orders. They are purchased with cash and are similar to cashier's checks. A few patients may use money orders to pay their bill.
- A **voucher check** is a type of check with a stub attached that can be used to indicate invoice dates, services provided, and so on. Many payroll checks are written on voucher checks; the voucher check is frequently used in the ambulatory care setting for accounts payable.
- **Traveler's checks** are available in most banks and are convenient and safer to use than cash when traveling. They are written in specific denominations ($20, $50, $100) and require a signature when purchased and when used. However, many banks today advise customers to use ATM machines for necessary cash if traveling to areas where ATM machines are readily available.

Depositing Checks

Deposits are usually made daily because they serve as another proof of posting and because leaving large sums of money in the facility overnight is unwise. A rubber endorsement stamp from the bank should be used to immediately imprint the back of all checks received directly from patients and in the mail. Be sure all checks are stamped before depositing them. Scanning or photocopying all checks before deposit is one way to ensure accuracy.

Because the endorsement transfers rights to whoever holds the check, it is important to take certain precautions. A blank endorsement consists of a signature only (whether in pen or with a stamp) and presents a danger in that, if the check is lost or stolen, someone else could endorse the check below the signature and cash it. A restrictive endorsement should be used on all checks received in the ambulatory care setting. Restrictive endorsements include the signature and the words "for deposit only" or "pay to the order of…" (include the name of bank and account number; in addition, all possible payees' names should be listed under the company name, with the practice address). This restricts the use of the check should it be lost or stolen.

Cash on Hand

Most medical practices need to have cash available on a daily basis. If it is the practice to collect co-payments and any coinsurance at the time of service, some patients will pay in cash and need change. Cash usually is kept in a locked change drawer that contains up to $200 in small bills at the beginning of each day. Any time a patient pays cash for the service, a receipt is prepared. Receipts are prenumbered, thus monitoring loss or theft. Cash amounts paid by patients must also be noted in their account or ledger. The terms *received on account (ROA) cash* is usually indicated in the description column. If payment is made by check, follow the same procedure except the word *check* is used instead of *cash*.

At the end of each day, the cash drawer is balanced. The amount of cash received will be noted on the deposit slip as "currency." The remaining amount in the cash drawer will be the same as the beginning amount. Also, the day's cash received must match the cash control on the daily sheet. It is a good idea for only one person to handle the cash in the cash drawer; thus, it is not necessary for more than one person to balance the cash drawer at the end of the day. The cash drawer is not to be confused with petty cash, which is discussed later in this chapter. Petty cash is used to purchase small items such as postage, office refreshments, and so on.

Checks are always written for major purchases, with the cash drawer used only to accommodate patient needs when payment is made in cash.

Most business accounts use deposit slips similar to the one in Figure 19-6. They are always completed in duplicate or a copy is made—one copy to accompany the deposit and one to be retained for office records. As shown, these deposit slips are longer than those generally used for personal accounts and have room for more entries and more information. If your manual day sheet has a built-in duplicate deposit slip, it will have been completed during posting.

A computerized system of financial records can provide deposit slips that may be used. The same procedure is followed as previously discussed. Procedure 19-7 outlines the steps in preparing a deposit.

Accepting Checks

When accepting checks from patients and other individuals, take a few minutes to inspect the check. This may eliminate checks returned from the bank for various reasons:

- Inspect the check for correct date, amount, and signature.
- Do not accept a third-party check (a check written to the patient from another person or company) unless it is from the insurance carrier.

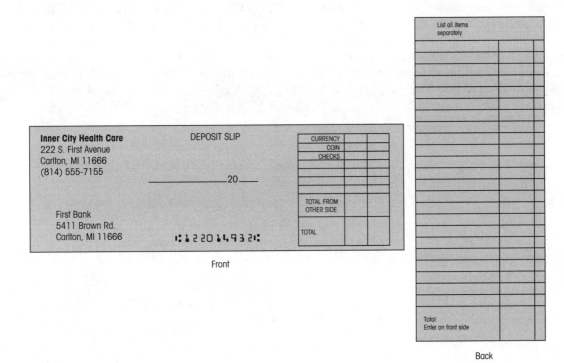

Figure 19-6   Sample deposit slip.

- If a deposited check is returned marked "nonsufficient funds" (NSF), call the bank that returned it and verify availability of funds. If funds are available, immediately redeposit the check for processing. If the check is returned a second time marked NSF, it is necessary to perform two bookkeeping functions. First, deduct the amount from the checking account balance of the practice. Second, add the amount back into the amount due by the patient in his or her account balance by entering the amount in the paid column in parentheses and increase the balance by the same amount. Place a brief explanation in the description column. Follow the office procedure for notifying the patient that the check was returned. See Procedure 19-8.

Lost or Stolen Checks

In the event that a check is missing and is thought to be lost or stolen, report this to your bank immediately. In some cases, you may be advised to stop payment to prevent unauthorized cashing of the check. In other situations, the bank may place a warning on the account, advising bank representatives to be especially careful about checking signatures to detect any attempt at a forged signature.

Writing and Recording Checks

Part of daily financial practices includes writing checks to pay bills (**accounts payable**), refunds of overpayment, and replenishment of petty cash. Writing the checks and paying the bills is usually done systematically. Chapter 21 discusses accounts payable and disbursement records in greater detail. It is important that checks be prepared either

electronically or written legibly to avoid bank errors. Checks should be dated and must include the name of the **payee** and the amount of payment entered both in figures and in words. It is also advisable that the "memo" line indicate what the check is for and include any account or invoice number for reference. Figure 19-7 shows a sample of a properly completed check.

Rules for Preparing Checks. Follow these rules to ensure that checks are properly prepared and recorded (see Procedure 19-9).

- Confirm that the numeric and written amounts agree.
- Confirm that everything is spelled correctly.
- Follow office procedure for having the provider or office manager approve all expenditures and sign all outgoing checks.
- Determine that the check has been signed by an individual with signature privileges.
- Confirm that the check is payable to the correct payee and that the current date is used.

    Chapter 21 provides information on electronic check writing.

Reconciling a Bank Statement

Each month the bank will send a statement for the checking account (Figure 19-8). With online banking, a bank statement can be accessed electronically at any time. It also can be printed and used similar to a standard printed bank statement. The statement will show the account balance according to the bank's records, a listing of all checks that have

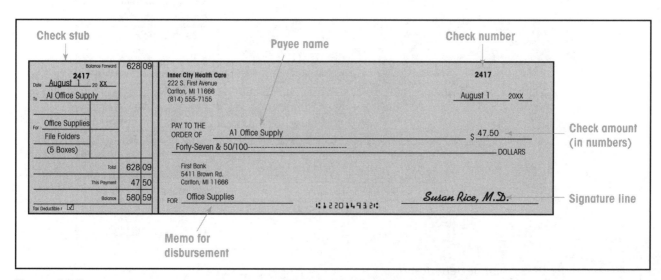

Figure 19-7 Sample of properly completed check and check stub.

Summary of Account Balance			Closing Date 1/15/XX		
Account # 1257-164013			Ending Balance $8,347.62		
Beginning Balance	$7,152.18				
Total Deposits and Additions	$8,643.86				
Total Withdrawals	$7,433.21				
Service Charge	$ 15.24				
Number	Date	Amount	Number	Date	Amount
201	12/18/XX	173.82	234	1/4/XX	96.31
223*	12/18/XX	44.12	235	1/4/XX	73.48
224	12/20/XX	586.00	236	1/6/XX	325.40
225	12/21/XX	24.15	237	1/7/XX	40.00
226	12/22/XX	33.90	238	1/8/XX	66.77
228*	12/23/XX	1250.00	241*	1/9/XX	15.55
229	12/24/XX	11.75	242	1/10/XX	12.45
230	12/24/XX	19.02	243	1/10/XX	4441.25
231	1/2/XX	43.80	244	1/10/XX	64.55
232	1/3/XX	39.00			
233	1/4/XX	71.50			

*Denotes gap in check sequence

Date	Deposit Amount	Date	Deposit Amount
18-Dec	361.75	4-Jan	825.00
19-Dec	586.00	5-Jan	1286.71
20-Dec	918.21	7-Jan	608.00
21-Dec	201.00	8-Jan	811.15
2-Jan	475.00	9-Jan	1092.68
3-Jan	1478.36		

1. Enter Ending Balance from the front of this statement
$ 8,347.62

2. Enter deposits not shown on this statement
$ 3,162.50

3. Subtotal (add 1 & 2)
$ 11,510.12

4. List outstanding checks or other withdrawals here

Check #	Amount
222	37.89
227	161.15
239	11.50
240	92.12
245	835.17
246	21.75
247	586.00

5. Total outstanding checks
$ 1,745.58

Balance (subtract #5 from #3)
$ 9,764.54
This should equal your checkbook balance

Front   Back

Figure 19-8   Sample bank statement with check reconciliation.

cleared the bank, deposits received by the bank, and any service charges deducted from the account. It is necessary to reconcile the entries in the checkbook against this statement to be sure there are no errors either in the checkbook or in the bank's records. Your bank statement is another means of ensuring that the accounts receivable is accurate for the previous month. If you use an accounting software package, this will also have a computerized option for reconciling.

Procedure 19-10 details the steps involved in reconciling the statement.

PURCHASING SUPPLIES AND EQUIPMENT

It is important to ensure proper control over purchasing of supplies and equipment for several reasons:

1. To avoid purchase of unnecessary items
2. To avoid duplication of items purchased
3. To provide a system for payment of only those items properly ordered and received

To accomplish these things, you should follow the first rule of purchasing: nothing is ordered or paid for without a purchase order or purchase order number. A copy of the purchase order is sent to the supplier and a copy is retained by the clinic for verification of shipment and payment of invoice.

Preparing a Purchase Order

Purchase order forms are available from office supply companies or can be ordered from a printer and customized to the needs of the ambulatory care setting. As an alternative to ordering preprinted purchase order forms, the clinic staff may choose to create their own forms using Microsoft Excel® software. This enables the clinic to have electronic access to the form with imbedded formulas. Figure 19-9 shows a typical purchase order form properly completed, which is reviewed here section by section.

The purchase order form can vary greatly; some have more or less information. The form shown in Figure 19-9 contains the usual information required. The important thing is that the purchase order is used consistently.

- *Date.* Day purchase order is made.
- *Purchase order number.* A preprinted number that is used on invoices and statements from the supplier and on the check used to pay the invoice. It is also

PURCHASE ORDER

NO. 1742

Date:

Bill To:	Ship To:	Vendor:
Inner City Health Care 222 S. First Avenue Carlton, MI 11666 (814) 555-7155	**Inner City Health Care** 222 S. First Avenue Carlton, MI 11666 (814) 555-7155	**AZ Medical Supply** 4721 E. Camelback Rd. Phoenix, AZ 85252 (602) 555-3246

REQ BY	BUYER	TERMS
Karen Ritter	Walter Seals	Net 30

QTY	ITEM	UNITS	DESCRIPTION	UNIT PR	TOTAL
10	427A	Box	Surgical Gloves - Sz 7	9.20	92.00
1	327DC	Case	2" gauze pads	60.30	60.30
5	1943C	Box	Tongue Depressors	5.80	29.00
15	7433	Ea	Examination Table paper (roll)	10.50	159.50

SUBTOTAL	338.80
TAX	28.80
FREIGHT	Prepaid
BAL DUE	376.60

Figure 19-9 Purchase order form.

important for tracking the status of the order. In smaller practices, the purchase order number may simply be the name of the person ordering with the date the order was placed immediately following.

- *Bill to address.* This is generally used when items are to be shipped to an address different from the address where the supplier will send the bill for goods or services.
- *Ship to address.* When items are to be sent by supplier, this must always be completed.
- *Vendor information.* The name and address of supplier where purchase order is to be sent.
- *Req. By.* States which individual or department has requested the item(s).
- *Buyer.* States the individual in the office who is authorized to issue a purchase order.
- *Terms.* Agreement between buyer and seller as to when payment is due.
- *QTY.* Quantity of item being ordered (number of units).

- *Item.* Vendor's catalogue part or item number.
- *Units.* How the item is sold—individually (ea.), by the box, case, or dozen. Many suppliers will not split units (i.e., sell less than a full case).
- *Description.* Brief description of item (helps as a cross-check for vendor in the event that an item number is entered incorrectly).
- *Unit price.* How much *one* unit (ea., box, case, dozen) costs.
- *Total.* Cost of one unit multiplied by the number of units being ordered.
- *Discount.* If any discount is allowed for quick and early payment, it is noted here. For instance, there might be a 10% discount for paying within 10 days. The discount amount is entered before the Total column is summed.
- *Subtotal.* Sum of the Total column.
- *Tax.* Sales tax required by the state.
- *Freight.* How much the customer must pay to have the order delivered (not always applicable).

- *Bal. Due.* The sum of the subtotal, tax, and freight charges; this is how much the office will be billed.

Verifying Goods Received

Proper purchasing procedure does not stop with the completion and mailing of the purchase order. When goods are received, it is necessary to verify that the correct items and quantities were shipped by the vendor. Chapter 21 discusses accounts payable.

PETTY CASH

Petty cash is money kept in the office for minor, routine, or unexpected expenses such as postage-due mail or coffee supplies. Keep petty cash totally separate from the cash drawer that is used to make change for patients paying their co-payment. Keeping this cash on hand eliminates the necessity of the provider or office manager having to sign checks for such items. Petty cash is not used to pay bills or make large routine purchases.

The amount of cash on hand for this purpose is small, usually $75 to $100, and is usually kept in small denominations. However, records must be as carefully maintained as for any other financial transactions and balanced each day before closing.

Establishing a Petty Cash Fund

If your clinic does not already have a petty cash fund or if you are in a new practice that has not yet established a fund, determine how much the fund should be and write a check to "Cash" for that amount. The amount should be enough to cover several days of incidental expenses.

Tracking, Balancing, and Replenishing Petty Cash

Tracking. Keep a supply of petty cash vouchers on hand to track how petty cash is used. When money is taken from petty cash, a voucher must always be completed and the receipt from the purchase attached. Vouchers and receipts are kept in the petty cash box with the money until the fund is replenished.

Balancing and Replenishing. When the fund gets low, write another check to "Cash" to bring it back up to the original amount. To determine the amount of the check, it is necessary to first balance the account. After the account is balanced, list how funds were spent in such a way that the bookkeeper can disburse the check properly.

Procedure 19-11 outlines the steps involved in establishing and maintaining a petty cash account.

DOCUMENTATION

Financial records of patients are to be kept separate from the patients' medical charts. Except for the attachment of the encounter form or superbill at the time of the visit, they rarely are seen together. Often, only the patient's medical record is necessary for documentation; other times, only the financial information is necessary. This policy also serves as a reminder that the care given to patients has nothing to do with their ability to pay ————

Procedure 19-1

Recording/Posting Patient Charges, Payments, and Adjustments in a Manual System

PURPOSE:
To record information including services rendered, fees charged, any adjustments made, and balances pertaining to a patient's visit to the provider and patient's account.

EQUIPMENT/SUPPLIES:
Calculator
Patient's account or ledger

PROCEDURE STEPS:
1. Check the patient's account before the patient's appointment to make certain it is current. The account will indicate any recent insurance payments, any amount received on the account, and any balance due. RATIONALE: Allows the medical office assistant to focus entirely on the patient at arrival time and gives a current picture of the patient's account.

continues

Procedure 19-1 (continued)

2. When the patient arrives, check for name, address, telephone numbers, and any changes regarding medical insurance. Make any changes in the account or on the ledger. RATIONALE: Ensures that information is current and up to date.

3. On the encounter form or superbill, complete any necessary items such as the date of service and the responsible party's name. Then attach it to the patient's medical chart that is now ready for the clinical medical assistant to take with the patient to the examination room. RATIONALE: The encounter form allows the provider to indicate appropriate procedure and diagnosis codes.

4. When the provider completes the treatment or examination, he or she will check the procedures and diagnosis on the encounter form. RATIONALE: Provider marks the appropriate codes and signs the encounter form, indicating it is correct. The provider or licensed caregiver is the only one authorized to select the appropriate procedure codes.

5. When the patient returns to the front desk, refer to the provider's fee schedule, enter the charge next to each procedure, and calculate the total. If the procedure description is not indicated, one is to be provided. A description is necessary for each service. Check to see if the codes match the services provided. If they do not match, refer it back to the provider or licensed caregiver for correction. RATIONALE: Medical office staff and the patient can identify the charge to the particular service given and know that the coding and charges will match.

6. In the *manual pegboard system,* post each service or procedure as a charge or debit. Post any payments received today in the payment column as a credit. RATIONALE: Clearly indicates charges made and payments received, creating an updated account.

7. If any adjustment applies to the account, enter the amount in the adjustment column. If there is no adjustment column and the adjustment will *reduce* the bill, enter the amount in the payment column enclosed by parentheses. If the adjustment will *increase* the bill, place the amount in the charge column (no parentheses) with an explanation in the description column. In the *manual system,* the adjustment amount will be either added or subtracted from the totaled figures. RATIONALE: Adjustment is shown as separate from basic charge so that the provider's fee profile is unaffected.

8. Determine current balance by adding credits and subtracting debits to the running balance and determine the amount in the current balance. Always use a calculator (one with a tape is recommended) to calculate and verify your mathematics. RATIONALE: Completes the recording of patient charges, payments, and adjustments.

9. If the recording is a payment from the patient, place a restrictive endorsement on the check. RATIONALE: Ensures that the check can only be cashed by the authorized party.

10. Enter the amount in the payment column. In the description column, identify as cash, check, or insurance payment. If payment is a check, enter the number of the check. RATIONALE: This information is necessary in making the bank deposit slip.

11. Place the cash or processed check in the appointed secure place awaiting deposit. RATIONALE: Keeps receivables together and ready for deposit.

Procedure 19-2

Balancing Day Sheets in a Manual System

PURPOSE:
To verify that all entries to the day sheet are correct and that the totals balance.

EQUIPMENT/SUPPLIES:
Day sheet
Calculator

continues

PROCEDURE STEPS:

1. *Column totals.* The first step in balancing a day sheet is to total columns A, B_1, B_2, C, and D, and enter the total for each column in the boxes marked "Totals This Page." The column totals are then added to the figures entered in the "Previous Page" column boxes to arrive at the "Month to Date" totals, which provide the total charges, credits, and so forth entered from the first working day of the month to the present. RATIONALE: Establishes column totals.

2. *Proof of posting.* This box is used to verify that entries have been made correctly and that the column totals are accurate. *All figures entered here are taken from the "Totals This Page" column boxes.*

   a. Enter today's column D total, which shows the sum of all the previous balances entered when the transactions were posted.

   b. Added to this is the column A total of all charges for that day, to arrive at a subtotal. Enter the amount where indicated in the box.

   c. Because columns B_1 and B_2 are both credit columns that reduce balances, they are added together and entered in the box labeled "Less Cols B_1 and B_2"; the total of credits is subtracted from the subtotal. If all entries and addition are correct in the posting area, the result should equal the amount in column C and the transactions for that day are balanced. RATIONALE: Verifies entries have been made correctly and that the totals are accurate.

   Overview: When an individual transaction is entered, the patient's previous balance (D) is added to the charges for the day (A). If there are any payments or adjustments made at that time, they are entered in the B columns and subtracted from the A + D amount to achieve the new balance (C). Because each transaction is actually D + A − B = C, the column totals of D + A − B will always equal the C total.

   $$
   \begin{array}{cccccccc}
   & D & & A & & B & & C \\
   & 10 & + & 5 & - & 2 & = & 13 \\
   & 2 & + & 7 & - & 1 & = & 8 \\
   \textbf{Column Totals} & 12 & + & 12 & - & 3 & = & 21
   \end{array}
   $$

3. *Accounts Receivable (A/R) Control.* This box simply adds the previous day's A/R balance to the current day's totals to include the current day's business and arrive at the new A/R total.

   a. The column A and column B totals are carried straight across from the Proof of Posting box to the corresponding blanks in the A/R Control box.

   b. Add the amount already entered in the Previous Day's Total space to the Column A amount to arrive at a subtotal.

   c. Subtract the amount carried over from the "Less Columns B_1 and B_2" box to find the new A/R amount. RATIONALE: Determines new accounts receivable balance.

4. *A/R Proof* verifies, or proves, the A/R balance in the A/R Control box. *The figure entered on the first line of this box will not change during a calendar month* because it shows how much the A/R balance was on the first working day of the month. *All other figures entered will be taken from the "Month-To-Date" column boxes.*

   a. Enter the amount from column A (month-to-date) where shown.

   b. Add the column A amount to the "A/R 1st of Month" figure and enter the sum in the subtotal space.

   c. Enter the B_1 and B_2 month-to-date amounts and subtract from the subtotal. This amount goes in the Total A/R space.

   If all posting and addition are correct, the Total A/R amounts in the A/R Control and A/R Proof boxes will match and the day is balanced. RATIONALE: Verifies the accounts receivable balance in the accounts receivable control box.

5. *Deposit verification* involves totaling the columns in Section 2 and entering the sum of the columns in the space marked "Total Deposit." *NOTE:* The Total Deposit and the Total of Payments Received in column B_1 should match. RATIONALE: Verifies deposit total.

6. *Business Analysis Summary.* If this section is used, total each column in the summary section. *NOTE:* If the Business Analysis Summary is used to break out charges by type or by provider, the sum of the columns should equal today's column A total. If it is used to credit payments to different providers, the sum of the columns will equal

continues

Procedure 19-2 (continued)

today's payment column. RATIONALE: The total deposit and the total of payments received in column B₁ should match to prove totals.

7. *After the day sheet is balanced,* there is one step remaining: the transfer of balances.

a. Take out a new day sheet for the next day.

b. Transfer the "Month-To-Date" column totals to the "Previous Page" columns boxes on the new sheet.

c. Enter the Total A/R amount from the last day sheet in the "Previous Day's Total" space of the A/R Control box on the new day sheet.

d. Enter the A/R 1st of Month Amount in the A/R Proof box on the new sheet. RATIONALE: Transfers balances to prepare a new day sheet for the next day's activities.

The new day sheet is now ready for posting.

Procedure 19-3

Posting Patient Charges Using Medical Office Simulation Software (MOSS)

PURPOSE:
To electronically post patient charges.

EQUIPMENT/SUPPLIES:
Computer
MOSS

POSTING PATIENT CHARGES EXERCISES:

1. Jordan Connell had an appointment on June 3, 2009, with Dr. Heath. Dr. Heath is billing for an established patient level 3 visit (99213) and a rapid strep test (87880). The diagnoses indicated by Dr. Heath are as follows: Strep Throat (034.0) and Otitis Media (382.9). Patient reference number is 100.

2. Ed Gormann came in for his physical with Dr. Heath on September 15, 2009. This visit will be billed using the preventive medicine procedure code 99396 and diagnosis code V70.0. Patient reference number is 101.

3. Elane Ybarra's appointment was on June 4, 2009, with Dr. Schwartz. Dr. Schwartz has submitted a superbill indicating that he is billing for an established patient level 4 visit (99214). He has also indicated the following diagnosis: Gastroenteritis (558.9). Patient reference number is 102.

MOSS PROCEDURE STEPS:

1. Open MOSS and select Procedure Posting from the main menu.

2. In the Search Criteria box of the patient list, type in "Con" and click on "Search". RATIONALE: This will show those patients whose last names begin with these letters.

3. Highlight the line with Jordan Connell's name and select "Add" at the bottom of the dialog box because you will be adding procedures.

4. The Procedure Posting window will open. In Field 1, enter the reference number for the patient, "100". RATIONALE: This is determined by each individual clinic and is used to help find accounts when posting payments, adjustments, etc.

5. Field 2 should have the name of the provider the patient saw on the day for which you are posting payments. If not, use the drop-down arrow to select the correct provider, "Dr. Heath."

6. In Field 3, select "Office" as the place of service where the patient was seen.

7. Field 4, leave blank. This is used only if the provider has seen the patient at another facility other than the office.

8. In Field 5, enter "06/03/2009," the date of service for the visit.

continues

9. Field 6, leave blank. This field would be completed with a date only if the "To" date was different from the date entered in Field 5, indicating that the service had been provided on consecutive days. RATIONALE: This is most commonly used when the provider performs hospital visits or nursing home visits.

10. Field 7 will automatically populate based on the entries in Fields 5 and 6.

11. In Field 8, click on the magnifying glass and in the Search Criteria box enter "99213." Highlight the code and click on "Select."

12. In Field 9, click on the drop-down arrow and select modifier "-25." RATIONALE: This is necessary because a separately identifiable service (the rapid strep test) was performed in addition to the visit.

13. Field 10 will automatically populate based on the patient's insurer and the fee schedules loaded into the database.

14. In Field 11, click on the radio button to the left of "Primary." RATIONALE: This procedure is being billed to the patient's primary insurer.

15. In Field 12a, click on the magnifying glass to the right of the data entry box and in the Diagnosis Code window "Search Criteria" box enter "034.0." Highlight this code and click on "Select."

16. In Field 12b, click on the magnifying glass to the right of the data entry box and in the Diagnosis Code window "Search Criteria" box enter "382.9." Highlight this code and click on "Select."

17. Fields 12c and 12d should be left blank because there are no additional diagnoses to report.

RATIONALE: Remember, only four diagnoses can be reported on a claim form.

18. Make sure that Field 13 has "No" checked, as this visit was not the result of an accident.

19. Check your work with Figure 19-10. At the bottom of the Procedure Posting window, in Field 14, click on "Post." RATIONALE: This will result in one line of information appearing in the "Procedure Detail" portion in the middle of the window.

20. Return to Field 1 and enter "100" for the patient reference number.

21. Field 2 should have the name of the provider the patient saw on the day for which you are posting payments. If not, use the drop-down arrow to select the correct provider, "Dr. Heath."

22. In Field 3, select "Office" as the place of service where the patient was seen.

23. Field 4, leave blank. This is used only if the provider has seen the patient at another facility other than the office.

24. In Field 5, enter "06/03/2009," the date of service for the visit.

25. Field 6, leave blank. This field would be completed with a date only if the "To" date was different from the date entered in Field 5, indicating that the service had been provided on consecutive days. RATIONALE: This is most commonly used when the provider performs hospital visits or nursing home visits.

26. Field 7 will automatically populate based on the entries in Fields 5 and 6.

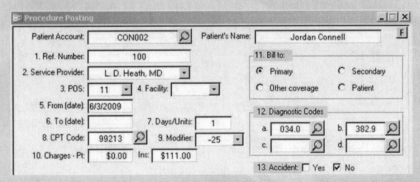

Figure 19-10   Top portion of procedure posting screen for Jordan Connell.

27. In Field 8, click on the magnifying glass and in the Search Criteria box enter "87880." Highlight the code and click on "Select."

28. Field 9, leave blank.

29. Field 10 will automatically populate based on the patient's insurer and the fee schedules loaded into the database.

30. In Field 11, click on the radio button to the left of "Primary." This procedure is being billed to the patient's primary insurer.

31. In Field 12a, click on the magnifying glass to the right of the data entry box and in the Diagnosis Code window "Search Criteria" box enter "034.0." Highlight this code and click on "Select."

32. Fields 12b, 12c, and 12d should be left blank because there are no additional diagnoses to report. RATIONALE: The otitis media diagnosis would not be linked to the rapid strep test.

33. Make sure that Field 13 has "No" checked, as this visit was not the result of an accident.

34. At the bottom of the Procedure Posting window, in Field 14, click on "Post." Now two lines of information appear in the "Procedure Detail" portion in the middle of the window, reflecting the two entries you have posted (Figure 19-11).

35. Click on "Close" in the bottom right corner of the screen and "Close" the patient listing screen.

36. Repeat the above steps, using the information provided in Posting Patient Charges Exercises 2 and 3.

37. Take screenshots of the complete Procedure Posting screen (the window shown in Figure 19-11) for Exercises 2 and 3 and submit to your instructor either as a printout or in an email file.

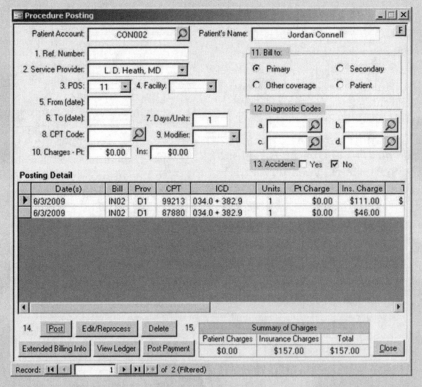

Figure 19-11   Completed procedure posting screen for Jordan Connell.

Procedure 19-4

Insurance Billing Using Medical Office Simulation Software (MOSS)

PURPOSE:
To prepare and simulate sending electronic insurance claim forms using MOSS.

EQUIPMENT/SUPPLIES:
Computer
MOSS

INSURANCE BILLING EXERCISE:
1. Process the bill for Jordan Connell's visit on 6/3/2009.
2. Process the bill for Edward Gormann's visit on 9/15/2009.
3. Process the bill for Elane Ybarra's visit on 6/4/2009.

MOSS PROCEDURE STEPS:
1. Open MOSS and select Insurance Billing from the main menu. RATIONALE: This will open the Claims Preparation window.
2. In Field 1, select "Patient Name" using the drop-down arrow as the sort order.
3. In Field 2, make sure the radio button for "Bill" is selected, use the drop-down arrow to select "Dr. Heath" because he is the provider who is billing for the service. In the "Service Dates From" input box enter "06/03/2009" and in the "Through" input box enter "06/03/2009." Select "Jordan Connell" from the drop-down menu next to Patient Name. Leave "Account Number" blank. RATIONALE: This would only be used if you were sorting by account number.

4. Field 3, select "Electronic" for the transmission type (unless your instructor requests paper claims).
5. Field 4, select "Primary" as the Billing Option; you are billing the primary insurer for these services.
6. Field 5, select "Consumer One HRA." RATIONALE: This is the patient's insurer. Check your work with Figure 19-12.
7. Click on the "Prebilling Worksheet" button at the bottom of the window. Verify that the information on the report is what was entered to be billed for the patient. RATIONALE: Checks the data entry against the patient bill. Print this by clicking the printer icon and give to your instructor.
8. Click "Close" in the upper left corner of the screen.
9. Back at the Claims Preparation screen, select "Generate Claims." This will open a window with a CMS-1500 form that you should scroll through to verify that correct diagnoses and procedures are given on the claim.
10. Select "Transmit EMC" at the bottom of the window. This will open a "Transmission Status" window. Once this has finished, click on "Close." This will bring you back to the main menu.
11. Repeat the above steps, using the information provided in Insurance Billing Exercises 2 and 3.
12. Submit the completed prebilling worksheets for all three scenarios to your instructor.

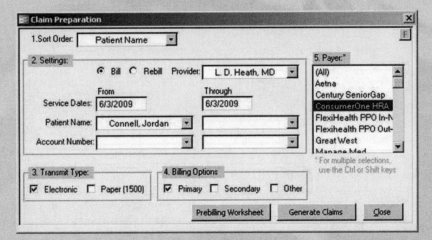

Figure 19-12   Claim preparation screen for Medical Office Simulation Software® (MOSS).

Procedure 19-5

Posting Payments and Adjustments Using Medical Office Simulation Software (MOSS)

PURPOSE:
To electronically post payments and adjustments.

EQUIPMENT/SUPPLIES:
Computer
MOSS

POSTING PAYMENTS AND ADJUSTMENTS EXERCISES:

1. FlexiHealth PPO In-Network reimbursed the practice on October 20, 2009, for Ed Gormann's physical performed on September 15, 2009. The plan allowable was $200.56 minus a $20.00 patient co-payment that was not collected at the time of service. The net amount the plan paid for the visit totals $180.56.

2. Payment is received from ConsumerOne HRA on July 31, 2009, for Jordan Connell's visit on June 3, 2009, in the amount of $71.76 for the office visit (99213) and $11.04 for the strep test (87880). Write off any remaining balance as an insurance adjustment.

3. For Elane Ybarra's visit on June 4, 2009, her insurer, FlexiHealth PPO In-Network, reimbursed the practice on August 10, 2009, in the amount of $89.06. The EOB indicates that the patient has a $22.26 coinsurance that was not collected at the time of the visit. Dr. Schwartz is not a participating provider in this plan. The patient will receive a bill for the balance due in a subsequent chapter exercise (Procedure 20-4).

MOSS PROCEDURE STEPS:

1. Open MOSS and select Posting Payments from the main menu.

2. In the Search Criteria box of the patient list, type in "Gor" and click on "Search." RATIONALE: This shows those patients whose last names begin with these letters.

3. Highlight the line with Edward Gormann's name and select "Apply Payment" at the bottom of the dialog box.

4. In Field 1 of the Posting Payments window there will be a list of all billed procedures. Highlight the line for the date of service "09/15/2009" by clicking in the box to the left of the date and click on "Select/Edit" at the bottom of the screen. RATIONALE: This will have to be done for each procedure individually, just as it appears on the EOB.

5. Field 2 is automatically populated with the patient's primary insurance.

6. In Field 3, enter "10/20/2009," the date the payment was received.

7. In Field 4, click on the drop-down arrow and select "Payment Insurance."

8. Field 5, leave blank. This field is used to indicate the payer's claim number, but for this exercise, this field is left blank.

9. In Field 6, enter "180.56," the actual amount paid by the insurer.

10. Leave Fields 7 through 9 blank at this time.

11. In Field 10, use the drop-down arrow and select "Adjustment Insurance." RATIONALE: Indicates what type of adjustment is being made to the account.

12. In Field 11, enter "65.44." This represents the difference between the charges minus the insurance allowable and any patient responsibility (co-payment, deductible, or coinsurance). RATIONALE: This is the amount the practice will be writing off.

13. Field 12, leave blank. This field would only be used if the EOB indicated that there was a patient deductible due.

14. Field 13 automatically calculates the balance based on the amounts entered in Fields 6, 9, 11, and 12.

15. Field 14 can be left blank. RATIONALE: This is used to make any notes pertinent to the payment or balance due.

16. Check your work with Figure 19-13. Click "Post." The screen will remain open to post any additional payments to the patient's account. Click "Close."

continues

Procedure 19-5 (continued)

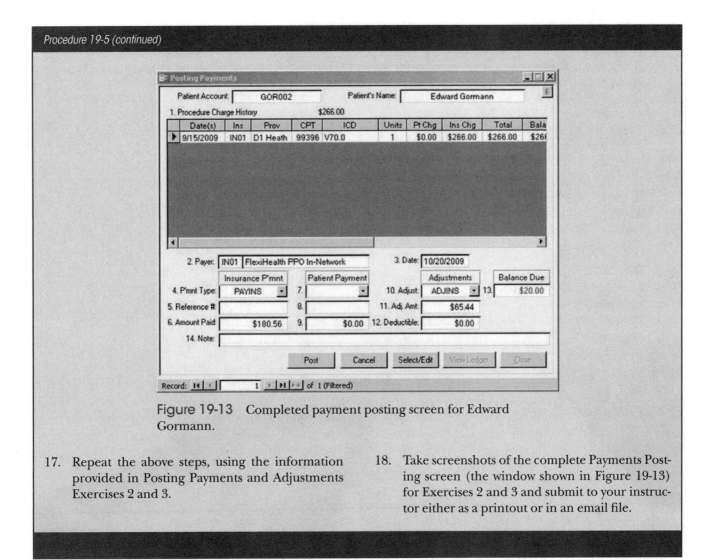

Figure 19-13   Completed payment posting screen for Edward Gormann.

17. Repeat the above steps, using the information provided in Posting Payments and Adjustments Exercises 2 and 3.

18. Take screenshots of the complete Payments Posting screen (the window shown in Figure 19-13) for Exercises 2 and 3 and submit to your instructor either as a printout or in an email file.

Procedure 19-6

Processing Credit Balances and Refunds Using Medical Office Simulation Software (MOSS)

PURPOSE:
To electronically process credit balances and refunds.

EQUIPMENT/SUPPLIES:
Computer
MOSS

PROCESSING CREDIT BALANCES AND REFUNDS EXERCISES:

1. Josephine Albertson came in for an appointment on July 10, 2009, and paid a $20.00 co-payment. Upon receipt of reimbursement by her insurance carrier, it is noted that she did not have a co-payment. She is now entitled to a $20.00 refund.

continues

2. Andrew Jefferson had an appointment on July 5, 2009, and paid his co-payment of $20.00 at the time of his visit. One week later, a check was received from Andrew's wife in the amount of $20.00 for his visit. He now must be refunded the $20.00 overpayment.

3. Alice Maxwell paid $15.00 for her co-payment when she came for her appointment on July 5, 2009. When the reimbursement for the visit was received from her insurance carrier, the co-payment was only $10.00. She is now entitled to a $5.00 refund.

MOSS PROCEDURE STEPS:

1. Open MOSS and select Posting Payment from the main menu.

2. In the Search Criteria box of the patient list, type in "Alb" and click on "Search." RATIONALE: This shows those patients whose last names begin with these letters.

3. Highlight the line with Josephine Albertson's name and click on "Apply Payment."

4. In Field 1 of the Posting Payments screen, highlight the line for the date of service "7/10/2009" and click on "Select/Edit" at the bottom of the screen.

5. Field 13 should have a balance of "-$20.00." RATIONALE: Shows the amount the patient should be refunded.

6. Click in Field 3 and enter "8/20/2009," the date you are processing the patient's refund.

7. Tab over to Field 10, click on the drop-down arrow, scroll down and select "REFUND."

8. In Field 11, enter "$20.00" as the amount of the refund.

9. Check your work with Figure 19-14. Click on "Post" in the bottom left-hand portion of the screen. RATIONALE: Completes the bookkeeping cycle for the refund.

10. Take screenshots of the complete Payment Posting screen (the window shown in Figure 19-14) for Exercises 2 and 3 and submit to your instructor either as a printout or in an email file.

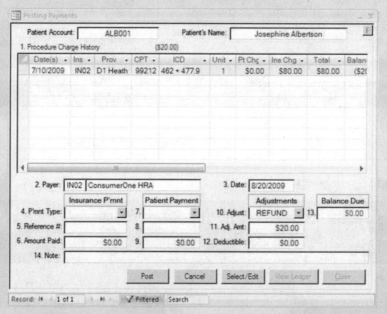

Figure 19-14   Completed payment posting screen for Josephine Albertson.

Procedure 19-7

Preparing a Deposit

PURPOSE:
To create a deposit slip for the day's receipts.

EQUIPMENT/SUPPLIES:
New deposit slip
Check endorsement stamp
Calculator
Cash and checks received for the day

PROCEDURE STEPS:

1. Separate all checks from currency (paper money). RATIONALE: Each must be entered as a separate total.

2. Count all currency to be deposited and enter the amount in the space provided. Gather bills facing the same direction in order (i.e., 50s, 20s, 10s, and so on). RATIONALE: Follows bank procedure.

3. Count all coins to be deposited and enter the amount in the space provided. Coins may need to be wrapped. RATIONALE: Follows bank procedure.

4. On the back of the deposit slip list each check separately. Include the patient name in the left-hand column and enter the amount of the check in the right-hand column. RATIONALE: Follows bank procedure.

5. Total the checks listed and copy the total on the front where it is indicated to place the total from the other side. RATIONALE: Follows bank procedure.

6. The sum of currency, coins, and checks should always equal the total in the Payments column on that day's day sheet. RATIONALE: Proof of accuracy.

7. Attach the top copy of the deposit slip to the deposit, leaving the carbon on the pad. RATIONALE: Provides the office and bank with record of deposit.

8. Enter the date and amount of the deposit in the space provided on the checkbook stubs. RATIONALE: Keeps checkbook register current with money in account.

9. Add the amount of the deposit to the checkbook balance. RATIONALE: Keeps checkbook register current with money in account.

10. Deposit at the bank, either in person or at the night deposit. In either case, be sure a record of deposit is received (it will be mailed if the night deposit is used). It is not recommended that deposits be made through ATMs; currency should never be deposited in an ATM. RATIONALE: Proof bank processed the deposit as indicated.

Procedure 19-8

Recording a Nonsufficient Funds Check in a Manual System

PURPOSE:
To perform bookkeeping functions that keep account in proper balance.

EQUIPMENT/SUPPLIES:
The practice's account balance
Manual day sheet
Manual ledger
Nonsufficient funds (NSF) check

PROCEDURE STEPS:

1. Follow the office policy for notifying the patient of the returned check. RATIONALE: Policy may vary from clinic to clinic.

2. When the NSF check has been returned the second time, deduct the check amount from the account balance of the practice. RATIONALE: The funds can no longer be counted as earnings received.

continues

3. Add the amount of the NSF check back into the patient's ledger. Place the amount in parentheses in the paid column and increase the total by the same amount. In a manual system, the entry and math are performed by the medical assis-

tant. RATIONALE: The amount is still owed by the patient, is not considered paid, and must be reflected in the amount due.

4. Place a brief explanation in the description of the column such as "NSF 12/09/XX."

Procedure 19-9

Writing a Check

PURPOSE:
To write a check to pay for expenses incurred and provide proof of payment. (Never written a check before? Go to http://www.thebeehive.org for practice.)

EQUIPMENT/SUPPLIES:
Checkbook and check register with balance of $7,298.35
Pen with black ink
Calculator

CHECKING WRITING EXERCISES:
Write checks for the following invoices using the current date:

1. $54.99 for case of printer paper to Landau Products

2. $450.00 for last month's janitorial services to MJB Services

3. $1,335.38 for clinical supplies to Redding Medical Supply House

4. $687.19 to Atlantic Electric for last month's heat and electricity

5. $350 to American Association of Medical Assistants for AAMA membership for the four medical assistants in the clinic

PROCEDURE STEPS:
1. Gather all invoices to be paid.

2. For the check register, use black ink:

   a. Enter check number 101 in the register if not preprinted.

   b. Enter the current date and year (usually in numbers, i.e., 02/14/XX).

   c. Enter the individual or company the check is to be paid to: Landau Products.

   d. Enter the amount to be paid on the check: $54.99.

   e. Subtract check amount from the present balance. Total $7,243.36 appears as the available balance. RATIONALE: These steps ensure that the check register is not overlooked when writing a check and establishes a well-recognized routine.

3. To write the check, use black ink:

   a. Enter check number 101 if not preprinted.

   b. Enter the current date and year (usually written out, i.e., February 14, 20XX).

   c. Enter the individual or company the check is to be paid to: Landau Products.

   d. Enter the amount to be paid on the check: $54.99. Do not leave spaces between numbers or between the dollar sign and the first number. RATIONALE: This helps to prevent any tampering of the check by adding numbers.

   e. Write out the amount to be paid by check (Fifty-four dollars and 99/100). Fill in any space left between the last number or word and draw a wiggly line over to the amount entered in numbers. RATIONALE: When the written amount and the number amount match, errors are prevented. The wiggly line makes it more difficult for anyone to tamper with the check.

   f. Describe what the check is written for in the bottom left corner (Printer paper, case).

continues

Procedure 19-9 (continued)

RATIONALE: Explains the purpose of the check.

g. If you have check-writing authority in the clinic, sign the check with your name the same as indicated on the bank's records. If you do not have check-writing authority, hold this check and the others to give to the individual with that authority. RATIONALE: The person responsible can review the checks with the invoices to verify valid expenses.

4. Continue writing checks for items 2 through 5 in the Check Writing Exercises, being certain to number checks consecutively and to subtract each check. Submit checks and check register with final balance to your instructor for evaluation.

Procedure 19-10

Reconciling a Bank Statement

PURPOSE:
To verify that the balance listed in the checkbook agrees with the balance shown by the bank.

EQUIPMENT/SUPPLIES:
Checkbook
Bank statement
Calculator

PROCEDURE STEPS:
1. Make sure the balance in the checkbook is current (all deposits and checks entered have been added or subtracted). RATIONALE: Ensures totals are accurate.

2. If a service charge is listed on the statement, subtract that amount from the last balance listed in the checkbook. RATIONALE: Reconciles current balance.

3. In the checkbook, check off each check listed on the statement and verify the amount against the check stub. RATIONALE: Verifies accuracy.

4. In the checkbook, check off each deposit listed on the statement. RATIONALE: Verifies accuracy.

5. The back of the statement contains a worksheet to be used for balancing.

6. Copy the ending balance from the front of the statement to the area indicated on the back.

7. Go through the check stubs and list on the back of the statement in the area provided any checks that have not cleared and any deposits that were not shown as received on the statement.

8. Total the checks not cleared on the statement worksheet.

9. Total the deposits not credited on the worksheet.

10. Add together the statement balance and the total of deposits not credited.

11. Subtract the total of checks not cleared. This amount should agree with the balance in the checkbook. If so, the checkbook is balanced and the statement should be filed in the appropriate place. RATIONALE: Following procedure steps 5 through 11 completes verification of accuracy.

Procedure 19-11

Establishing and Maintaining a Petty Cash Fund

PURPOSE:
To establish and maintain a petty cash fund for incidental expenses, making certain that receipts match the difference between the beginning and ending balance of the fund.

EQUIPMENT/SUPPLIES:
Petty cash box with cash balance
Vouchers
Calculator

Petty Cash Exercises:
1. Write a check for $100 cash at the bank.
2. Vouchers are made for the following incidentals:
   a. $20 to staff employee to purchase coffee supplies. Actual amount for supplies is $13.87; employee returns $6.13 cash.
   b. $2.24 for postage due to postal employee
   c. $3.18 to postal employee for guaranteed forwarding address
   d. $35.00 to Shannon's Pizza delivery for staff meeting lunch

PROCEDURE STEPS:

Establish the Fund:
1. Write a check at the bank to "Cash" for $100 (or other predetermined amount). Receive the cash in denominations of 1s, 5s, 10s, and 20s. Place the cash in the cash box. RATIONALE: The amount establishes petty cash and provides bills for the incidental purchases.
2. When cash is need for an incidental expense, such as postage due, prepare a voucher for the amount needed. No cash is taken from the fund without a voucher. RATIONALE: The written voucher indicates what money is used for.
3. After the purchase, attach the receipt for the purchase to the voucher. RATIONALE: This step provides proof of the purchase.

Balance Petty Cash Fund:
1. After the activity identified in the Petty Cash Exercises, count the money remaining in the box. RATIONALE: Verifies the amount of cash remaining in petty cash.
2. Total the amounts of all vouchers in the petty cash box. RATIONALE: Determines amount of expenditures.
3. Subtract the amount of receipts from the original amount in petty cash. This should equal the amount of cash remaining in the box. RATIONALE: Proves that the amount of expenditures deducted from the beginning amount equals the amount left in the box.
4. When the cash has been balanced against the receipts, write a check *only for the amount that was used*. RATIONALE: Brings dollar amount back to original petty cash amount.

Petty Cash Check Disbursement:
1. Sort all vouchers by account.
2. On a sheet of paper list the accounts involved.
3. Total vouchers for each account and record individual totals on the list.
4. Copy this list with its totals on the memo portion of the stub for the check written to replenish petty cash.
5. File the list with the vouchers and receipts attached, after noting the check number on the list.

Case Study 19-1

Review the scenario at the beginning of the chapter. As you consider the discussion of patient fees, determine what steps to take in the following situations.

CASE STUDY REVIEW

1. The clinic's patient has been diagnosed with non-Hodgkin's lymphoma (diffuse large B-cell) in stage 3. Surgery and aggressive chemotherapy are in process. The patient has Medicare and a small Medigap policy. You know there are expenses coming soon that neither insurance will cover. What can you suggest?

2. This patient has been with the clinic for 11 years and was covered most of the time by excellent private insurance. The circumstances have changed significantly, however. Today the patient works part time, has only Medicaid insurance, and has very few private funds. The provider's diagnosis is severe depression, and the provider instructs the patient to make two appointments weekly until the medication prescribed begins to make a significant difference in this patient's life. You know there are severe limitations to reimbursement from the state regarding this diagnosis. What steps will you take?

Case Study 19-2

Joann Crier has completed her 3-month probation period with Drs. Lewis and King. She is doing quite well and has demonstrated skill in accurate financial documentation. She has been asked to take over reconciling the monthly bank statements and managing all the accounts payable, including getting the checks ready for the provider's signature. She has difficulty, however, completing these tasks until after hours when the office is closed and quiet. Marilyn Johnson has told her that it must be done within normal working hours unless special permission is granted.

CASE STUDY REVIEW

1. What suggestions can you make to Joann to allow her to complete these tasks during normal working hours?

2. What impact does the time of day, day(s) of the month, or place where the tasks are completed have on your suggestions?

3. Are there any circumstances you can identify when overtime might be warranted to allow Joann to complete the tasks after hours?

SUMMARY

In this chapter, we discussed the daily financial duties in an ambulatory care setting: patient bookkeeping, working with the checkbook, purchasing supplies and equiment, and petty cash. By becoming proficient in these functions, you will be prepared to handle the day-to-day financial aspects of any ambulatory care setting.

Patient bookkeeping involves not only a responsibility to your employer (you are keeping track of income) but also to the patient, to be certain that charges for services rendered are correct and that payments are properly credited. The pegboard system is a comprehensive manual system for posting and tracking these data. Computerized bookkeeping offers many advantages of speed, high accuracy, and elimination of some routine tasks while providing the same important financial data.

It is important to maintain a scrupulous accounts payable system to ensure that bills are paid on time and that payments are properly documented for tax purposes. To accomplish this, checks are prepared properly, prepared on time, and recorded to effectively track expenditures.

Accuracy is important at all times. To ensure maximum accuracy in all bookkeeping functions, observe a few rules: record all charges and receipts immediately; make deposits of checks and currency the same day they are received; always verify and recheck totals of all deposits and expenditures; stay current with all checking account duties such as account reconciliation; and be prompt with all accounts payable.

┌─────────────────────────────┐
│ **STUDY FOR SUCCESS**   │
└─────────────────────────────┘

To reinforce your knowledge and skills of information presented in this chapter:

- Review the Key Terms
- Practice any Procedures
- Consider the Case Studies and discuss your conclusions
- Answer the Review Questions
  - Multiple Choice
  - Critical Thinking
- Navigate the Internet and complete the Web Activities
- Practice the StudyWARE activities on the textbook CD
- Apply your knowledge in the Student Workbook activities
- Complete the Web Tutor sections
- View and discuss the DVD situations

REVIEW QUESTIONS

Multiple Choice

1. The debit column of a ledger is:
   a. the column to the right of the balance column
   b. the column on the left; used to enter charges, procedure codes, and description of services
   c. the column at the far right that records the difference between the debit and credit columns
   d. the column that indicates the patient's debt to the practice

2. The use of debit/credit cards by patients to pay for services in ambulatory care settings is:
   a. never done
   b. unethical
   c. sure to compromise the integrity of the office
   d. a financial arrangement increasingly being used

3. The first section of the manual day sheet is used:
   a. to record deposits
   b. for business analysis
   c. to post individual transactions
   d. to total transactions

4. Good working habits for bookkeeping functions include:
   a. double-checking all entries for accuracy
   b. keeping the bookkeeping tasks current and up to date
   c. allowing the computer to create all the entries
   d. a and b

5. Petty cash
   a. is necessary to give patients change when they pay in cash.
   b. is used by the provider when taking a colleague to lunch
   c. pays for routine and unexpected minor expenses of the clinic
   d. comes from the provider's personal account

6. Encounter forms:
   a. can be ordered to fit the practice
   b. provide a separate ledger for each patient household
   c. list common services provided, procedural code, and diagnosis code
   d. a and c

7. Receipts:
   a. are used for payments on accounts
   b. are not given unless services are rendered the same day
   c. are mailed to patients when payment is made by mail
   d. are unnecessary, especially in the computerized system

8. When accepting checks from patients:
   a. inspect for correct date, amount, and signature
   b. immediately stamp with a restrictive endorsement
   c. third-party checks are acceptable
   d. a and b

9. A check with an attached stub for recording information is called a:
   a. certified check
   b. cashier's check
   c. voucher check
   d. money order
10. It is important to ensure proper control over purchasing of supplies and equipment for the following reasons:
   a. to avoid purchase of unnecessary items
   b. to avoid duplication of items purchased
   c. to provide a system for payment of only those items properly ordered and received
   d. all of the above

Critical Thinking

1. Discuss the types of checks identified in the text. Give an example of how each might be used or seen in the ambulatory care medical setting.
2. Check with a local bank or two to determine how after-hours deposits are made. Are any special supplies necessary? What is the bank's responsibility? What is the responsibility of the office staff?
3. When you reconcile the practice bank statement, you see that a check written almost 30 days ago to one of your supplier's has not been deposited. What course of action do you take, if any?
4. Even when a computer software system is used for the management of the practice's finances, discuss why following the bookkeeping guidelines for a manual system still has merit.
5. Check for the current interest rates on both business regular savings and money market accounts. If you had $5,000 to keep in a liquid (quickly turned into cash) account for the practice, how much interest would you earn in 1 month through a regular savings account? Through a money market account?

WEB ACTIVITIES

1. Using your favorite Internet search engine, determine how many medical or ambulatory care computerized bookkeeping systems might be available. One popular computerized system is called Medisoft. What does your research tell you about their prescription processing? Discuss the advantage or disadvantage of such a process.
2. Search online for a Web-based computer billing software such as AdvancedMD. What is the main difference between a Web-based system and a system complete within a particular medical facility? What are the advantages and disadvantages?
3. Search online for pegboard or write-it-once bookkeeping systems. Can you identify reasons why some medical practices might prefer this system? What are they? Some financial managers believe that a thorough understanding of a manual bookkeeping system makes it much easier to understand the rationale and processes of a computerized bookkeeping system. Do you agree? Explain your response.

REFERENCES/BIBLIOGRAPHY

Centers for Medicare & Medicaid Services. (2007). *CMS clarifies guidelines for national provider identifier (NPI) deadline implementation.* Retrieved April 12, 2007, from http://www.cms.hhs.gov.

Electronic Prescriptions. Retrieved February 2008, from http://www.medisoft.com.

Fordney, M. T., French, L., & Follis, J. (2008). *Administrative medical assisting* (6th ed.). Clifton Park, NY: Delmar Cengage Learning.

How to write a personal check. Retrieved February 2008, from http://www.thebeehive.org.

Chapter 20

Billing and Collections

KEY TERMS

Accounts Receivable Ratio

Collection Ratio

Fair Debt Collection Practice Act

Probate Court

Statute of Limitations

Truth-in-Lending Act

OUTLINE

Billing Procedures

Credit and Collection Policies

Payment at Time of Service

Truth-in-Lending Act

Components of a Complete Statement

    Computerized Statements

Monthly and Cycle Billing

    Monthly Billing

    Cycle Billing

Past-Due Accounts

Collection Process

    Collection Ratio

    Accounts Receivable Ratio

Aging Accounts

    Computerized Aging

Collection Techniques

    Billing Insurance Carriers

    Telephone Collections

    Collection Letters

Use of an Outside Collection Agency

Use of Small Claims Court

Special Collection Situations

    Bankruptcy

    Estates

    Tracing "Skips"

Statute of Limitations

Maintain a Professional Attitude

OBJECTIVES

The student should strive to meet the following performance objectives and demonstrate an understanding of the facts and principles presented in this chapter through written and oral communication.

1. Define the key terms as presented in the glossary.
2. Analyze the importance of billing and collections to the ambulatory care setting.
3. Describe the advantages of billing at least the co-payment and co-insurance at time of service.
4. Discuss the Truth-in-Lending Act.
5. Compare computerized billing and manual billing.
6. Recall the components of a complete statement.
7. Differentiate between monthly and cycle billing.
8. Explain the process of aging accounts.
9. Describe the importance of a courteous manner in telephone collections.
10. Restate legal and ethical guidelines for telephone collections.
11. Describe the process of sending a series of collection letters.

OBJECTIVES (continued)

12. Recall points to consider when using a collection agency.

13. Recall three special collections problems encountered in the ambulatory care setting.

14. Explain the ramifications of the statute of limitations on collections.

15. Explain the merits of a professional attitude in collections.

Scenario

At Drs. Lewis and King, patient billing is typically done at time of service, and a charge slip noting date, description of charges, and fees is given to the patient on leaving the office. Office policy states that, if possible, patients should pay their part of the fee, or their co-pay, at time of service. Marilyn Johnson, the office manager, has found that this is the most efficient way to ensure timely payment and eliminates the need to mail a separate statement. However, the office is flexible, and if the patient cannot pay all or part of the charge at the visit, Marilyn works out a payment schedule that is acceptable to both office and patient.

INTRODUCTION

In the ambulatory care setting, patient billing is a critical administrative function that helps to maintain a healthy, viable practice. Timeliness is essential in billing, because the ambulatory care setting depends on its accounts receivable to pay its bills in a responsible manner. Billing need not be a complex activity, but it must be completely accurate. In the few offices still using pegboard accounting, billing and collection procedures are done manually, often using the patient's ledger as the basis for the statement. When the facility is computerized, patient bills and collection notices are computer generated.

The best method of patient billing and collections is a method that is customized to the practice and that regards the patient as a consumer who should be respected. Patients appreciate knowing in advance what charges and fees to expect. Many facilities include these in their informational brochures or post them in a prominent place on the premises.

BILLING PROCEDURES

The ambulatory care setting's cash flow and collection process are dependent on up-to-date and accurate billing techniques. The financial status of the practice is reflected in monthly statements indicating unpaid patient balances, which, if they persist, are reviewed for appropriate action, including possible referral to a collection agency. Copies of all billing forms will be retained in the patient account record.

Timeliness and accuracy have a significant influence on prompt payment and how soon collection of the patient account will be finalized. In other words, billing performance can be measured

Spotlight on Certification

RMA Content Outline
- Financial and bookkeeping

CMA (AAMA) Content Outline
- Professional communication and behavior
- Legislation
- Bookkeeping systems
- Computer applications

CMAS Content Outline
- Fundamental financial management
- Patient accounts

by the time it takes to generate and submit a complete statement, that is, a statement with full documentation. If a facility is experiencing problems generating patient bills, a billing timeliness analysis worksheet can be constructed to identify internal delays that affect how quickly an account is billed, and thus paid. By focusing on inefficiencies in the revenue cycle, processes may be identified that need to be streamlined. For example, the date of service and insurance verification, the date the bill was generated, and the date the bill was submitted to the patient or third party can determine the efficiency of the billing process.

A billing efficiency report is another instrument that may be used to monitor efficiency. This report lists the previous month's billing backlog, which is added to the number of new accounts. The number of processed accounts is then subtracted. The weekly number of accounts that were rebilled also is noted, and the amount of time billing personnel spent on billing accounts is recorded. Production efficiency is calculated from these data. Inherent to this system is the careful monitoring of follow-up bills: whether they were paid, whether the insurance paid, and assessment of the patient's responsibility for payment.

CREDIT AND COLLECTION POLICIES

It is important that patients understand the billing policy and are educated about their accounts, how they are paid, and what their responsibility is toward payment. This is most easily accomplished in a patient-information brochure (see Chapter 45) identifying all aspects of the medical practice, including how bills are paid. The office staff also must have a well-defined policy related to patient billing and collecting.

Even uncomplicated patient billing should be done according to credit and collection policies established by the provider–employers of the ambulatory care setting. Having a formalized policy makes decision making easier and gives the medical assistant or office manager responsible for billing and collections authority to act. For example, some questions the providers and office manager may want to address include:

- When will payment be due from the patient?
- What kind of payment arrangements can be made if the patient does not pay at time of service?
- At what point should a patient be reminded of an overdue bill?

- How is that reminder initially managed: by telephone, note on statement, or letter?
- At what point will a patient bill be considered delinquent?
- Will a collection agency be used? Who decides?
- If exceptions to the policy are to be made, who makes these exceptions and what steps are taken?

By answering these and other questions, a straightforward credit and collection policy can be devised that is a guide to both patients and the medical assistant in charge of billing.

PAYMENT AT TIME OF SERVICE

The best opportunity for collection is at the time of service. This process begins with the medical assistant who schedules appointments. Make certain all patients have the information they need. After determining the urgency and reason for the appointment, collecting information regarding a chief complaint, and assigning a time for the appointment, it is appropriate to discuss the financial concerns of patients (Procedure 20-1). Patients may be shy in asking certain questions, but they have questions about most of the following issues:

- Whether the providers contract with their insurance carrier
- How payment is made if insurance does not cover certain procedures
- Whether they can be billed for co-payments and coinsurance
- How payment is made for services if they have no insurance
- An approximate cost of a particular service

Patient Education

Patients appreciate knowing their responsibility in terms of payment. Whoever schedules the first appointment with a new patient should diplomatically inform the patient of office policy on payment of fees. If the patient anticipates a problem in paying promptly, a schedule can be established that is agreeable to both parties.

Do not tell a patient, "We do not take your insurance." It is much better to make a statement such as, "Our providers do not contract with that insurance. However, we can work with you on a fee-for-service basis and help make finances workable for you." The atmosphere has now been created to ensure prompt collection and increased cash flow for the practice. To accommodate patients, offices now increasingly accept debit and credit card payments. Remember, also, that if your facility does use a sign-in method as patients arrive (see Chapter 8), then the all-important personal contact may be missed. With that missed opportunity also goes the opportunity to discuss finances.

Most insurance contracts require the provider to bill the insurance company *before* billing the patient, except for the co-payment. It is critical to abide by each contract to protect the provider. If the patient is a member of a health maintenance organization (HMO) and the ambulatory care center is a participating provider, it is bound to the terms of that agreement. If not restricted by the insurance contract, be certain to explain to patients at the time of service that any payment made will be adjusted according to their insurance and the terms of that policy. Also remember that all patients must be treated the same and charged the same for services.

With the knowledge of what portion of the fee can be collected at the time of service, the medical assistant says to the patient prior to leaving the facility, "The fee for your services today is $85. Will you be paying by cash, check, or credit/debit card?" When the policy for collecting fees is shared when the appointment is made, patients are not surprised by this approach. Allow the patient to be the next person to speak in response to the question asked. If for some reason a fee cannot be immediately paid, the patient will respond by asking what kind of arrangements might be made. Even if financial arrangements are necessary, the discussion of the day's fee for the service is in process.

TRUTH-IN-LENDING ACT

In those situations where a payment schedule is arranged, clinic policy will dictate if any interest is charged. Although it is not illegal to charge interest on patient accounts, many providers still prefer not to assign any interest on installment payments or past-due accounts.

For installment payments (such as prenatal care or surgery), medical assistants need to be aware of the conditions of the **Truth-in-Lending Act,** Regulation Z of the Consumer Protection

Act of 1967 (see Chapter 7). If there is bilateral agreement between providers and their patients for payment of medical services in more than four installments, that agreement must be in writing and must provide information on any finance charge. The information must be in writing even if there are no finance charges made (Figure 20-1). The patient is given the original copy of the disclosure statement; a second copy is kept in the office.

COMPONENTS OF A COMPLETE STATEMENT

Once a patient has been accepted for treatment, it is important to maintain accurate and timely records of his or her account and payment history.

CAPITAL AREA HEALTH CARE
839 Sycamore Park
Boise, ID 83725
(208) 863-4210

FEDERAL TRUTH-IN-LENDING STATEMENT
For Professional Services

Patient _____ Cari R. Jacobson _____

Address _____ 913 Swanson Street _____

_____ Boise, ID 61820 _____

Parent _____

1. Cost of services rendered	$ 1,500.00
2. Down Payment	225.00
3. Unpaid Balance	1,275.00
4. Amount Financed	1,275.00
5. Finance Charge	-0-
6. Annual Percentage Rate of Finance Charge	-0-
7. Total of Payments (4 + 5 above)	1,275.00
8. Total Amount After Payments	1,500.00

Total payment due is payable to __Dr. Leslie Swaggert__ at above address in __5__ monthly installments of $__255__. The first installment is payable on __August 1 20XX__, and each subsequent payment is due on the same day of each consecutive month until paid in full.

__07-24-XX__   _____
Date of Agreement   Signature of Patient;
                      Parent if Patient is Minor

Figure 20-1   Truth-in-Lending Act document showing installment and interest agreement.

That information is just as vital to the healthy management of the practice as the patient's medical record. Invoice patient services promptly according to the office policy, send statements regularly, and make certain they are complete and accurate. Statements to patients must be professional looking, neat, inclusive of all services and charges, and easily understood. Procedure and diagnosis codes are necessary for insurance and reimbursement, but they usually mean nothing to patients. Make certain patients can understand the terminology used to explain the procedures they received.

Billing occurs in a number of different ways, with the computer-generated statement the most widely used. As mentioned in Chapter 19, an encounter form may be used as the statement, especially if payment is made at the time of the service (Figure 20-2). Typewritten statements will likely use the continuous-form billing statement that is printed on a roll with perforated edges for separation. Photocopied statements are often used with a pegboard system. The ledger cards are coordinated with the same size copy paper. These photocopied ledgers are placed in a window envelope so that the address on the ledger card shows through the window.

If the statement is to be mailed, an enclosed self-addressed envelope is appreciated by the patient and may result in a faster turnaround of payment. Stamp the words "Address Service Requested" on the envelope just below the return address. When this statement is stamped on the envelope, a valuable tool in collections is available at minimum cost. If the statement cannot be delivered as addressed (the patient has moved or "skipped" and has left no forwarding address), the post office researches this information and returns the envelope to you with a yellow sticker providing the new address and any other updated information. If the patient has ordered that mail be forwarded, the post office will forward the statement to the patient and send the medical facility a form with the new address. There is a fee for this service.

A well-prepared patient statement should contain not only information for the patient but information needed to process medical insurance

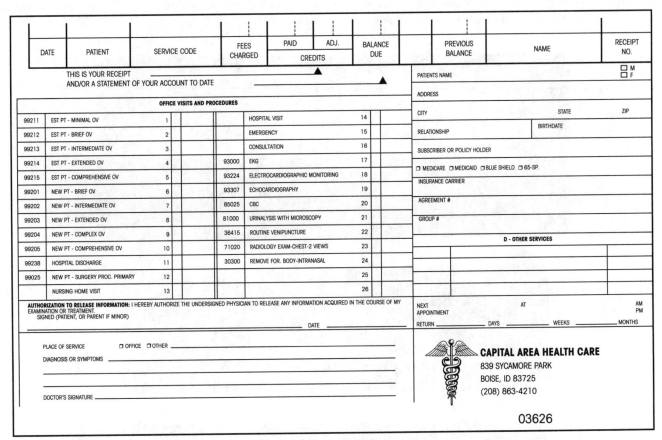

Figure 20-2   This sample encounter form (charge slip) is a multipurpose form used to document information for insurance claims as well as to provide the patient with a receipt and documentation of procedures, diagnoses, and fees. It can be used as the patient's first bill.

claims as well. The following information should be included (see Procedure 20-2):

- Patient's name and address
- Patient's insurance carrier and identification number
- Date and place of service
- Description of service and fee for each service
- Accurate procedure and diagnosis codes for insurance processing (see Chapters 17 and 18)
- Provider's signature and identification code or National Provider Identifier (NPI)
- Clinic name, address, telephone number, fax number, and Web site when applicable

Computerized Statements

By far the most common statements are computer generated. Typically, the medical assistant keys the computer command to search the patient database for outstanding balances and directs the computer to print statements.

Financial management software will age accounts (see Aging Accounts section) and can generate collection letters that have been specifi-

cally designed for the practice, allowing the medical assistant to key in the appropriate specific information (Figure 20-3).

All provider orders, prescriptions, recommendations, and a copy of the visit and health summary can be waiting for the patient at the time of checkout if desired. With a single key entry, an electronic invoice is generated with appropriate diagnostic and procedural codes already applied. If insurance is to be billed, the claim is automatically placed in the insurance queue to be uploaded electronically to third-party payers.

Any payments made can be posted electronically and statements printed for the patient. The collection portion of the financial management software keeps up with the daily billing tasks. Procedures 20-3 and 20-4 identify accounts receivable and itemized accounts for billing using an electronic system.

MONTHLY AND CYCLE BILLING

The billing schedule is often determined by the size of the medical practice. Monthly billing is a system in which all accounts are billed at the same time each month. In a smaller ambulatory care

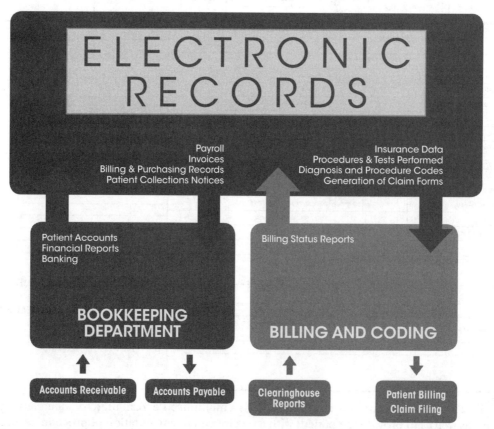

Figure 20-3   Total practice management system diagram illustrating billing and collections activities.

setting, monthly billing may be the most efficient method. Cycle billing staggers bills during the month and is a flexible system for larger practices.

Monthly Billing

In a monthly billing system, 1 or 2 days are devoted to billing and mailing all statements. Typically, statements should leave the office on the 25th of the month to be received by the first of the month. The major disadvantage of monthly billing is that a medical assistant may neglect other activities during this time-consuming period. To avoid these problems, billing statements may be prepared intermittently over a 1- or 2-week period and stored until the mailing date. To avoid confusion caused by delays in mailing, a message to "Disregard if payment has already been made" should be printed on the form. Patients become annoyed and the practice appears disorganized if a statement arrives several days after payment has been made.

Cycle Billing

In a cycle billing system, all accounts usually are divided alphabetically into groups, with each group billed at a different time. In this way, administrative personnel with numerous bills to process each month will be able to handle them in a more efficient manner. Statements are prepared on the same schedule each month. They can be mailed as they are completed, or held and mailed at one time. A typical cycle billing schedule is shown in Figure 20-4. The system can be varied to suit the needs of the individual practice.

Sample of Cycle Billing

1. Divide the alphabet into four sections: A–F, G–L, M–R, S–Z.
2. Prepare statements for patients whose last names begin with A through F on Wednesday and mail them on Thursday of Week 1.
3. Prepare statements for patients whose last names begin with G through L on Wednesday and mail them on Thursday of Week 2.
4. Prepare statements for patients whose last names begin with M through R on Wednesday and mail them on Thursday of Week 3.
5. Prepare statements for patients whose last names begin with S through Z on Wednesday and mail them on Thursday of Week 4.

Figure 20-4   Typical schedule for cycle billing system.

PAST-DUE ACCOUNTS

As efficient and effective as the billing process may be, there will still be collections on some accounts. The most common reasons for past-due accounts include:

- *Inability to pay.* People may have financial hardships from time to time (see Chapter 19).
- *Negligence.* People may forget to make a payment because they have been away or dealing with a family emergency.
- *Unwillingness to pay.* When a patient complains about a charge or refuses to pay, it may have nothing to do with finances. Often, they are dissatisfied with the care or treatment they have received. These patients should be referred to the provider or office manager for immediate attention.
- *Third-Party Payers.* Past-due accounts may result because of inaccurate or insufficient insurance information. Claims can be rejected because of many varied reasons, and time limits must be observed.
- *Minors.* Minors who are not legally emancipated may seek and receive treatment, but they are not responsible for paying the bill (see Chapter 7). If the medical practice treats minors who are not emancipated, an office policy should determine how minors pay for their services. Many facilities ask for cash at the time of the service. Emancipated minors are responsible for their bills.

COLLECTION PROCESS

The process of collecting delinquent accounts begins with first establishing how much has been owed and for how long.

Ideally, collection of accounts receivable should be prompt and conducted in a timely fashion. Management consultants recommend collecting at least a portion of the fees at the time of service and that a **collection ratio** of 90% or better should be maintained. Another important factor is the **accounts receivable ratio** that measures the speed with which outstanding accounts are paid. The desirable accounts receivable ratio is less than 2 months for collection of accounts receivable.

Collection Ratio

A collection ratio is a method used to gauge the effectiveness of the ambulatory care setting's billing practices. This ratio shows the status of collections and the possible losses in the medical facility. It is a good idea to obtain the ratio monthly, quarterly, and yearly. Typically, the collection ratio is calculated by dividing the total collections by the net charges (gross or total charges minus any adjustments). This yields a percentage that is referred to as the collection ratio. See the following example:

$$\frac{\text{Total Amount Collected this Month}}{\text{Total Monthly Charges Minus Adjustments}} = \text{Monthly Collection Ratio}$$

$$\frac{\$34,650}{\$44,928} = .7712 \text{ or } 77\%$$

In this sample, you can determine that more time and energy needs to be spent in collecting accounts. The practice is losing almost 25% of its income potential. Not only is the income potential being lost but the ability to invest that income is also lost, making the potential loss even greater.

Accounts Receivable Ratio

An accounts receivables ratio indicates how quickly outstanding accounts are paid. It can also be a measure of how effective the collections are. To calculate the accounts receivable ratio, divide the current accounts receivable balance by the average monthly gross charges. This yields the typical turnaround for collecting accounts receivable. See the following example:

$$\frac{\text{Current Accounts Receivable}}{\text{Average Monthly Gross Charges}} = \text{Accounts Receivable Ratio}$$

$$\frac{\$145,048}{\$44,928} = 3.2$$

Because the goal of the accounts receivable ratio is payment in less than 2 months, you can quickly observe that this practice is over 1 month behind in collections. Chapter 21 gives additional information on accounts receivable and collection ratios.

The longer a practice delays attempting to collect delinquent accounts, the less chance there is of receiving payment. Statistics show that the value of the dollar decreases rapidly in the collection process. The more time and energy put into collections, the less value received in return. That is, you may manage to collect the full amount due, but when you consider the time and expense involved, it may not have been worth the effort and expense. Therefore, the value of the debt to be received after successful collection must be considered when determining how aggressive to be in debt collections.

AGING ACCOUNTS

Account aging is a method of identifying how long an account has been overdue. This means that past-due accounts are identified according to the length of time they have been unpaid. When using a pegboard bookkeeping system, color-coded strips are attached to the ledger cards to show the age of an account, or the cards can be stored behind a color-coded divider in a separate file labeled "Unpaid." For example, a red strip might be used for accounts 1 month overdue, a blue strip for accounts 2 months overdue, and other colors for additional months overdue. A written code such as "OD3/2/23" should be written on the ledger card to indicate when the overdue notice was mailed, meaning "Overdue notice No. 3 mailed on February 23."

Depending on the type of patient served, different aging systems are used. In a computerized billing system, the accounts are automatically aged, and the aging schedule or process is shown on the computerized ledger.

Computerized Aging

Aging accounts using a computer software system is simple. Before printing billing statements, the medical assistant keys the appropriate commands to age the accounts. The program can age accounts according to several criteria: for example, by past due balance, zero balance, or credit balance accounts. Accounts can also be aged by government agency category or by insurance carrier. All Medicare or Medicaid accounts might be aged separately from other accounts. Sorting out Medicare and Medicaid accounts may also be done when computing the accounts receivable ratio and the collection ratio.

The computer can also generate and print an accounts receivable report showing each overdue account, the balance overdue, and a breakdown showing how long the account has been overdue. This breakdown is usually divided into accounts 0 to 30 days overdue, 31 to 60 days overdue, 61 to 90 days overdue, and 90 days or more overdue. Additional reports can be generated from the accounts receivable report. For example, the clinic staff may wish to print a report showing accounts that have been delinquent for more than 90 days or accounts that are delinquent by more than a certain dollar amount.

COLLECTION TECHNIQUES

Ambulatory care settings use both telephone and written communications in their collection techniques. Although both have some measure of effectiveness, some practices prefer to call the patient with a past-due account before officially initiating collection proceedings. The patient may have misplaced the statement, forgotten a payment, or been away on an extended vacation; a quick telephone call can often resolve the situation without the time and expense involved in collections. Also, the patient usually appreciates the courtesy and personal approach.

Many patients work part or full time, sometimes making telephone calls difficult to complete. It is often beneficial for providers to ask the office manager or the medical assistant in charge of collections to work 2 or more hours one evening a week for the purpose of making collection telephone calls. Calls are more likely to be answered in the time period from 5 to 8 PM than during the middle of the day. Figure 20-5 shows a sample collections policy.

Billing Insurance Carriers

Many patients have some form of medical insurance (see Chapter 17). Make it a practice to send each computer claim within 2 days or less of the patient account data being entered into the computer. Batches of claims to insurance carriers should be forwarded at the end of each day. In the era of electronic claims processing, much time is saved in not having to prepare hard copies of the forms for mailing. Electronic claims transmission (ECT; also known as electronic medic claims, or EMC, and electronic claims submission, or ECS) dictates that the practice's computer system must be able to communicate with the insurance carrier's computer. This paperless process yields less errors than the manual process because ECT software includes some built-in checks to determine any invalid codes, sex or age conflicts, and correct procedure and diagnostic code linkages to the services provided. Sending insurance claims via the paper process will take more time to process, and the turnaround time for payment is also longer. Most claim departments of insurance carri-

SAMPLE COLLECTION POLICY SCHEDULE

- Encounter form (if used) given to patient at time of visit
- Itemized statement sent no later than the end of that month
- Itemized statement with overdue notice no later than the end of the second month
- Telephone call reminding the patient of the bill. "We've sent two statements and we haven't received payment. Do you need more information from us?" Offer help at this point in establishing a payment schedule, and seek to get a commitment from the patient.
- If a financial schedule is to be established, prepare it and mail to the patient within a day of the phone conversation. Follow up on that commitment within 15 days. The follow up message may be a thank you for sending the first payment. Carefully monitor payments and their timeliness.
- If no payment schedule is made by the patient, send a letter stating the amount due before the account is past due three months. Discuss with office manager and/or physician regarding the merit of continued collection at this time.
- If collections are to continue, notify the patient one more time of their responsibility and ask for payment.
- If no payment is received, send a letter stating that "Your account has been turned over to a collection agency" if outside collectors are used. Make no more phone calls.*

*Some physicians send a letter of discharge to patients at this time via certified mail. (See Chapter 7.)

Figure 20-5   Sample collection schedule.

ers and government agencies have large numbers of employees with varying levels of experience. Payment can be delayed because of an overburdened claim department, a form that has been lost in transit, a misfiled form, an inexperienced employee, or numerous other reasons.

The medical assistant should maintain an up-to-date claims register or insurance-pending report and take firm control of the practice's collection procedures to ensure that claims are paid promptly.

This claim register or insurance-pending report may be a part of the computerized billing system. If so, the printout will show how much the practice charged insurance carriers and how much was received. This clearly shows which carriers are slower than others and where other problems might arise. For any claim pending more than 45 days, it is a good idea to make a call to the carrier to find out whether the claim has been received, where it is in the process, and whether the office staff might have done something to delay the process. Such phone calls can become carefully cultivated personal contacts with insurance representatives to pave the way for cooperation in the future.

In clinics where the medical assistant files claims for patients, a follow-up collection policy is important to maintain strong cash flow. When carriers do not pay in full or question or deny a claim, the medical assistant should determine the nature of the problem and rebill or appeal the decision, whichever action is appropriate.

Telephone Collections

The medical assistant is likely to use the telephone for collection procedures. Telephoning is often an effective measure because a patient may respond to a call more than to a bill received in the mail.

A successful telephone collection call is enhanced by keeping to the facts and being tactful, pleasant, and diplomatic. When making calls to patients regarding past-due accounts, there are some things to keep in mind to maintain the desired relationship with patients. Always remain courteous and respectful. Do not treat patients with suspicion or threats. Remember, the health profession is dedicated to helping people; avoid antagonizing patients.

Most people do not let their bills become past due on purpose or out of spite. Keep this in mind when making calls. Work with patients to encourage and enable them to pay any fees they owe.

Certain legal rules and ethical guidelines govern telephone collections:

- When making collection calls, callers must identify themselves and ascertain that they are talking to the person who is responsible for the account.

- A collection call could be embarrassing to the patient; therefore, it should not be made to the patient's place of employment.

- In most states, a debtor may be contacted only between 8 AM and 8 PM.

- Do not make telephone calls at odd hours or make repeated calls to the debtor's friends, employers, or relatives.

- If a contact must be made to the debtor's place of business, do not reveal to any third party the nature of the call. Patients have a right to confidentiality and privacy.

- Do not threaten to turn the person's account over to collection agencies.

Violating these rules makes the caller vulnerable to charges of harassment under the **Fair Debt Collection Practice Act.** (For additional information, search the Internet for Fair Debt Collection Practice Act.)

When collecting by telephone, it is helpful to keep complete, accurate records of the process indicating who said what and how much was promised as payment. If after 2 weeks nothing has been resolved as a result of the calls, then another course of action may be the solution, especially for large sums of money owed. Collection letters may be necessary.

Collection Letters

Collection letters are sent to encourage patients to pay overdue balances. After two statements are mailed to patients and the charge slip or encounter form has brought no response, the ambulatory care setting begins sending collection letters.

Lack of payment from a patient may not be considered serious until after 60 days. When the patient fails to respond to the encounter form, to the statement, or to a 60-day statement with an "Overdue" remark, a series of collection letters begins. One typical collection letter series is shown in Figure 20-6A through C. Collection letters and notes are kept separate from a patient's chart.

USE OF AN OUTSIDE COLLECTION AGENCY

Occasionally, the ambulatory care setting turns over highly delinquent accounts to an outside collection agency. Discretion is always advised here, however, because the expense of collection may not justify the fees to be collected. For unpaid accounts with large balances, however, this is often a viable solution.

One service provided by a collection agency is an intercept letter. For a nominal fee, this letter may be sent from the agency as the last resort before the account is turned over to collection. This communication alerts patients to the fact that if a response is not received, their account will go to collection. This often is the only action needed for the patient to pay the outstanding bill. Another service of a credit bureau or collection agency is to provide credit ratings of patients at the provider's request. Provider's who pay for this service are able to monitor patients' ability to pay their bills, as well as to trace a "skip," someone who leaves with an outstanding bill and no forwarding address.

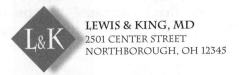

LEWIS & KING, MD
2501 CENTER STREET
NORTHBOROUGH, OH 12345

June 14, 20XX

Mr. John O'Keefe
12 Gravers Lane
Northborough, OH 12345

Dear Mr. O'Keefe:

Your account with our office is three months past due, and you have not responded to our previous requests for payment. Please pay your balance of $852 at this time, or contact us with a plan for payment.

Please call me at 312-824-6925 if you have a question about your account or a plan for payment. Otherwise, we expect your payment immediately.

Sincerely,

Marilyn Johnson
Office Manager

NORTHBOROUGH
FAMILY MEDICAL GROUP

A

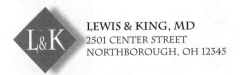

LEWIS & KING, MD
2501 CENTER STREET
NORTHBOROUGH, OH 12345

July 15, 20XX

Mr. John O'Keefe
12 Gravers Lane
Northborough, OH 12345

Dear Mr. O'Keefe:

Your son, Chris, was seriously ill in March when he was seen by Dr. King. Dr. King used her experience and education to treat Chris, believing you would pay your account within a reasonable amount of time.

Four months have passed and you have still not remitted the $852 outstanding balance on your account. We cannot continue to keep your unpaid account on our books. If you are experiencing financial difficulties, please call the office at 312-824-6925 so we can arrange a payment schedule that is agreeable to both of us.

Sincerely,

Marilyn Johnson
Office Manager

NORTHBOROUGH
FAMILY MEDICAL GROUP

B

Figure 20-6   Sample collection letters: (A) First letter. (B) Second letter.

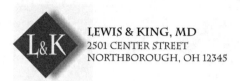

August 17, 20XX

CERTIFIED MAIL

Mr. John O'Keefe
12 Gravers Lane
Northborough, OH 12345

Dear Mr. O'Keefe:

This is our final attempt to collect your account of $852, which is five months past due. You have not responded to all our previous letters [or letters and phone calls], so we have no alternative but to turn over your account to a collection company.

Your account is being assigned to Ambler Medical Collection Service, which will pursue whatever legal means is necessary to collect this debt. If you contact me at 312-824-6925 within seven days, we can prevent the account from this assignment and resolve the balance.

Sincerely,

Marilyn Johnson
Office Manager

NORTHBOROUGH
FAMILY MEDICAL GROUP

C

Figure 20-6   (continued) (C) Third letter.

When selecting a collection agency, be certain to hire one that is compatible with the medical practice's philosophy. Questions that might be asked of potential collection agencies include the following:

- Does the agency handle only medical and dental accounts?
- What methods are used to make collections?
- Is the agency fee a flat charge per account or a percentage of the account recovered?
- How promptly does the agency settle accounts?
- Will the agency supply a list of satisfied customers or references?
- What ability does the medical practice have to end the agency's collection efforts?

Once a collection agency has been selected, carefully follow their instructions about any contact patients make to the medical office regarding their account and any other guidelines in their contract with the practice. Keep a record of accounts given to the agency, as well as their rate of return. Hopefully, the agency will be able to motivate patients to pay for the health care services they have received while still maintaining the practice's good reputation and increasing your profit margin. Medical collections lets your patients know that the practice is serious about collecting past-due accounts.

There is often a question about how payments from collection agencies are posted. This is one purpose of the adjustment column. Place the amount received in the adjustment column because it is a subtraction from the amount due. If there is no adjustment column, put the amount in the charge column and put red parentheses around it or circle in red so the amount is actually subtracted from the balance. The remaining balance after collections is paid is written off (Procedures 20-5 and 20-6).

USE OF SMALL CLAIMS COURT

 In certain circumstances, a clinic's office manager may consider bringing a case to small claims court. Typically, small claims courts handle cases that involve only limited amounts of debt (these vary from state to state), they usually do not permit representation by an attorney, and they are generally efficient and streamlined in their proceedings. Nonetheless, preparing for small claims courts and taking time to appear will require a certain investment of staff. It is important to note that, if the court finds in the clinic's favor, the clinic still must collect the money from the defendant. An account assigned to a collection agency cannot be filed in small claims court.

SPECIAL COLLECTION SITUATIONS

In patient billing and collections, a number of special situations may arise.

Bankruptcy

If a patient has declared bankruptcy, statements may no longer be sent nor any attempt be made to collect delinquent accounts. A patient declaring bankruptcy usually does so under Chapter 7 or Chapter 13 bankruptcy law. In Chapter 7 bankruptcy, a patient declares bankruptcy to all debtors and is allowed to clear all debts and start fresh. The medical office should file a proof-of-claim form and provide a copy of the patient's outstanding account to the bankruptcy court. In Chapter 13 bankruptcy, also known as "wage-earner's bankruptcy," patients (wage-earners) are protected from bill collectors and are allowed to pay their bills over a specified time. The court determines a monthly amount that the debtor can pay, collects that sum, and parcels it out to the creditors over a period as long as 5 years. The clinic must file a claim as directed by the debtor's attorney to collect any fees outstanding. Because a provider's fee is an unsecured debt, it is one of the last to be paid. Bankruptcy laws are federal and are subject to the Federal Wage Garnishment Law of attaching property to satisfy debt.

Estates

Collection of fees when a patient has died must be directed to the executor of the estate or the one responsible for overseeing the estate. Some general guidelines to follow include:

- Show courtesy by not sending a statement in the first week or so after a death.
- Prepare an itemized statement of the deceased patient's account. (In some cases, a special form is required for this.)
- Mail the account information via certified mail with a return receipt requested to the administrator of the estate. The name can be obtained by calling the probate department of the superior court.

- If there is no known or identified administrator, send a copy of the itemized statement to the "Estate of (name of patient)" to the patient's last known address. Often, a family member has assumed the responsibility for paying the patient's account balances.
- If unsure of how to proceed, contact the office's attorney or the clerk of the **probate court** for advice.

Tracing "Skips"

 A "skip" is a patient with an unpaid bill who has apparently moved with no forwarding address. If a statement is returned to your office marked "no forwarding address," first determine if any internal errors were made in addressing the envelope. If the address is determined to be correct, the medical assistant may try to call the patient at the telephone number on the patient ledger; it is possible that the patient has retained the same number, or there may be a new number given. If the medical assistant is unable to secure a telephone number, the facility needs to decide whether to pursue the unpaid debt. This will depend on office policy and the amount that is owed. If it is decided to pursue an unpaid account, it can be turned over to a collection agency. If the medical assistant attempts to trace the skip by calling employers or relatives, it is important not to violate any laws in doing so and maintain the patient's confidentiality.

STATUTE OF LIMITATIONS

 A **statute of limitations** is a statute that defines the period in which legal action may take place. When applying this concept to collections, the time period is usually defined by the class into which the account falls. These include open book accounts, which may have periodic charges against them; written contracts; and single-entry accounts, which have only one charge against them. The time period in which legal action must take place against any of these accounts varies from state to state. If an unpaid account is more than 3 years old, it is wise to investigate the statute of limitations in your state before spending time and effort in collections. (For state-by-state information on the statute of limitations on debts, see http://www.creditinfocenter.com under Debts.)

MAINTAIN A PROFESSIONAL ATTITUDE

Collecting past-due accounts is one of the most difficult tasks delegated to medical assistants. Not everyone is able to perform the task. Placing calls can be discouraging, especially if the results seem less than anticipated. Not all accounts can be collected. Identify these accounts early, write them off, and save the medical practice time and money. Keep any bias and your emotions out of the process. Rely only on your information, the aged account, and the realization that the office policy is well thought out and provides a win-win solution for both the patient and the provider as much as possible. When dealing with a "true dead-beat" who has no intention of paying the bill, be proud of your provider's attention to that patient's need, but discuss with the provider the possibility of discharging the patient. Staff may need additional training and education from time to time to update skills on patient service and how to maintain good-will during the collection process.

Procedure 20-1

Explaining Fees in the First Telephone Interview

PURPOSE:
To establish rapport with patients, to discuss providers' fees, and to identify the patient's responsibility before the first visit.

EQUIPMENT/SUPPLIES:
Provider's fee schedule
Appointment schedule
Telephone

PROCEDURE STEPS:

1. Place the providers' fee schedule and the appointment schedule close to the telephone. RATIONALE: The office staff that is prepared does not have to search for something vital to the phone conversation.

2. Answer the phone before the third ring. Identify the name of the clinic and yourself. RATIONALE: The person calling feels attended to and knows the call has been correctly placed.

3. Offer assistance; for example, a comment such as "How can I help you?" RATIONALE: Sets the tone for the patient to continue with the request.

4. After the patient is identified as a new patient and the nature of the visit is determined appropriate, discuss possible dates for the appointment. A statement such as, "Our next available appointment is Thursday at 11:30 AM. Can you make it then?" is a good way to begin.

5. Tell the patient that you will be discussing clinic policies briefly now and will mail the Patient Information Brochure before the appointment. RATIONALE: The patient brochure details some of the information discussed in the telephone conversation and further verifies the clinic's policies.

6. Ask about medical insurance. If insured get the identification number, the name of the subscriber, employer, and a telephone number of the insurance carrier if possible. RATIONALE: This allows you to check for any preauthorization required and for the currency of the plan.

7. Explain that the clinic policy requires any co-payment and coinsurance to be paid at the time of the visit. RATIONALE: Establishes patient's financial responsibility immediately.

8. Check to see if the patient has transportation and knows how to get to the clinic, and provide directions if necessary. RATIONALE: Ensures that there is no confusion about location and accessibility.

9. Request that the patient arrive about 15 minutes before the appointment to complete some forms. RATIONALE: Ensures that the patient has time to complete information and can ask any questions that might occur.

10. After closing the telephone interview, promptly mail the Patient Information Brochure.

Procedure 20-2

Prepare Itemized Patient Accounts for Billing in a Manual System

PURPOSE:
To notify patients of the fees for services rendered and collect on those accounts.

EQUIPMENT/SUPPLIES:
Typewriter
Calculator
Patient account or ledger cards
Billing statement forms

PROCEDURE STEPS:

1. Gather all accounts and ledgers with outstanding balances. RATIONALE: Everything in one place saves time and energy.

2. Separate any accounts that are labeled as overdue. RATIONALE: Individual decisions on these accounts are necessary before taking action.

3. For each account, perform the following:

   a. Verify the name and address of the patient and the person responsible for payment.

   b. Place current date on the statement.

   c. Scan the account information for any possible errors.

   d. Itemize the procedures in terms patients understand and indicate charges.

   e. Identify and subtract any payments (copayment, coinsurance, down payment) that have been made.

   f. Use the calculator to verify the unpaid balance that is carried forward and is due.

4. Discuss with the office manager any action to be taken on past-due accounts. Follow through with those instructions. RATIONALE: More than one person is involved in the collection process.

5. Place statements in envelopes and mail. RATIONALE: Ensures timely delivery of statements.

Procedure 20-3

Identify Accounts Receivable Using Medical Office Simulation Software (MOSS)

PURPOSE:
To determine credit balances for patient billing.

EQUIPMENT/SUPPLIES:
Computer
MOSS

PROCEDURE STEPS:

1. Open MOSS and select "Report Generation" from the main menu.

2. Select the report labeled "Billing and Payment Report" on the Reports Panel. Enter 06/01/2009 and 09/15/2009 as the start and end dates.

3. Print the resulting report for use in the remaining steps of this procedure (Figure 20-7 is a sample of a billing and payment report). RATIONALE: To easily identify accounts with a balance due.

4. Using the hard copy that was just printed, locate the first patient. Note that each claim line that was submitted for this patient is listed with any payment activity. Look at the "Balance Due" column to determine if the patient has any outstanding balances. At the end of the patient listing is the total balance due.

continues

Insurance Billing & Payments for Student1

Account / Insurance Provider	Date of Service	Submitted By	Total Claim	Patient Payment	Payment Code	Insurance Payment	Dis-count	Adjust. Code	Adjust. Amount	Deduct-ible	Balance Due
ALB001 Josephine Albertson											
IN02 ConsumerOne HRA	10-Jul-09	Electronic	$80.00	$20.00	PAYINS	$64.00	0	ADJINS	$16.00	$0.00	$0.00
								Josephine Albertson Balances:		$0.00	$0.00
BLA002 Donald Blair											
IN08 Aetna	12-Jun-09	Electronic	$130.00	$0.00		$0.00	0		$0.00	$0.00	$130.00
IN08 Aetna	12-Jun-09	Electronic	$1,702.00	$0.00		$0.00	0		$0.00	$0.00	$1,702.00
								Donald Blair Balances:		$0.00	$1,832.00
CON002 Jordan Connell											
IN02 ConsumerOne HRA	03-Jun-09	Electronic	$111.00	$0.00	PAYINS	$71.76	0	ADJINS	$39.24	$0.00	$0.00
IN02 ConsumerOne HRA	03-Jun-09	Electronic	$46.00	$0.00	PAYINS	$11.04	0	ADJINS	$34.96	$0.00	$0.00
								Jordan Connell Balances:		$0.00	$0.00
GOR002 Edward Gormann											
IN01 FlexiHealth PPO In-Network	15-Sep-09	Electronic	$266.00	$0.00	PAYINS	$180.56	0	ADJINS	$65.44	$0.00	$20.00
								Edward Gormann Balances:		$0.00	$20.00
JEF001 Andrew Jefferson											
IN01 FlexiHealth PPO In-Network	01-Jul-09	Electronic	$111.00	$20.00	PAYINS	$88.80	0	ADJINS	$2.20	$0.00	$0.00
								Andrew Jefferson Balances:		$0.00	$0.00
MAX001 Alice Maxwell											
IN03 Signal HMO	02-Jul-09	Electronic	$111.00	$15.00	PAYINS	$88.80	0	ADJINS	$2.20	$0.00	$0.00
								Alice Maxwell Balances:		$0.00	$0.00
YBA001 Elane Ybarra											
IN07 Flexihealth PPO Out-of-Netw	04-Jun-09	Electronic	$180.00	$0.00	PAYINS	$89.06	0	ADJINS	$68.68	$0.00	$22.26
								Elane Ybarra Balances:		$0.00	$22.26

Figure 20-7   A sample billing and payment report from MOSS.

5. The data on this report can be confirmed by comparing the patient ledger for each patient. This can be done while the report is still on the screen by using the pull-down menu "Billing" and selecting "Patient Ledger" (Figure 20-8). Select the patient whose ledger you wish to review using the "Search" icon, select the patient name, and click on "View." RATIONALE: Can compare the information and balance due in the ledger to the balance due on the report.

6. Look at the patient's insurance information in Field 6 of the patient ledger. RATIONALE: Will verify that no secondary billing is necessary. Make a notation in the margin of the printed report to help you remember the details later (e.g., bill patient, bill secondary, etc.)

7. Continue to analyze the Billing and Payment Report, making notes as necessary.

8. When finished analyzing the report, close all windows and return to the main menu. RATIONALE: Prepares for the next step, which is to create electronic patient statements.

continues

Procedure 20-3 (continued)

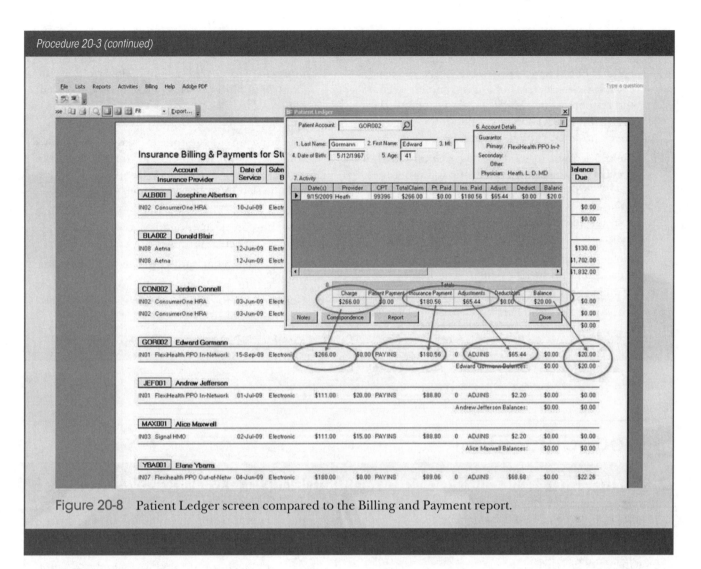

Figure 20-8   Patient Ledger screen compared to the Billing and Payment report.

Procedure 20-4

Preparing Itemized Patient Accounts for Billing Using Medical Office Simulation Software (MOSS)

PURPOSE:
To notify patients of the fees for services rendered and collect on those accounts.

EQUIPMENT/SUPPLIES:
Computer
MOSS
Billing & Payment Report generated in Procedure 20-3

PROCEDURE STEPS:

1. From the MOSS main menu, select "Patient Billing."

2. In Field 1, select the radio button next to "Remainder Statement." This will generate a statement for all patients who have a balance due.

3. In Field 2, use the drop-down arrow and select "ALL" to generate patient statements for patients of all providers in the practice.

4. Field 3 Service Dates: enter 06/04/2009 for both the "from" and "through" service dates. Enter 08/10/2009 as the Report Date.

5. Field 3, Patient Name, select Elane Ybarra. The account number field can be left blank.

continues

6. Field 4 should have "Preview on Screen" selected. Print can be selected, but it is recommended that the statements be viewed on screen before they are printed. RATIONALE: Allows for one final check prior to printing statements.

7. Field 5 is used to send messages to all patients receiving statements. Type in the following message: "Your insurance has been billed. The balance shown on this statement represents your responsibility. Thank you for your prompt payment."

8. Field 6 is used to type in a message that will appear only on specific patient statements.

9. If Field 6 is used, in Field 7, select the patients who will receive the message in Field 6. To select more than one patient, hold down either the Control or Shift key while clicking on the patient name.

10. Click on the "Process" button. RATIONALE: This will bring up an "Output to" screen that allows you to save your statements. If you do not wish to save the statements, click on the "Cancel" button and the statement preview screen will open.

11. Review Elane Ybarra's statement to make sure that the correct message is shown and the balance is correct.

12. Print the statements and turn in to your instructor.

13. Now create a Patient Statement for Edward Gormann, who had a physical on 8/10/2009 (report date of 10/20/2009).

Procedure 20-5

Post/Record Collection Agency Adjustments in a Manual System

PURPOSE:
To keep track of financial adjustments.

EQUIPMENT/SUPPLIES:
Manual bookkeeping system
Patient's account
Black, blue, and red ink pen for use in manual bookkeping system

PROCEDURE STEPS:

1. With the daily schedule of services/charges in front of you (the manual daily sheet), enter amount received from the collection agency on a patient's account and a note such as "Payment from ABC Collection Agency" in the explanation section. RATIONALE: Indicates funds received on a collection contract.

2. Record the amount received and the explanation in the patient's account as well. The amount received is *subtracted* from the account balance. The balance amount of the account is placed in the "adjustment" column. If there is no adjustment column, put the amount in the charge column with parentheses around it or circle the amount in red. These data are copied to the patient's account in the write-it-once system. RATIONALE: Demonstrates the activity and amount from the collection agency on a patient's account in the patient account documents.

3. Subtract the amount paid by the collection agency from the total charges to create the new balance. RATIONALE: Clearly indicates what portion of the account the patient has paid and the amount that is not collectible.

4. Write off this balance, indicating a zero balance on the patient's account. In the daily sheet, the difference between the amount collected and the amount paid by the collection agency (plus the agency's fee) is entered as a negative adjustment. RATIONALE: At the end of the year, totals can be obtained indicating the amount of uncollected charges for the practice's income tax preparation.

Procedure 20-6

Post/Record Adjustments Using Medical Office Simulation Software (MOSS)

PURPOSE:
To keep track of financial adjustments.

EQUIPMENT/SUPPLIES:
Computer
MOSS

POST/RECORD ADJUSTMENTS EXERCISES

1. Megan Caldwell was seen on December 15, 2008, but she never paid her $20.00 co-payment. The account was sent to collections, and they have forwarded a $10.00 payment for this collection. The remaining $10.00 must be written off.

2. Justin McNamara had an office visit on December 18, 2008, and his claim was processed, indicating the balance of $64.00 to be applied to his deductible. He did not pay, and his account was forwarded to the collection agency. They recently forwarded a payment on the account in the amount of $49.20. The remaining balance should be written off.

3. Evan Lagasse had his annual physical on November 21, 2008. His insurance carrier processed the claim, indicating a patient deductible amount of $208.00. Attempts to collect were unsuccessful, and his account was forwarded to collections. The agency has forwarded a payment in the amount of $144.53. The remaining balance must be written off.

PROCEDURE STEPS:

1. Open MOSS and select Posting Payment from the main menu.

2. In the Search Criteria box of the patient list, type in "Cal" and click on "Search." RATIONALE: This shows those patients whose last names begin with these letters.

3. Highlight the line with Megan Caldwell's name and click on "Apply Payment."

4. In Field 1 of the Posting Payments screen, highlight the line for the date of service "12/15/2008" and click on "Select/Edit" at the bottom of the screen.

5. Click in Field 3 and enter "09/30/2009." RATIONALE: This is the date you are processing the collection and write-off.

6. In Field 7, click on the drop-down arrow and select "Other Payment."

7. In Field 9, enter "$10.00." RATIONALE: Indicates amount paid.

8. Field 10, click on the drop-down arrow, scroll down, and select "ADMINISTRATIVE ADJUSTMENT."

9. In Field 11, enter "$10.00" as the amount of the adjustment. RATIONALE: Indicates the amount to be written off.

10. Check your work with Figure 20-9. Click on "Post" in the bottom left-hand portion of the screen.

11. Take screenshots of the complete Payment Posting screen (the window shown in Figure 20-9) for Exercises 2 and 3 and submit to your instructor either as a printout or in an email file.

12. Close all windows and return to the main menu.

continues

Procedure 20-6 (continued)

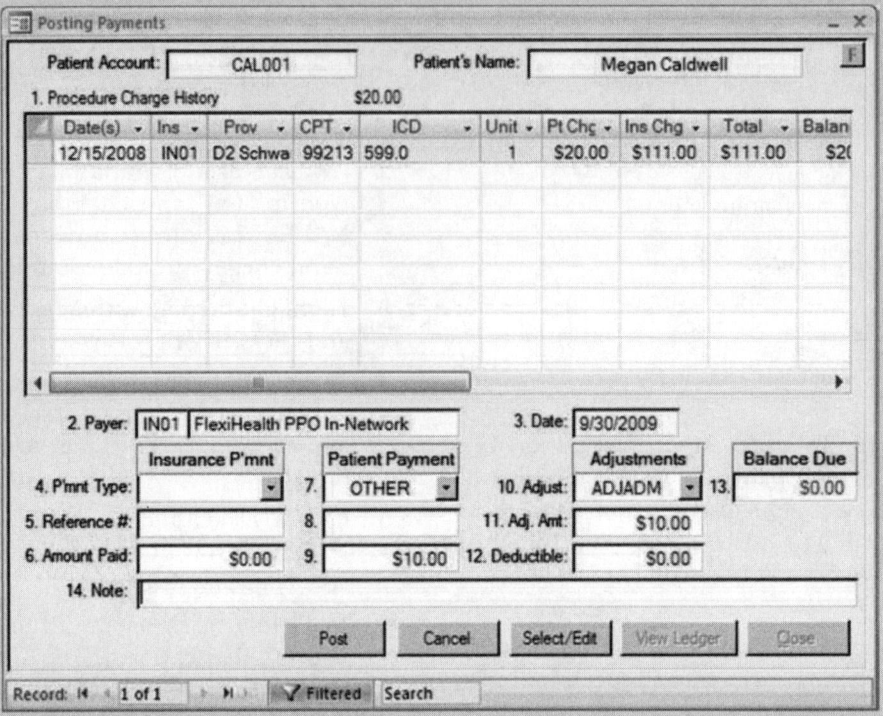

Figure 20-9 Completed Payment Posting screen in MOSS showing the financial adjustment.

Case Study 20-1

Refer to the scenario at the beginning of the chapter. For patient accounts more than 60 days overdue, the offices of Drs. Lewis and King begin a series of collection proceedings to attempt to collect the monies. Initially, they place a telephone call to the patient to determine whether a billing problem might be present that can be clarified over the telephone. If they cannot reach the patient or the patient does not respond to the call, then collections begin. Marilyn has assigned this function of the billing process to Ellen Armstrong, because Ellen has a warm telephone manner and is good with patients.

CASE STUDY REVIEW

1. Why is Ellen's telephone manner important in the collection process?

2. In addition to telephone collections, what patient letters might Ellen send?

3. Ellen has come across an account that is delinquent and discovers that the patient has declared bankruptcy. What can Ellen do now?

Case Study 20-2

Morgan Bryant is the custodial parent and single mother of her 5-year-old son Custer, who has been a patient in the Valley Pediatric Clinic since his birth. Custer's father's insurance covered his medical expenses. During a separation and the resulting divorce, the medical bills continued to go to Custer's father. Morgan comes to the reception desk to discuss the collections letter she received. Her parenting plan requires her former husband to provide medical coverage for their son. However, it appears he canceled his policy coverage on his son 4 months ago and Morgan did not know until she received the letter. Morgan is in tears.

CASE STUDY REVIEW

1. What is the first step the administrative medical assistant should take?

2. Is there anything the clinic staff might have done differently in collecting this account?

3. What might be done for Morgan now? Are any resources available to Morgan?

SUMMARY

Billing and collection activities in the ambulatory care setting are intricately linked to daily financial practices and claims processing, and the medical assistant responsible for billing should also be well aware of these other functions. Billing need not entail a complex or elaborate system, but whether accomplished by manual or computer methodology, it needs to be precise, professional, and comprehensive, as all communications with patients should be. If collections become necessary, courteous and straightforward letters and telephone exchanges are the most effective. The goal of all billing and collections is to maintain the relationship with the patient, while ensuring good cash flow and payment of accounts receivable in the ambulatory care setting.

STUDY FOR SUCCESS

To reinforce your knowledge and skills of information presented in this chapter:

- Review the Key Terms
- Practice any Procedures
- Consider the Case Studies and discuss your conclusions
- Answer the Review Questions
  - Multiple Choice
  - Critical Thinking
- Navigate the Internet and complete the Web Activities
- Practice the StudyWARE activities on the textbook CD
- Apply your knowledge in the Student Workbook activities
- Complete the Web Tutor sections
- View and discuss the DVD situations

REVIEW QUESTIONS

Multiple Choice

1. The Truth-In-Lending Act:
   a. is designed to place limits on the amount of debt for which consumers are liable
   b. is also known as the statute of limitations
   c. is also known as Regulation Z
   d. does not apply to medical facilities
2. Cycle billing is a system of billing:
   a. completed every fourth month
   b. done only by computer
   c. completed by the 25th of the month
   d. in which accounts are divided into sections for billing purposes
3. One of the most common reasons patient bills go unpaid is:
   a. inability to pay because of financial hardship
   b. patients consider the cost of medical care too high
   c. patients think their insurance should cover all medical bills
   d. patients think providers make too much money
4. Aging accounts:
   a. is a process of identifying overdue patient accounts
   b. describes patients who have a long-term relationship with the ambulatory care center
   c. describes older adult patients with Medicare
   d. applies to accounts considered inactive
5. If an unpaid account goes to small claims court:
   a. the medical clinic must engage an attorney representative
   b. the medical clinic is still responsible for collecting even if the court finds in its favor
   c. there is no need to show up at court
   d. a large sum of money must be at issue
6. A collection ratio:
   a. shows status of collections and possible losses
   b. divides the current accounts receivable by the average monthly gross charges
   c. should be 90% or better
   d. a and c
7. A claims register:
   a. identifies how many past-due claims have been collected
   b. may also be called the insurance-pending report
   c. is maintained by each insurance carrier for the provider
   d. is a tickler file that maintains all patients' insurance information
8. Telephone collections:
   a. are best made after 8 PM when patients are home
   b. must abide by the Fair Debt Collection Practice Act

   c. are usually successful after numerous calls at the patient's place of employment
   d. will require overtime pay for the medical office staff
9. A "skip" is defined as:
   a. the time period when legal action cannot be taken
   b. an estate involved in probate
   c. one who moves without a forwarding address and leaves an unpaid bill
   d. one who has paid a portion of a debt
10. For patient accounts, a collection agency:
    a. is better if it handles only medical and dental accounts
    b. creates a bad feeling between patients and providers
    c. cannot possibly do as good a job as the medical office staff
    d. seldom describes its methods for collections

Critical Thinking

1. An elderly widow covered only by Medicare Parts A and B is a patient in your clinic. You know her resources are limited. She receives a very small pension and Social Security benefits. She is facing hip replacement that will involve surgery, hospital care, rehabilitation care prior to her return to her apartment, and outpatient physical therapy. Describe what steps your clinic might take to ease her financial burden for this much needed care.
2. You are making a collections call. You follow all the rules and you are gracious in your approach. Before you realize what is happening, however, you have listened to a tale of woe, the patient is in tears, and you want to write your own check for the unpaid balance due. What happened? What will you do now?
3. Collections are an activity that many medical assistants shy away from and prefer not to do. What factors contribute to that feeling?
4. When the office manager calls a patient regarding a past-due account, she is told by the patient, "I'm not about to pay that bill. The treatment made my pain worse, not better." What steps might be taken now?
5. Seymore Storme's original medical bill is $356. He has no insurance but keeps his account active by paying $25 per month. To date, he has made four payments of $25 in 4 months. Should a Truth-in-Lending Statement be prepared? Why or why not?
6. With another student, role-play a telephone collections call. One student can be the medical assistant, the other student can be the patient. Have a third student observe and evaluate the call. Discuss.

WEB ACTIVITIES

1. Research the Internet for information on debt collections. Consider keywords such as "credit law," "collections," and "debt recovery." What sources of information are found that might be helpful to an ambulatory care facility?
2. Research the statute of limitations in your state. How much time is allowed for legal action to take place in collecting a past-due account?
3. Go to http://www.whowhere.com and http://www.searchbug.com. Did you find any information that might help you locate a patient who appears to have skipped out on a major bill for elective surgery? What services are free to you? What services require payment? How much is the fee?

REFERENCES/BIBLIOGRAPHY

Fordney, M. T., French, L. L., & Follis, J. J. (2008). *Administrative medical assisting* (6th ed.). Clifton Park, NY: Cengage Delmar Learning.

Lewis, M. A., & Tamparo, C. D. (2007). *Medical law, ethics, and bioethics for health profession* (6th ed.). Philadelphia: F. A. Davis Company.

Chapter 21

Accounting Practices

OUTLINE

Bookkeeping and Accounting
Systems
   Single-Entry System
   Pegboard System
   Double-Entry System
   Total Practice Management
   System
   Computer and Billing Service
   Bureaus
Day-End Summary
   Tips for Finding Errors
Accounts Receivable Trial
   Balance
Accounts Payable
   Disbursement Records

The Accounting Function
Cost Analysis
   Fixed Costs
   Variable Costs
Financial Records
   Income Statement
   Balance Sheet
Useful Financial Data
   Accounts Receivable Ratio
   Collection Ratio
   Cost Ratio
Legal and Ethical Guidelines
   Bonding
   Payroll

KEY TERMS

Accounting
Accounts Payable
**Accounts Receivable
(A/R) Ratio**
Accrual Basis
Assets
Balance Sheet
Cash Basis
Check Register
Collection Ratio
Cost Accounting
Cost Analysis
Cost Ratio
Financial Accounting
Fixed Cost
Income Statement
Liability
Managerial Accounting
Owner's Equity
Trial Balance
Utilization Review (UR)
Variable Cost

OBJECTIVES

*The student should strive to meet the following performance objectives and
demonstrate an understanding of the facts and principles presented in this chapter
through written and oral communication.*

1. Define the key terms as presented in the glossary.
2. Understand the purpose and range of the accounting function
   in the ambulatory care setting.
3. Describe the four different types of bookkeeping and accounting
   systems.
4. Recall the importance of the day-end summary and the accounts
   receivable trial balance.
5. Compare and contrast financial, managerial, and cost accounting.
6. Explain the use and validity of the income statement and the
   balance sheet.
7. Recall three useful financial ratios and explain.
8. Identify proper steps in accounts payable management.
9. Discuss the impact of utilization review on reimbursement.
10. Discuss legal and ethical guidelines in accounting practices.

When James Whitney, one of the owners at Inner City Health Care, and Jane O'Hara, CMA (AAMA), the office manager, decided to add a new medical assistant to the staff, they first reviewed the financial records for the previous year. Although the volume of work in the center generated the need for an additional employee, Whitney and O'Hara had to be sure it was financially feasible. In addition to past records, they also had to make some projections for the upcoming year; with certain new managed care fees, they had to be sure that anticipated revenues would be sufficient to sustain the salary of a new employee.

INTRODUCTION

Medical financial management in the ambulatory care setting is most important in the daily functioning of the office business because it directly affects overall bookkeeping and accounting procedures. Accounting generates financial information for the ambulatory care setting and is defined as a system of monitoring the financial status of a facility and the specific results of its activities. It provides financial information for decision making.

Previous chapters have included the topics of proper daily bookkeeping financial practices (see Chapter 19), the accurate coding and the specific processing of insurance forms (see Chapters 17 and 18), and the efficient management of collecting on accounts (see Chapter 20). All of these functions are essential to obtain maximum reimbursement and create profitability for the practice.

This chapter ties many of these elements together and creates a total picture of their interdependence. Each element is critical to accurate accounting practices in the ambulatory care setting.

Spotlight on Certification

RMA Content Outline
• Financial bookkeeping

CMA (AAMA) Content Outline
• Computer applications
• Bookkeeping systems
• Accounting and banking procedures
• Employee payroll

CMAS Content Outline
• Fundamental financial management
• Patient accounts

BOOKKEEPING AND ACCOUNTING SYSTEMS

Medical practices use a variety of ways to monitor their financial accounts and the total financial operations of the business. Although a few offices still use the single-entry bookkeeping and peg-board systems, the majority prefer double-entry or computerized systems, or a combination.

Financial records should provide the following information at all times:

• Amount earned in a given period
• Amount collected in a given period
• Amount owed in a given period
• Where the expenses incurred in a given period

The financial records can show these data as often as you like, usually on a monthly, quarterly, or yearly basis. Comparisons can be made with similar periods. Analysis of the financial data can help to determine if some services are not profitable, whether the practice is experiencing a healthy growth, or why a loss might be realized. The accounts receivable and accounts payable data are vital to this information.

Single-Entry System

The single-entry system has been used in medical practices for many years. This includes a daily journal or log, patients' statements or accounts, ledgers, checks, and disbursement (expenditure) records. Information is first recorded in the journal, which provides a chronological record of financial transactions. Information from the journal is then transferred to the ledger through the process of posting. All amounts entered in the journal must be posted to the accounts kept in the ledger to summarize the results. This system has been used because of its simplicity and inexpensive nature. However, it is difficult to find errors, for there are no internal controls, and financial analysis information is inadequate.

Pegboard System

As discussed in Chapter 19, the pegboard, or "write-it-once," system is easier to use than the single-entry system and has greater internal controls. The pegboard system provides control over collections, payments, and charges. It uses No Carbon Required (NCR©) forms that are layered or shingled on pegs on the left of the board so that both income and disbursement entries need to be written only once. Many pegboard plans include a charge slip or encounter form, which simplifies third-party payment processing for both the medical practice and the patients. The charge slip is used to record the input needed during the patient's visit, while serving as the patient's receipt for services performed and fees charged. An advantage of the pegboard system is its accuracy, because data are entered at the time of service and not recopied, so fewer errors can creep in.

Double-Entry System

The double-entry system is based on the fact that each transaction has two aspects, that is, a dual effect on the accounting elements. This system is based on the accounting principle that assets equal liabilities plus owner's equity.

$$Assets = Liabilities + Owner's\ Equity$$

Assets are the properties owned by the business (supplies, equipment, accounts receivable, and so on). **Liabilities** include what is owed to creditors. **Owner's equity** is the amount by which the business assets exceed the business liabilities. Net worth, proprietorship, and capital are often used as synonyms for owner's equity.

The double-entry system requires that the two aspects involved in every transaction be recorded on each side of the equation and that the two sides always be in balance. Although this accounting system requires time and skill, it provides a comprehensive financial picture and has built-in accuracy controls. It is orderly, fairly simple, flexible, and accurate, making it impossible for certain types of errors to remain undetected for long. For example, if one aspect of a transaction is properly recorded but the other aspect is overlooked, the records are out of

balance. This occurrence may be easily discovered and subsequently corrected.

Total Practice Management System

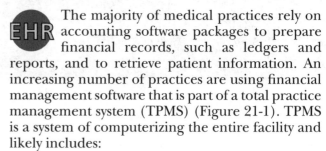 The majority of medical practices rely on accounting software packages to prepare financial records, such as ledgers and reports, and to retrieve patient information. An increasing number of practices are using financial management software that is part of a total practice management system (TPMS) (Figure 21-1). TPMS is a system of computerizing the entire facility and likely includes:

- Patient information data and scheduling
- Electronic medical records (EMRs) and electronic health records (EHRs)
- Insurance coding and billing; processing claims electronically
- Management and human resources; payroll, purchases, personnel records
- Bookkeeping and accounting; generation of financial records including business income and expenses.

A computerized accounting system is most likely to be based on the principles of either the pegboard (write-it-once) or a double-entry bookkeeping system, or a combination of both.

A computer financial system can be customized to meet the needs of the practice. Most large multispeciality clinics have a computer system designed particularly for their needs. TPMS has the capability of including the most common procedure and diagnostic codes within a database to be recalled when completing insurance claim forms. The software will assist in matching the charges with the appropriate diagnosis codes.

TPMS has the flexibility of assigning codes in other categories to indicate whether a bill has been paid with cash, a check, or by a third-party payer. Codes may also be assigned to place and type of service and the professional performing the service. This facilitates the tracking of payments and also allows for the analysis of specific sources that generate income for the practice. Adjustments to reflect discounts or reduced fees may also be entered into the computer. The software is used in the preparation of billing statements, insurance forms, collection letters, and a number of financial ratios and statements to assist in monitoring the practice's financial stability.

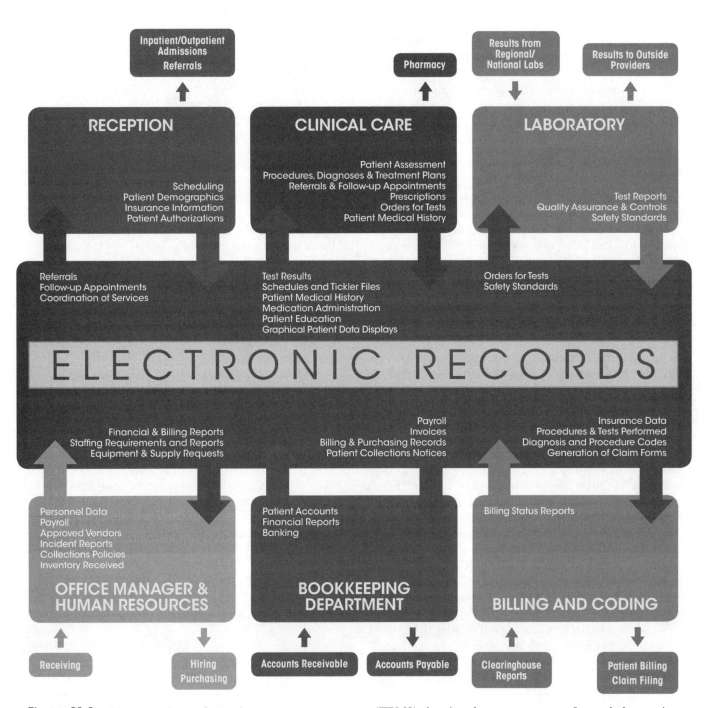

Figure 21-1   Diagram of a total practice management system (TPMS) showing the many aspects of a total electronic medical clinic system.

Computer and Billing Service Bureaus

An option for ambulatory care settings that choose not to purchase accounting software or a TPMS in their practice is to use a computer service bureau for billing purposes and the creation of many financial records. In this case, the ambulatory care setting provides the data, and the bureau provides basic billing and accounting services, furnishing financial statements, completed insurance forms, payroll materials, and checks.

Service bureaus handle accounts from the medical facilities in one of three ways:

1. Through the office's own computer terminal, online sharing occurs where the office is tied directly to the bureau's mainframe computer

2. Through online servicing, where the office has its own terminal, which allows direct communication with the service bureau's computer

3. Through off-line batch processing, where the medical assistant or bookkeeper sends daily batches of data to the bureau to process

 Many facilities, however, prefer to have their own computerized financial system or TPMS because dealing with a computer bureau can compromise patient confidentiality and limit control over computer usage. A proper contract should be negotiated and signed with any computer and billing service bureau to ensure confidentiality, HIPAA compliance, and strict privacy of all patient information.

DAY-END SUMMARY

The financial summary at the end of the day is a helpful tool for a quick financial analysis. Computer accounting systems automatically create the day-end summaries. Pegboard systems require the administrative medical assistant to total the summaries that are shown at the bottom of the day sheet.

The first section of the day sheet identifies all the financial transactions of the day. The second section includes the month-to-date totals. This is where today's totals are added to the month-to-date totals; this must be in perfect balance. The third section identifies the year-to-date accounts, which includes all accounts to obtain the year-to-date total. A deposit slip included with most systems enables the assistant to verify the cash receipts with the checks received. This is helpful in preparing the day's bank deposit.

When the totals do not balance at the end of the day, the medical assistant must begin the search for errors.

Tips for Finding Errors

Some tips for finding errors are as follows:

- Check the addition of each column, both horizontally and vertically. If a calculator is used, check the tape for entry errors.
- Compute the difference in the totals that are out of balance. Search the day sheet and patient accounts for that exact amount.
- If the amount of the error is divisible by 9, there may be an error in transposition of numbers.
- If the amount of the error is divisible by 2, the amount may have been posted in the wrong column.

- Check your entries when manually carrying forward previous balances. It is quite easy to carry forward an incorrect amount or to place numbers incorrectly. For example, the number $750 might be carried forward as $75.

Anyone who has worked with a manual pegboard system can report horror stories of chasing errors around for several days before finding them. It might be one error in one patient's account that creates the havoc. Also, a search can be made for an error for such length that the assistant keeps seeing and missing the error. Set the problem aside for a bit, or even a day if you are not pressed with month-end billing deadlines. Have another person check for you. Often that individual sees the error in just a few minutes.

Errors in an electronic financial system can create almost as much havoc but often can be caught earlier. If all data are entered accurately and kept up to date, an error that occurs when keying in certain data will create a warning notice that indicates the data are incorrect. Computers do not automatically update all information when fees for services are changed, reimbursement adjustments are changed, salaries are increased, or new data from the laboratory or clinical area are determined. Any time there is a person who is entering data into the system, errors can occur. All medical professionals entering any data into the system must be reminded not to rush through the process and to carefully check for accuracy.

ACCOUNTS RECEIVABLE TRIAL BALANCE

Before preparing monthly statements, a **trial balance** should be done on the accounts receivable in either a pegboard system or a computer system. The trial balance is created by totaling debit balances and credit balances to confirm that total debits equal total credits. The trial balance will indicate any problem between the daily journal and the ledger. Use the following steps to create the trial balance:

1. Pull all patient accounts that have a balance.
2. Total the balance of those accounts.
3. Create an accounts receivable total.
   a. Enter the accounts receivable at the first of the month.
   b. Add the total charges for the month and subtotal.

c. Subtract the total payments for the month and subtotal.

d. Subtract the total adjustments for the month.

e. The final total is the accounts receivable at the end of the month.

This final total, the end of the month accounts receivable, must be the same as the figure received when adding all the patient account balances. If they match, the accounts are then in balance. If they do not balance, the error must be found (see Procedure 21-1).

ACCOUNTS PAYABLE

Accounts payable are an unwritten promise to pay a supplier for property or merchandise purchased on credit or for a service rendered. Accounts payable are the most common liability or financial obligation in a provider's office. These include expenses such as medical and office supplies, salaries, equipment, and services. Payments for these expenses are made by check to ensure complete, accurate records of all money received and disbursed.

Supplies and equipment purchased usually come with a packing slip that describes the items purchased and their cost. An invoice may also be enclosed that serves as a bill for the items ordered; however, another invoice is sent to the business later as well. Take time to note on the invoice if there is a discount for early payment. Some financial managers suggest attaching the invoice and packing slip to the purchase order (see Chapter 19). File in your tickler file or reminder file on the computer so that payment is made in a timely fashion to receive any discount. Some vendors prefer that payment not be made until a statement (or request for payment) is received from them. This is particularly the case if the practice uses that vendor more than once a month. When the statement arrives, check the invoice for accuracy before sending payment. Prepare the check for the accounts payable as appropriate, either monthly or as necessary to receive a discount (see Chapter 19). Write the check number on the invoice, as well as the amount paid, and place in a file for accounts paid according to the practice's filing system.

Disbursement Records

 Computerized accounts payable systems track the disbursements and post to appropriate established accounts similar to a manual system. Computer accounts payable systems have a **check register** that records all checks written and categorizes them into separate columns, such as rent, insurance, office supplies, utilities, and so forth. These categories can be designed as detailed or general as preferred. The computer system also can create entries for bank deposits and payroll records.

The computer software has a check-writing file that presents checks on the screen. The information necessary to complete the check is entered at the keyboard; the computer stores it and prints out the check. Printing the checks can be done individually or by batch if several bills are being paid. The amount is automatically subtracted from the account's balance. The computer system also can recall data that need to be entered on the checks each time there is a payment. For example, the name of the company where most supplies are purchased can be recalled from the database; thus the assistant does not have to key in that information again. This feature is a particular timesaver when payroll checks are prepared (see Chapter 45).

The manual or pegboard system uses a check register page to record checks written. The check is aligned on the pegboard over the check register before completion. The pegboard checks have an NCR transfer strip that copies the date, the payee, the check number, and the amount to the check register. Pegboard checks can be designed so that the address is entered beneath the payee line and mailed in a window envelope. This check register has a number of columns to categorize expenses. All entries are totaled on the check register when completed, and these totals carried forward. A balanced check register provides a way to verify the bank statement when it arrives. The check register can also be used for bank deposits and for payroll records.

THE ACCOUNTING FUNCTION

Accounting is a system of monitoring the financial status of a facility and the financial results of its activities. Accounting may be divided into two major categories: financial and managerial. **Financial accounting** provides information primarily for entities external to the organization such as the government. In contrast, **managerial accounting** generates financial information that can enable more efficient internal management. **Cost accounting** helps to determine what it costs the ambulatory care setting to perform particular services and is an integral part of managerial accounting. A hospital cost report for Medicare is essentially part of financial accounting because the report is generated for an external user—the Centers for Medicare & Medicaid Services (CMS), which administers the Medicare program. However, it is also a part of cost accounting because a cost report on Medicare will show what it costs to care for patients on Medicare.

COST ANALYSIS

An important aspect of the practice is **cost analysis.** The purpose of the analysis is to determine the costs of each service. There are two factors to consider: fixed costs and variable costs.

Fixed Costs

Fixed costs are costs that do not vary in total as the number of patients vary. For example, the annual depreciation cost of the equipment is fixed because it will remain the same regardless of the number of patients who use it.

Variable Costs

Variable costs are those that vary in direct proportion to patient volume, such as clinical supplies and laboratory procedures. Average costs to treat patients decline because of fixed costs, not variable costs. The greater the volume, the more widely the fixed costs are spread and the less cost any one unit is responsible for.

Patient cost factors include administrative costs, such as the cost of billing and collections, personnel costs for office staff providing patient care, equipment costs, and costs for clinical supplies. The provider cost will include costs for interpreting tests, diagnosing illnesses, and maintaining professional liability insurance.

Calculating and reviewing costs provide the ambulatory care setting with data to set fees, market the practice, determine profit, and monitor the practice's performance.

FINANCIAL RECORDS

Indicators of the financial status of the medical facility include financial statements that reflect the daily operations of the business. These records comprise an accounting information system that is maintained for numerous reasons, one of which is to provide source data for use in the preparation of various reports. Two financial statements common to the ambulatory care setting are the income/expense statement and the balance sheet.

Income Statement

Figure 21-2 shows a sample **income statement,** the most commonly generated year-end report. The sample shows the profit and expenses for a given month. The income statement shows the cumulative profit and total expenses by reporting patient income, outside revenue sources, and overhead expenses such as office and medical expenses. Provider's compensation and benefits and employees' compensation, benefits, and withholding taxes can be itemized as well.

Balance Sheet

Sometimes called the statement of financial condition or statement of financial position, the **balance sheet** is an itemized statement of the assets, liabilities, and owner's equity of a medical facility as of a specified date. Its purpose is to provide information regarding the status of these basic accounting elements.

The balance sheet is made possible through the double-entry system of accounting because every transaction is recorded by two sets of entries made in a ledger or journal. Increases in assets are recorded as debits; decreases are recorded as credits. Increases in liabilities and owner's equity are recorded as credits; decreases are recorded as debits.

Debit and credit entries to one or more accounts make up the system. In any recording, the total dollar amount of the debit entries must equal the total dollar amount of the credit entries. Each ledger or journal entry should have the elements:

1. Date of transaction
2. Journal or ledger account names involved
3. Dollar amount of the charges
4. Brief explanation of the transaction

USEFUL FINANCIAL DATA

A business must determine how and when it will report income earned. There are two systems for doing this. The **accrual basis** reports income at the time charges are generated. This is used mainly in commercial environments. The **cash basis** is most often used in medical practices. In the cash basis, income is recognized when money is collected.

A few financial ratios can help evaluate how the practice is doing. Data from the current year and the previous year's financial statements can be converted into ratios to highlight different financial characteristics. Ratios should always be viewed in relation to the total financial picture, however.

Ratios are not difficult to calculate, but they can be time consuming when using a manual system. They are quick to create in a computer system because all the data are readily available, already totaled, and sometimes created automatically. It is helpful to understand the concept, however, and not rely too heavily on computer-generated reports. Data that have been entered incorrectly at some point will be reflected in reports generated. The user of accounting software must train his or her mind to think about the sensibility of the report.

Although two of these ratios were discussed in Chapter 20, some elaboration is in order in the context of this chapter.

INNER CITY HEALTH CARE
INCOME STATEMENT

	Month of , 20XX	Year-to-Date	Budget for Year	Overhead Percentages
A. Revenue:				
1. Office #1	$	$	$	
2. Office #2	$	$	$	100%
B. Total Revenue:	$	$	$	
C. Expenses:				
1. Non–provider (staff) salaries—gross	$	$	$	%
2. Staff fringes				
– Payroll taxes	$	$	$	
– Empl. benefits	$	$	$	
– Empl. seminars	$	$	$	
– Uniforms	$	$	$	
– Retirement plan	$	$	$	
	$	$	$	%
3. Occupancy costs:				
– Rent—Off. #1	$	$	$	
– Rent—Off. #2	$	$	$	
– Property taxes	$	$	$	
– Insurance	$	$	$	
– Utilities	$	$	$	
– Janitor/Grounds	$	$	$	
	$	$	$	%
4. Medical expenses:				
– Medications	$	$	$	
– Supplies	$	$	$	
– Lab fees	$	$	$	
	$	$	$	%
5. Office expenses:				
– Office supplies	$	$	$	
– Postage	$	$	$	
– Telephone	$	$	$	
	$	$	$	%
6. Malpractice ins.	$	$	$	%
7. Professional expenses:				
– Auto expenses (Providers')	$	$	$	
– Dues/subscriptions	$	$	$	
– Books and videos	$	$	$	
– Dues/memberships	$	$	$	
– Entertainment	$	$	$	
– Professional development	$	$	$	
– Travel	$	$	$	
	$	$	$	%

(continues)

Figure 21-2   A sample income statement that can show profit and expenses for 1 month.

	Month of , 20XX	Year-to-Date	Budget for Year	Overhead Percentages
8. Equipment costs:				
– Depreciation/amortization	$	$	$	
– Rent	$	$	$	
– Service/maintenance	$	$	$	
– Interest (if on equipment purchase loans)	$	$	$	
	$	$	$	%
9. Marketing expenses				
– Advertising	$	$	$	
– Other fees	$	$	$	
	$	$	$	%
10. Professional expenses:				
– Accounting	$	$	$	
– Legal	$	$	$	
– Consulting	$	$	$	
– Ret. Plan Admin.	$	$	$	
	$	$	$	%
11.				
12.				
13.				
14.				
D. Total Non–Provider Expenses:	$	$	$	%
E. Operating New Income Before Provider's Costs (B minus C)	$	$	$	%
F. Associate Provider's Costs:				
– Salaries—gross:	$	$	$	
– Benefits	$	$	$	
–	$	$	$	
–	$	$		
G. Total Non–Owner Provider's Costs	$	$	$	%
H. New Income Available to Owner– Providers (E minus G)	$	$	$	%
I. Owner–Providers' Costs:				
1. Salaries—gross:				
–Dr. A	$	$	$	
–Dr. B	$	$	$	
2. Bonuses—gross:				
–Dr. A	$	$	$	
–Dr. B	$	$	$	
3. Retirement contributions:				
–Dr. A	$	$	$	
–Dr. B	$	$	$	
4. "Semi-personal" expenses:				
–Dr. A	$	$	$	
–Dr. B	$	$	$	
J. Total Owner–Providers' Costs	$	$	$	
K. Net Income (H minus J)	$	$	$	

Figure 21-2   (continued)

Accounts Receivable Ratio

The **accounts receivable (A/R) ratio** formula measures the speed in which outstanding accounts are paid. The accounts receivable ratio provides a picture of the state of collections and probable losses. The longer an account is past due, the less the likelihood is of successfully making the collection.

$$\frac{\text{Total Accounts Receivable}}{\text{Monthly Receipts}} = \text{Turnaround Time}$$

Example:

$$\frac{\$120,000}{\$60,000} = \text{2 Months Turnaround Time for Payment on an Account}$$

The goal of an efficient billing and collecting policy should be a turnaround time of 2 months or less.

Collection Ratio

The **collection ratio** shows the percentage of outstanding debt collected. The goal should be a 90% collection ratio. Total receipts divided by total charges give the unadjusted collection ratio, but adjustments may include federal and state insurance programs (Medicare and Medicaid, Workers Compensation), managed care adjustments, and any other adjustments as directed by the provider.

Total Receipts	= $40,000
+ Managed Care Adjustments	$3,000
+ Medicare Adjustments	$2,000
TOTAL	$45,000
Total Charges	$52,000

$$\frac{\text{Total Receipts } \$45,000}{\text{Total Charges } \$52,000} = \begin{array}{l}\text{86.5\% Collection Ratio} \\ \text{after Adjustments}\end{array}$$

Cost Ratio

The **cost ratio** formula shows the cost of a procedure or service and can help in determining, for instance, the cost effectiveness of maintaining a laboratory in the ambulatory care setting. The ratio is:

$$\frac{\text{Total Expenses}}{\text{Total Number of Procedures for 1 Month}}$$

$$\frac{\text{Total Laboratory Expenses for September}}{\text{Total Number of Procedures Performed for September}}$$

$$\frac{\$48,000}{240} = \$200 \text{ per Procedure}$$

A conclusion might be reached that the laboratory is too costly because each procedure is not billed at $200.00.

LEGAL AND ETHICAL GUIDELINES

It is hoped that a careful hiring process (see Chapter 46) results in the best employees whose credentials, ethics, and personal actions are above reproach. However, embezzlement does occur in medical practices, partly because of the way in which the financial aspect of the practice is designed and managed. To decrease the opportunity for embezzlement:

- The accountant and the managing provider(s) should conduct regular and irregular audits of the practice accounts. Seek an accountant who is available at any time, not just when it is time to report wages or compute the yearly taxes. The accountant also becomes a valuable asset to the practice in providing essential information to the clinic staff.

- Separate duties among several employees. Consider having one employee open the mail and post checks received. A second employee handles all the cash transactions and prepares the deposit slips. A third employee might order the supplies and prepare all the checks. Many providers choose to sign the checks; however, this is also a task that can be assigned to the office manager.

- Only one person should use the signature stamp; better yet, consider not using a signature stamp at all.

- The signature card on file at the bank must include the names of each individual authorized to sign the checks.

- Seek employees whose personal honesty sets a good example for everyone.

Providers who demonstrate the same personal honesty and integrity expected of their staff are less likely to be victims of embezzlement.

Bonding

There is another recommended step to take. To protect the practice from embezzlement or other financial loss, providers can purchase fidelity bonds. These bonds reimburse the practice for any monetary loss caused by the practice's employees. There are three types of bonds to consider, and perhaps reason to have more than one type. These bonds include:

1. Position-schedule bond covers the position rather than a specific individual. For instance, the bookkeeper, office manager, and receptionist might be covered.

2. Blanket-position bond covers all employees. If the staff members often share duties, cover for one another when there are absences, or work really well together as a team during busy periods, this type of bond might be most beneficial.

3. Personal bond is designed to cover specific individuals by name and generally requires a personal background investigation. This type of bond may give the most assurance.

Bonding not only protects the providers and the practice, but it assures employees that they are

UTILIZATION REVIEW

In the present health care climate where there are many managed care plans, more attention has been focused on how the billing and financial management process should proceed. Because of the influence of governmental mandates in the practice of medicine and the growth of the **utilization review (UR)** industry, more accurate recordkeeping and documentation in all facets of the ambulatory care setting have become necessary. There are numerous UR firms throughout the country. These companies aggressively sell their services to employers and to insurance carriers. UR is actually a review of the patient service required before it may be performed. If the reviewer determines that the procedure or treatment is not needed, then it will not be approved or covered under the patient's insurance plan. Policies that once permitted medical decisions to be made solely by the provider often are now made by other health professionals who are employed by UR firms. Some clinics may find it beneficial to have one medical assistant whose main responsibility is to present procedures to UR for acceptance or denial. Because of the increasing concern for quality of health care at low cost, more providers also are realizing they need more documentation of both medical and financial information with more accessible means for retrieval.

covered by a bond should there be a problem with the finances during their shift. Bonding service companies will require implementation of certain procedures and security measures as outlined in their contracts. Costs depend on risk levels, but they are well worth the protection.

Payroll

The administrative medical assistant is likely to be involved in making certain the W-4 form, the Employee's Withholding Allowance Certificate, is completed by all employees. However, salary calculations, withholding taxes, and Social Security calculations are the responsibility of the office manager. Payroll tasks usually are assigned to the office manager because of the privacy of salary issues, Social Security numbers, and confidentiality of the employees' tax information. Manual systems for managing payroll are available, but the most efficient systems are computerized. The financial management of the payroll responsibilities in the ambulatory care setting is detailed in Chapter 45.

Procedure 21-1

Preparing Accounts Receivable Trial Balance in a Manual System

PURPOSE:
A trial balance will determine if there is any problem between the daily journal and the ledger or patient accounts.

EQUIPMENT/SUPPLIES:
Patient accounts
Calculator

PROCEDURE STEPS:

1. Pull all patient accounts that have a balance due.
   RATIONALE: Provides only amount due information.

2. Enter the balance of those accounts into the calculator.

3. Add the balances and total. (A calculator with tape can make it quicker to check for errors.)
   RATIONALE: Gives you the total amount due to date.

4. Create an accounts receivable total:

   a. Enter the accounts receivable total from the first of the month into the calculator.

   b. Add total charges for this month and subtotal.

   c. Total the amount of all payments received this month.

   d. Subtract the total of payments from subtotal of "b" above and subtotal.

   e. Total the amount of the month's adjustments and subtract from the subtotal in "d" above.

   f. This total is the accounts receivable amount.

   RATIONALE: The end-of-the month accounts receivable total ("f") above must match the total in Step 3. If these totals do not match, an error has been made. If they do match, the trial balance is in order.

Procedure 21-2

Preparing Accounts Receivable Trial Balance Using Medical Office Simulation Software (MOSS)

PURPOSE:
A trial balance will determine if there is any problem between the daily journal and the ledger or patient accounts.

EQUIPMENT/SUPPLIES:
Computer
MOSS

PROCEDURE STEPS:

1. Open MOSS and select "Report Generation" from the main menu.

2. From the Reports Panel select "Monthly Summary."

3. This report will automatically generate and indicate, by payer and for each month, what was billed, what was paid by the patient and by insurance, and any adjustments and deductibles. The remaining balances will also be reflected. RATIONALE: This is your accounts receivable.

4. Review the report for any possible errors. The grand total at the end of the report will be your accounts receivable balance. RATIONALE: Allows a summary of accounts receivable for the requested time period.

5. Print the report for submission to your instructor.

6. Close all windows and return to the main menu.

Case Study 21-1

Review the scenario at the beginning of the chapter.

CASE STUDY REVIEW

1. Identify the financial records most likely reviewed by James Whitney and Jane O'Hara.

2. What information will be considered when projecting future income?

3. Identify other concerns to consider when hiring an additional medical assistant.

Case Study 21-2

Richard Saxton is a newly licensed acupuncturist who has been in practice for less than a year. He is renting space for his procedures and services with an established doctor of osteopathy. Richard is using a simple pegboard system, makes his own appointments, and collects for most procedures at the time services are rendered unless the patients have medical insurance covering acupuncture. Richard has done fairly well, likes working in the environment the facility offers, and is beginning to show some profit. He would like to purchase a new table, chair, and stool for his acupuncture room.

CASE STUDY REVIEW

1. What facts might Richard want to consider before making the purchases?

2. Consider the variable costs versus the fixed costs of the practice of acupuncture. (You may need to do a little research to determine supplies and other factors.)

3. What information will his pegboard system give him?

SUMMARY

Medical financial management is crucial to the profitability of the ambulatory care setting. It is necessary for each medical facility to decide on which accounting system best serves the individual practice. Careful monitoring of billing procedures and aging accounts, and accurately documenting both the medical and financial record, will help in providing a sound financial analysis and a strong financial foundation for the ambulatory care setting. Just as it is essential that patients receive the best of care and that accuracy be maintained in all patient records, so too must the accuracy of all financial records be maintained in the ambulatory care setting.

STUDY FOR SUCCESS

To reinforce your knowledge and skills of information presented in this chapter:

- Review the Key Terms
- Practice any Procedures
- Consider the Case Studies and discuss your conclusions
- Answer the Review Questions
  - Multiple Choice
  - Critical Thinking
- Navigate the Internet and complete the Web Activities
- Practice the StudyWARE activities on the textbook CD
- Apply your knowledge in the Student Workbook activities
- Complete the Web Tutor sections

REVIEW QUESTIONS

Multiple Choice

1. If a number has been transposed in financial reports:
   a. the error is divisible by 4
   b. the error is divisible by 2
   c. the error is divisible by 9
   d. none of the above

2. An example of a fixed cost is:
   a. salaries
   b. cost of supplies
   c. depreciation of equipment
   d. cost of treating patients

3. An itemized statement of financial position is the:
   a. income statement
   b. balance sheet
   c. trial balance
   d. collection ratio

4. A check register:
   a. records all checks and categorizes them into separate columns
   b. is used when taking cash from patients

   c. is an accounts receivable record
   d. a and c

5. Utilization review:
   a. looks at the utility of all personnel
   b. examines how useful the ambulatory care center is to patients
   c. is a review of a procedure before it is performed to determine if it is necessary
   d. only affects hospitals

6. Assets include:
   a. equipment and supplies on hand
   b. building or property
   c. accounts receivable
   d. all the above

7. A computer billing and service bureau:
   a. is the service you hire to care for the office computer system
   b. may compromise patient confidentiality
   c. can function through linkage of computers, online servicing, or off-line batch processing
   d. b and c

8. In a medical facility where the total receipts including any adjustments are $83,500 and the total charges equal $97,750, the collection ratio:
   a. would be great at 94%
   b. would be quite good at 88%
   c. shows a fair return at 85%
   d. shows a modest return at 75%
9. Money can be saved with accounts payable when:
   a. bills are paid promptly
   b. discounts are realized
   c. supplies are not purchased in bulk
   d. a and b
10. Bonding:
   a. binds providers to the safe caretaking of their patients
   b. protects medical office staff and providers if embezzlement occurs
   c. can be purchased in three different types
   d. b and c

Critical Thinking

1. Discuss the pros and cons of an on-site complete computer system and a computer service bureau.
2. The accounting equation can be reported in more than one formula. It can be stated as:

$$\text{Assets} = \text{Liabilities} + \text{Owner's Equity}$$
$$\text{or}$$
$$\text{Assets} - \text{Liabilities} = \text{Owner's Equity}$$

   Is one easier to interpret? Why or why not? Add some totals of your choice to illustrate.

3. Recall from previous chapters and other studies in which you may be involved some basic guidelines for using computers in the medical facility. Identify these. What is one critical procedure that is done quite regularly, especially at the end of a project or the end of the day?
4. Where and how are financial records and reports kept? Who is responsible for their storage? Is there a length of period that the records might be kept?

WEB ACTIVITIES

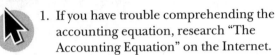

1. If you have trouble comprehending the accounting equation, research "The Accounting Equation" on the Internet. What helpful sites did you find? Are there any examples that show how the equation relates to a medical practice? Give an example of what you find.
2. Research "Medical Practice Management" for software packages that include the accounting reports described in this chapter. Identify at least two that seem to have the broadest coverage of how computers are used in a medical practice. Identify the pieces in the package and what they cover.

REFERENCE/BIBLIOGRAPHY

Droms, W. G. (2003). *Finance and accounting for nonfinancial managers* (2nd ed.). Cambridge, MA: Perseus Publishers.

CERTIFICATE OF COMPLETION

has completed *Medical Office Simulation Software (MOSS) 2.0 Procedures*

Evaluator Signature

Date

Patient Name

Medications

Date	Progress

Patient Name _____   **Medications** _____

Date	Progress
_____	_____
_____	_____
_____	_____
_____	_____
_____	_____
_____	_____
_____	_____
_____	_____
_____	_____
_____	_____
_____	_____
_____	_____
_____	_____
_____	_____
_____	_____
_____	_____
_____	_____
_____	_____
_____	_____
_____	_____
_____	_____
_____	_____
_____	_____
_____	_____
_____	_____
_____	_____
_____	_____
_____	_____
_____	_____
_____	_____
_____	_____
_____	_____
_____	_____
_____	_____

Patient Name _____   **Medications** _____

Date	Progress

Patient Name

Medications

Date	Progress

Patient Name _____   **Medications** _____

Date	Progress

Patient Name _____   **Medications** _____

Date	Progress

Patient Name _____   **Medications** _____

Date	Progress

Patient Name

Medications

Date	Progress

Patient Name   **Medications**

Date	Progress

272

Patient Name _____   **Medications** _____

Date   **Progress**